Reverse
diabetes

Reverse diabetes

A Simple Step-by-Step Plan to Take Control of Your Health

Reader's Digest

The Reader's Digest Association, Inc.
Pleasantville, New York / Montreal

PROJECT STAFF

Executive Editor
Marianne Wait

Senior Art Director
Rich Kershner

Cover Designer
Elizabeth Tunnicliffe

Contributing Editor
Sarí Harrar

Copy Editor
Marcia Mangum Cronin

Indexer
Cohen Carruth Indexes

READER'S DIGEST HOME & HEALTH BOOKS

President, Home & Garden and Health & Wellness
Alyce Alston

Editor in Chief
Neil Wertheimer

Creative Director
Michele Laseau

Executive Managing Editor
Donna Ruvituso

Associate Director, North America Prepress
Douglas A. Croll

Manufacturing Manager
John L. Cassidy

Marketing Director
Dawn Nelson

THE READER'S DIGEST ASSOCIATION, INC.

President and Chief Executive Officer
Mary Berner

President, Global Consumer Marketing
Dawn Zier

First printing in paperback 2010

Address any comments about *Reverse Diabetes* to:
The Reader's Digest Association, Inc.
Editor in Chief, Books
Reader's Digest Road
Pleasantville, NY 10570-7000

Visit our online store at **rdstore.com**

Printed in China

1 3 5 7 9 10 8 6 4 2 (hardcover)
1 3 5 7 9 10 8 6 4 2 (paperback)

Library of Congress Cataloging-in-Publication Data is available upon request.

ISBN 978-1-60652-991-1 (hardcover)
ISBN 978-1-60652-149-6 (paperback)

Note to Readers
The information in this book should not be substituted for, or used to alter, medical therapy without your doctor's advice. For a specific health problem, consult your physician for guidance. The mention of any products, retail businesses, or Web sites in this book does not imply or constitute an endorsement by the authors or by The Reader's Digest Association, Inc.

Cover photos © Jupiter Images

DI · A · BE · TES

(noun): a disorder of carbohydrate metabolism
characterized by inadequate
production or usage of insulin and
causing excessive levels of glucose
in the blood and urine

RE · VERSE

(verb): to turn in the opposite direction or send on
the opposite course

contents

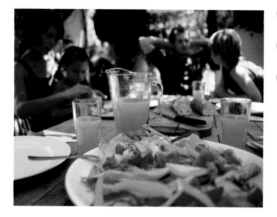

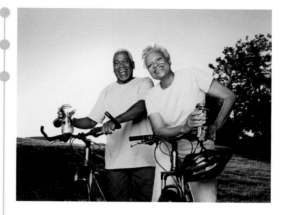

PART ONE

EAT
to reverse diabetes

PART TWO

MOVE
to reverse diabetes

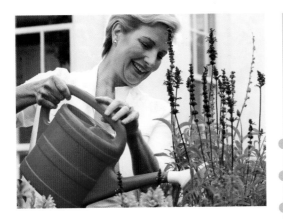

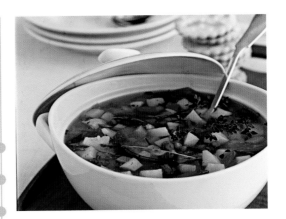

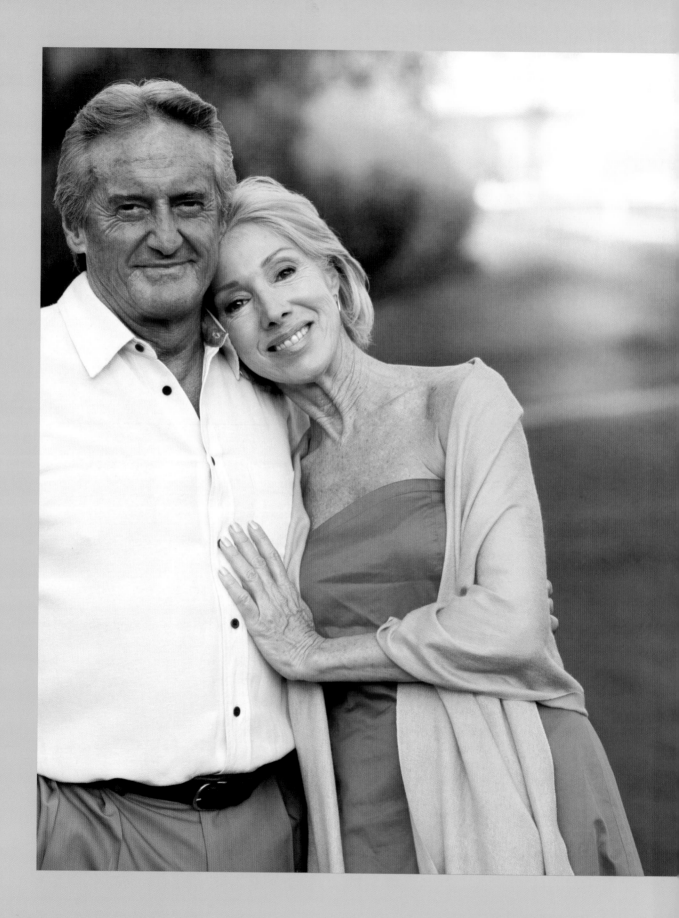

Introducing the Eat, Move, Choose Plan

Is there a cure for type 2 diabetes? Just a year or two ago, doctors would have emphatically answered "no." But since then, groundbreaking studies on real patients have shown that it's possible to send the disease into complete remission—to erase all signs of it.

Doctors accomplished this through weight-loss surgery on obese people, but even without surgery, it's now clear that *you* have the power to reverse the course of your disease—to turn back the clock on insulin resistance, the metabolic problem at the core of the condition, and see better blood sugar levels again, along with vastly improved overall health. All with far less hassle than you might think.

A wave of recent studies shows that by making easy, manageable changes to your daily habits you can achieve remarkable improvements in your A1C level (an indirect measure of your blood sugar levels over the last three months), your weight, and other health markers. If you take diabetes medications or use insulin, you may be able to reduce your dose or even tear up your prescription, depending on where you are in the course of your disease.

Powerful new research shows that even modest lifestyle changes can have profound benefits. For instance, simply taking a brisk walk three times a week can significantly lower blood sugar. Eating a bit less every day, but *not* dramatically cutting calories, can lead to long-term weight loss, a vital goal for most people with type 2 diabetes. Swapping certain foods for healthier choices can not only improve your body's sensitivity to the hormone insulin— essentially reversing the course of your diabetes—but can also keep a lid on your risk for heart disease, without punishing your palate. Scientists have even discovered that reining in stress can lower blood sugar and decrease the amount of deadly fat, known as visceral fat, that you carry deep in your belly, fat that makes blood sugar control more difficult.

Reverse Diabetes incorporates all the newest findings about the best ways to manage this condition and translates these revelations into simple, clear goals and easy-to-follow advice. But first, a bit more about the new cutting-edge science upon which this book is based.

The New Thinking on Reversing Diabetes

RESEARCHERS ARE LEARNING more and more every day about what it takes to control and even reverse diabetes and the complications that may eventually develop as a result of it. Recently, important discoveries have been made in five areas: weight, diet, exercise, mood, and sleep.

WEIGHT MANAGEMENT
Cutting Calories Is Crucial

Imagine you had a life-threatening infection that caused you to develop a fever. What if your doctor ignored the infection and sent you home with an aspirin for the fever? You would probably find a new doctor—fast. Yet many physicians make a similar mistake when they treat patients with type 2 diabetes, says Osama Hamdy, MD, of the Joslin Diabetes Center in Boston. The problem: Doctors tend to focus solely on lowering blood sugar. However, it's excess body fat that helped trigger the disease. "Treating obesity is treating the core of the problem," says Hamdy. We now know that dropping even modest amounts of weight can improve blood sugar control and protect you from diabetes-related problems.

One of the most crucial steps you can take to shed pounds is the simplest: cut a small number of calories from your daily diet. In his study, Hamdy found that patients with type 2 diabetes who trimmed 250 to 500 calories from their daily diets for a year lost 7.6 percent of their body weight, on average, or about 18 pounds. (The patients exercised regularly, too.) The payoff? An impressive 82 percent of the patients lowered their A1C below the all-important 7 percent threshold. (Only about 37 percent of diabetes patients nationally reach this goal.) By the end of the study, most of the patients also had fewer risk factors for heart disease, the number one killer of people with diabetes. Their blood pressure and cholesterol improved, while their blood and arteries showed less evidence of inflammation, now considered a major contributor to heart attacks.

Cutting 250 to 500 calories is as simple as swapping a fast-food burger and cola for a turkey sandwich and sparkling water. "We didn't ask patients to significantly cut calorie intake. That makes it easier to maintain the diet for a long time," says Hamdy. We won't ask you to, either.

THE *NEW* DIABETIC DIET
Better Carbs, Healthy Fats

The old thinking about diabetes and diet could be summed up in two words: avoid sugar. That seemed logical; if diabetes causes high blood sugar, why would you want to add to the problem by gobbling chocolate bars and guzzling soda pop?

But sugar is just one ingredient in the nutritional pie. While it's still a great idea to eat less of it, other dietary tweaks are proving just as powerful or even more powerful when it comes to managing and reversing diabetes.

The new advice? Quit focusing on forbidden foods. Instead, think about *adding* to your diet foods that help maintain steady blood sugar levels and simultaneously lower your risk for heart disease.

For instance, studies show that eating fruit and vegetables—nature's all-purpose disease fighters—appears to combat diabetes. People who eat three servings of fruit per day cut the risk for developing type 2 diabetes by 18 percent, according to a 2008 study. The same researchers found that every serving of leafy green vegetables you eat per day—such as lettuce, spinach, broccoli, and others—may lower the risk by 9 percent.

How does eating produce help? First, these healthy foods tend to be low in calories. Second, the carbohydrates in most fruits and vegetables have only a modest effect on blood sugar levels, making them "low-glycemic" foods. (The glycemic index rates foods based on how high they raise blood sugar in the two hours after they're eaten.) High-glycemic foods, on the other hand, tend to send blood sugar soaring. They include highly processed foods such as refined grains (like white bread and white rice), candy, desserts, and soft drinks. Starchy vegetables, especially potatoes, are high-glycemic foods, too.

Replacing high-glycemic carbs with low-glycemic choices keeps blood sugar levels under control

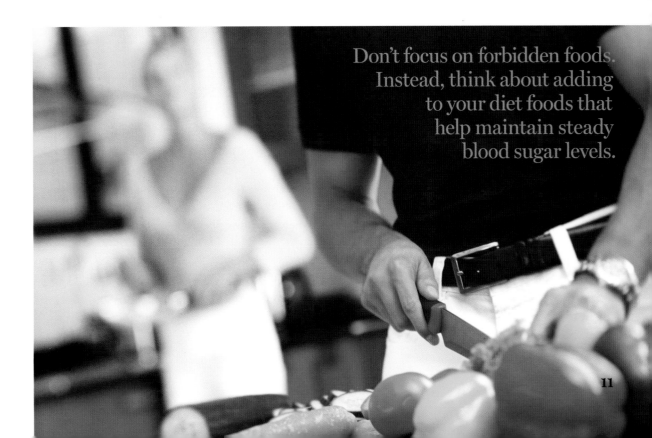

Don't focus on forbidden foods. Instead, think about adding to your diet foods that help maintain steady blood sugar levels.

at a critical time—immediately following a meal. Post-meals spikes in blood sugar are dangerous for several reasons, not least of all because they help to produce destructive molecules called free radicals, which damage healthy cells and cause inflammation and other problems that raise the risk of heart disease and other chronic conditions (including diabetes).

Amazingly, a low-glycemic diet can chill inflammation by up to 30 percent, according to a 2008 study by University of Toronto scientists. Other new research shows that eating a low-glycemic diet helps the heart by lowering levels of LDL ("bad") cholesterol and triglycerides while raising HDL ("good") cholesterol.

Other simple, tasty swaps can work wonders on diabetes, too. How about snacking on a handful of peanuts instead of cookies? Holding the grated cheese and adding some avocado slices to a salad? Skipping the butter and drizzling fruity extra-virgin olive oil over steamed vegetables? Nuts, avocados, and olive oil are all top sources of monounsaturated fat. Unlike artery-clogging saturated fat (found in full-fat dairy and in meats) and trans fat (the fat in many snacks and fast foods), "monos" appear to fight heart disease. Even better, researchers have recently discovered that replacing "bad" fats with the monounsaturated variety combats insulin resistance, which we've already described as the key metabolic problem at the core of type 2 diabetes.

A high-mono diet can help people with type 2 diabetes control their A1C and weight, according to a 2008 study at the University of Cincinnati. The study's lead author, nutritionist Bonnie Brehm, PhD, says the key to successfully re-crafting your diet is "to start with small, achievable goals"— exactly what you'll be doing on the plan we're about to introduce.

Accepting the Obvious

Many doctors who treat diabetes are giving a new answer when patients ask: What should I eat? In the 1970s, most major medical organizations began advising diabetes patients to eat low-fat, high-carbohydrate diets. "That was a really big mistake," says Osama Hamdy, MD, of the Joslin Diabetes Center in Boston. The problem with a high-carb diet seems obvious, he says. People with diabetes have problems processing carbohydrates, so it doesn't make sense for them to eat *more* carbs, especially at the expense of good-for-you fats.

Hamdy's studies show that people with diabetes fare better if they cut their carb intake to 40 percent of calories. Plenty of other research supports this moderately low-carb approach. Researchers at Wake Forest University reviewed 13 studies and found that low-carbohydrate diets were consistently superior to high-carb plans for improving blood sugar. In one study, low-carb dieters cut their A1C by 2.2 percent—a drop that would absolutely thrill your doctor.

EXERCISE
Revving Your Metabolic Engine

Play a few sets of tennis. Take a long hike. Spend an afternoon planting perennials. What do these enjoyable activities have in common? Like all forms of exercise, they burn up blood sugar. Fabulous! But they do even more: They tame insulin resistance, making cells more sensitive to the hormone and thereby putting your disease into reverse.

Here's how it works. Normally, in people who don't have diabetes, insulin easily "unlocks" muscle cells so they let in glucose (blood sugar) from the blood stream to use as fuel. But if you have type 2 diabetes, your body has become less responsive to insulin, and your cells remain "locked up" to glucose, leaving it to build up in the blood. That can cause damage to tiny blood vessels and nerves. Over time, chronically elevated blood sugar can lead to a long list of diabetes complications: vision loss, serious skin ulcers, kidney disease, and others.

Exercise forces the body to become more sensitive to insulin again. Hard-working muscle cells that desperately need glucose during your workout will go to extreme measures to get it, producing chemicals that lower their resistance to the hormone. The effects of a single walk or workout session fades within a day, but *regular* exercise makes muscle cells permanently more sensitive to insulin.

It turns out that even modest amounts of exercise can help stop diabetes in its tracks. Dutch researchers showed in a 2008 study that patients with type 2 diabetes lowered their A1C by an average of 0.5 percent—a tremendous improvement—over a six-month period simply by walking briskly for 60 minutes three times a week. In fact, the thrice-weekly walkers improved their blood sugar as much as another group of patients who worked out in a gym.

Walking, swimming, cycling, and dancing are all great forms of aerobic exercise. Want to lower your blood sugar even more? Most experts agree that adding strength training to your weekly routine is essential, too. A 2007 Canadian study found that combining strength, or resistance, exercise with aerobic exercise reduces A1C by an additional 0.46 percent on average compared to aerobic exercise alone. Turned off by the thought of pumping iron? You don't have to. In *Reverse Diabetes* we'll show you how to get your strength training without lifting a single weight.

The benefits of regular exercise go beyond lowering blood sugar, of course. Bigger muscles burn more calories, which helps maintain healthy weight. Exercise is critical for heart health, too.

MOOD MANAGEMENT
Diabetes and Your Emotions

Did you know that chasing away the blues can actually fight diabetes and add years to your life? Doctors have known for years that emotional distress is bad for your body. Now mounting evidence shows that stress and other mood wreckers can be a double whammy when you have diabetes. For starters, feeling anxious or depressed often leads to bad habits. You know the usual suspects: eating junk food, skipping exercise, drinking too much alcohol. You may forget to take your medications or just decide you can't be bothered with them. Any of these behaviors can throw good blood sugar control out the window.

But feeling stressed or down in the mouth does more than sap our will to take good of ourselves, according to Wayne Katon, MD, University of Washington professor of psychiatry and a leading authority on the link between diabetes and depression. His 2008 study found that depression may increase death rates by up to 38 percent in people with type 2 diabetes. Four out of five other studies since 2005 reached similar conclusions.

How can mood have such a powerful effect on diabetes? Chalk it up to hormones, such as the "stress hormone" cortisol. Stress makes us produce more of this hormone. And depressed people tend to respond to stress in their life by producing large amounts of it.

Cortisol helps to mobilize your "fight or flight" response in the event of a crisis—a fire, for instance. But it also raises blood sugar. That means that over the long-term, chronic stress can pose a serious

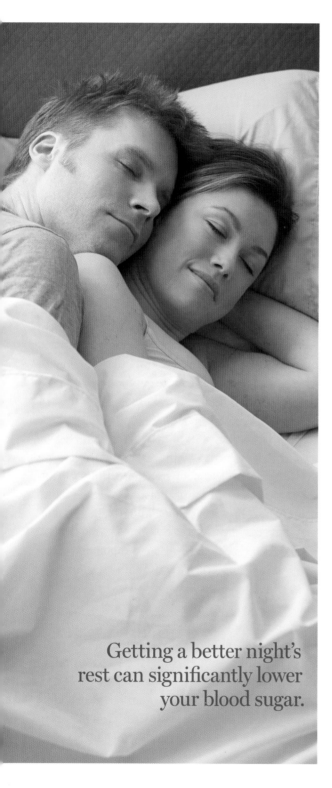

Getting a better night's rest can significantly lower your blood sugar.

problem. "High levels of cortisol and other stress hormones can put your diabetes out of control," says Katon.

Over time, stress can also increase the amount of fat you accumulate around your internal organs. So-called visceral fat is the worst kind—it produces dangerous chemicals that damage the arteries and increase the risk for heart attacks. To make matters worse, chronic stress raises your heart rate, too. An elevated heart rate makes you more likely to eventually suffer a fatal heart attack.

Soothing your psyche could prove to be a lifesaver. In one recent study, people with type 2 diabetes who learned to de-stress by meditating dropped their A1C scores by a nifty 0.48 percent, on average. Big bonus: Their blood pressure fell, too, by six points. Will you learn how to tame stress in *Reverse Diabetes*? It's a given.

AT THE END OF THE DAY
Why Sleep Matters

Here's a piece of news that you should take lying down: Getting a better night's rest can significantly lower your blood sugar and help you reverse your diabetes. A University of Chicago study found that type 2 diabetes patients who get by on just five hours a night may be able to lower their A1C numbers by more than 1 percent by stretching their nightly slumber time to eight hours.

Why is sleep so important when you have diabetes? No one is sure, but a few facts are clear. Studies show that sleep deprivation triggers insulin resistance. It also causes many other key hormones to go haywire. For instance, hormones that turn down your appetite plummet. At the same time, other hormones that make you hungry—especially for carbohydrates—shift into high gear. That's a setup for weight gain, which makes insulin resistance even worse.

Eat, Move, and Choose to Reverse Diabetes

BY LOSING WEIGHT and lowering your blood sugar and your resistance to insulin, you can put your disease in reverse. That simple, stunning fact was the inspiration behind *Reverse Diabetes* and the plan we call the Eat, Move, Choose Plan. This unique program, based on the best new science, is designed to help you—step by step and day by day—make the small changes in your life that will add up to better health, along with greater energy, a slimmer silhouette, and happier moods. The time to start it? Today. In fact, you can start right this second if you wish by putting down this book and going for a walk or eating a carrot. Yes, it's that easy!

A Comprehensive Three-Part Plan

Dealing with diabetes can feel overwhelming at times. But bringing the disease under control is an important task, and there's no one better qualified to do it than you. (Your doctor can prescribe medicines if you need them, but he can't cure or even manage the disease for you.) If you take the right steps, you can live a full and active life and even feel healthier than you have in years. We've charted the path for you with the Eat, Move, Choose Plan. It leaves nothing to chance—and if you follow it closely, we guarantee you'll see improvements in your blood sugar readings and probably your cholesterol profile, too.

In each of the three parts of the plan, we've spelled out crystal-clear goals along with the concrete steps you'll take to achieve them. On the Eat plan you'll discover surprising truths about what you should and shouldn't pile onto your plate when you have diabetes. For instance, taking in more fruits and vegetables is more important than ever, while the message about cutting back on fat has changed; researchers now know that eating "good" fats can help you improve your sensitivity to insulin. The carbohydrate message is also new. Slashing your intake of processed grains such as white rice and starchy vegetables like mashed potatoes and replacing them with "low-glycemic" carb foods that raise blood sugar more modestly is now job one. Portion control is also key, of course, and we've found a way to make it truly easy—no calorie counting required.

One of the most effective ways to reverse insulin resistance is to get off the couch and move your body. You may not think of yourself as the exercise "type," but don't write off this critical portion of the plan. You'll start the Move plan with a 10-minute walk. What able-bodied person can't do that? We'll also help you build up your muscle mass right at home, no equipment required, with a strengthening program we call the Sugar Buster Routine. Again, you can do it in just minutes a day, and there's no fitness prerequisite, so there really are no good excuses for skipping it. On the Move plan we'll also encourage you to sneak more "everyday" exercise into your life by spending some time yanking weeds in the garden, washing the car by hand, or simply taking the stairs instead of the elevator. These small choices may not seem like much, but the cumulative effect is much greater than you might think.

Speaking of choices: When you have diabetes, you can choose to let it takes it course, allowing it to get progressively worse every year, or you can choose to fight it. Choosing to fight means being willing to tweak your daily habits—and not just what you eat or how much you exercise. Getting enough sleep, finding ways to combat stress, and keeping a positive attitude are all vitally important aspects of good diabetes management, and they're all part of the Choose plan, along with planning well for sick days and travel.

Tracking Your Progress

Reversing diabetes isn't something that happens overnight (although getting a good night's sleep really does help keep blood sugar levels in check!). It's something you do every day—starting today. We're here to help you every step of the way. For every single day over the next 12 weeks, you'll record your progress toward each of your Eat, Move, and Choose goals in the 12-Week Planner section of the book.

Like a personal trainer, motivational life coach, and nutritional consultant rolled into one, the 12-Week Planner will suggest weekly goals, provide helpful tips, and let you record daily feedback to yourself on your eating choices, physical activity levels, stress reduction efforts, and sleep. You'll also record your weight, waist size, and blood sugar levels and watch them change over the course of the 12 weeks.

At the beginning of each week, you'll plan your meals for the next seven days, a powerful and important strategy for keeping you on top of your Eat goals. Use the more than 100 diabetes-friendly recipes in the Recipes section to help you. Then write a shopping list that sets you up for success. Knowing what you'll eat during the week translates into knowing exactly what you'll buy at the supermarket. That means you'll come home with shopping bags full of smart, delicious, healthy foods for weight loss and better blood sugar control—instead of high-calorie, high-fat treats that are so easy to buy on a whim at the grocery store.

By tracking your progress over 12 weeks of the plan, you'll notice and celebrate every success, discover areas that need improvement, feel inspired

Complications Are Not Inevitable

It was once thought that just about everyone with diabetes would eventually develop complications of the disease, such as nerve damage, foot problems, and vision problems. That's simply not true. By keeping your blood sugar in the normal range, you can slash your risk of these health problems and live a healthy life like anyone else.

to get up and do it all again tomorrow, and build motivation to get back on track if you've had a setback. You'll learn new things about yourself and your body—such as how daily stress reduction and exercise influence your blood sugar, how a few minutes of advance planning makes grabbing a healthy snack a snap, and how a week or a month of healthy choices pays off in lower numbers on the bathroom scale, on the tape measure you wrap around your middle, and on your blood sugar meter.

At the end of each week, there's room to note successes and confessions. We recommend spending a few moments on Sunday evening to look back at the previous week (and ahead to your goals for the coming week). Mull over how you did against the goals on the Eat, Move, Choose Plan. Be sure to give yourself a nice pat on the back for anything

and everything you've worked so hard to achieve, whether it was eating more vegetables, adding five minutes to your walks, or trying out one of our instant stress-buster strategies. Also note instances when you slipped up. Think about what got you off track and what you'd do differently the next time.

Why the Plan Works

Lots of plans offer good ideas about what *should* work when it comes to weight loss and diabetes management. Here's what makes the Eat, Move, Choose Plan so uniquely effective.

It doesn't rely on calorie-cutting alone. This plan corrects fundamental errors that people make while trying to lose weight, such as skipping

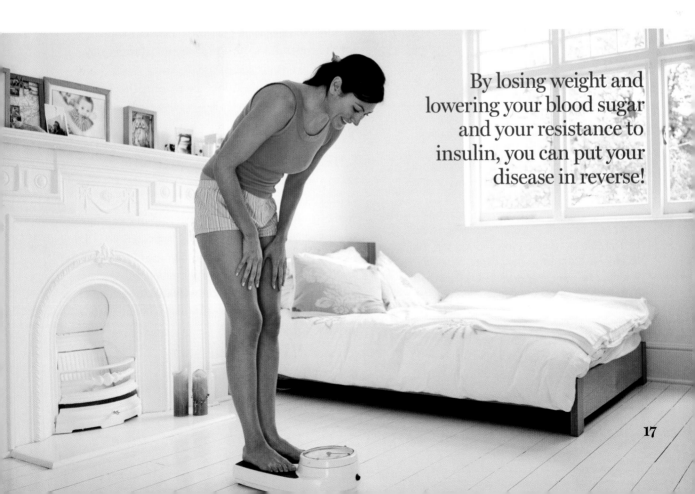

By losing weight and lowering your blood sugar and your resistance to insulin, you can put your disease in reverse!

breakfast, attempting to cut too much fat from their diets, and eating the wrong carbohydrate foods. Another common mistake: trying to lose weight by cutting calories alone. If you're not exercising, which you'll do on the Eat, Move, Choose Plan, you'll find it tough to shed the pounds you want to lose and keep them off. Stress and sleep deprivation also contribute to weight gain, and the plan helps you tackle both problems.

You can eat foods you like. This plan never restricts *what* you can eat, although you may need to eat favorite foods less often or in smaller portions or prepared in different ways. It won't feel like a diet, just a healthier way of eating.

It's a plan you can live with. Doctors and dietitians find that many people have an extremely tough time staying on diets that are radically low in either carbohydrates or fat. People give up on these diets because they're just too restrictive. This is a plan you can live with for life.

It's gradual. We won't ask you to change your life overnight. You can incorporate the steps in the Eat and Choose plans as quickly or as slowly as you wish. And the Move plan was designed to start you off slowly and gradually build you up to doing more exercise as you get fitter and fitter.

It's easy to follow, at home and away from home. There's no calorie or carbohydrate counting (except for an initial assessment of your current diet and check of your target calorie range), you don't have to try to make sense of the confusing glycemic index, and we won't ask you to eat your burger without a bun or pass up potatoes. You're allowed to eat bread and pasta, and even dessert, in reasonable amounts. Yes, you will need to make some changes—for instance, fill your plate with more vegetables, eat fewer French fries and potatoes, cut back a bit on portion sizes overall, and get off the couch for some exercise almost every day—but they aren't big ones. And we know you're ready for change, or you wouldn't be reading this book.

Don't Put This Book Away!

Unlike other books you own, this book is not meant to sit on your shelf for reference when you need it. It's meant to be used every day—so keep it at your bedside, on the coffee table, or on the kitchen table. Look at it at least once a day and be reminded of which foods to buy and eat, which snacks to have when hunger hits, what exercise to do in a given week, and how to deal with stress when you find yourself ready to explode or throw up your hands. Write in the Planner every day to keep yourself honest and motivated. Also, let your family, your friends, and your doctor know you're on the Eat, Move, Choose Plan so you'll get support and encouragement from every corner. The more faithfully you use this book, the more benefits you'll reap.

Our Promise

By the end of 12 weeks on the Eat, Move, Choose Plan, you'll be well on your way to losing 10 percent of your body weight—a goal that in one major study, the Diabetes Obesity Intervention Trial (DO IT), led to a significant drop in fasting blood sugar levels and to a reduction in medication use for many study volunteers. You will also have reaped a number of other important health benefits. Our promise to you:

Weight loss that works. We'll never ask you to follow a gimmicky diet, to eat special "diabetic" foods, to weigh or measure every morsel, to deprive yourself of your favorite edibles, or to sign up for a boot-camp level exercise routine. Radical overhauls may produce short-term results but can't stand up to the test of real-world living. That's the beauty and the power of the Eat, Move, Choose Plan. You'll follow clear, simple steps to success that are proven to work no matter what daily living has in store for you. We'll show you which changes have the most impact and how to fit them into your life. For example, you'll learn how to use your dinner plate to eat perfectly sized portions, how to fit walking and strength-training exercises into the busiest days, and how to get more sleep for automatic weight loss and effortless blood sugar benefits.

Less abdominal fat. The Eat, Move, Choose Plan uses a one-two-three strategy (the right foods, the right exercise, plus lifestyle tweaks including stress reduction) to trim belly fat—something that losing weight by simply cutting calories cannot accomplish. All weight loss is good, but it's especially important to get rid of fat deep in your abdomen, the stuff that wraps around internal organs, pumping blood sugar-raising compounds into your bloodstream around the clock. This plan shrinks it.

Better blood sugar control. Losing a fairly modest amount of weight can lower your blood sugar by a whopping 25 percent, enough to let some people reduce the dosage of their diabetes medications or stop them entirely. In the DO IT study, people who shed 10 percent of their body weight (that's 17 pounds if you weigh 170) saw their fasting blood glucose levels fall from an average of 170 mg/dl—well into dangerously elevated territory—to 125 mg/dl, a level considered "pre-diabetic." They also lowered their A1C levels from an average of 8 (normal for people with diabetes, but considered a risk for diabetes complications),

to 6.7—below the 7 target recommended by the American Diabetes Association.

Improved insulin sensitivity. People with type 2 diabetes are insulin resistant. Exercise, trimming deep belly fat, reducing stress, and eating a healthy diet—all of which you'll do on the Eat, Move, Choose Plan—work together to restore insulin sensitivity. In the DO IT study, sensitivity improved by two- to five-fold—enough that 18 of 25 study volunteers who took diabetes medications were able to stop.

Protection from diabetes complications. By following the research-tested strategies in this book, you will lower your blood pressure, reduce heart-threatening LDL cholesterol and triglycerides, and raise heart-protecting HDL cholesterol. The Eat, Move, Choose Plan also helps cool chronic inflammation, a potent risk factor for heart disease. The result: powerful protection against heart attacks, strokes, congestive heart failure, and other forms of cardiovascular disease.

But that's not all. Lowering your blood sugar will also protect you from major diabetes complications including vision loss due to diabetic retinopathy, kidney failure, and amputation due to nerve damage and poor circulation.

Involving Your Doctor and Dietitian

To get the most out of the Eat, Move, Choose Plan, it's important for you to talk with your doctor and with a registered dietitian or certified diabetes educator before you begin. These members of your diabetes care team can help you adjust and adapt the elements of the plan to your unique needs—by assessing your readiness for exercise, recommending a blood sugar testing strategy that will help you avoid highs and lows, and a medication strategy that will keep your blood sugar within a healthy range. Here's what your conversation should cover.

The best exercise for you. Most people with diabetes will be able to start the gentle, progressive Move plan just as it is. But if you take insulin or oral diabetes drugs called insulin secretagogues, you will need to discuss how to time exercise, medication doses, and perhaps a carbohydrate-rich snack so that exercise doesn't lead to dangerously low blood sugar.

If you've already experienced diabetes complications, your doctor may recommend adjusting your exercise routine. For example, if you have nerve damage called peripheral neuropathy, she may recommend activities like swimming, biking, or arm exercises instead of walking to avoid damage to your feet that could lead to infection. Your doctor may also recommend heart tests, such as an exercise stress test, before giving you the green light to exercise.

Meal adjustments. If you use carbohydrate counting to help control blood sugar, a dietitian can help you fit that eating strategy into the Eat guidelines. Your doctor, certified diabetes educator, or registered dietitian can also help you customize the Eat portion of the Eat, Move, Choose Plan so that the calories and food choices fit your needs.

A blood sugar testing schedule. Your diabetes management team can help you decide how often to perform blood sugar checks as you embark on the plan. Regular checks will show you how changes in your food choices, exercise level, stress, and sleep alter your blood sugar and will help your doctor decide whether you can reduce medication dosages. (Never alter your dosage or stop taking a drug on your own.)

Can You Get Off Your Meds?

For some people on the Eat, Move, Choose Plan, one of the biggest payoffs will be taking less diabetes medication or even getting off diabetes medication altogether. We can't make promises. You need to make treatment decisions with your doctor, especially when it comes to any changes in medication. And diabetes is a progressive disease—the longer you have it, the more likely you'll need pharmaceutical help to manage it. But here's what you might expect if you succeed in bringing your blood sugar down to the following levels:

126 to 140 or 150 mg/dl: While still above normal, these levels are low enough that you may be able to stop taking medication.

150 to 200 mg/dl: The chances are good that continuing to follow the plan may allow you to get off medication. For now, however, you may still need medication and perhaps occasional doses of insulin.

Above 200 mg/dl: You may need medication or full-time insulin coverage, and possibly both, but the plan may let you reduce your doses or make other adjustments. What's more, it will most likely lower your blood pressure and improve your cholesterol numbers. And of course, you'll enjoy a greater sense of control over your health.

A checkup plan. Expect your blood sugar to become easier to control and to move closer to a normal range as you progress through the 12-week Eat, Move, Choose Plan. If you're using medication, ask your doctor how often you should check in or make appointments to reassess your dosages and prescriptions. You may need to change one or both as your body becomes more sensitive to insulin.

Personal Contract

Keep this contract as a reminder of your commitment to the Eat, Move, Choose Plan and reversing your diabetes.

I vow that over the next 12 weeks I will learn and follow the steps to better blood sugar control and weight loss presented in the Eat, Move, Choose Plan.

MY GOALS

My weight loss goal over the next 12 weeks (up to 1 pound a week is an appropriate target for most people): _____

My blood sugar goals over the next 12 weeks (discuss what goal is reasonable for you with your doctor or certified diabetes educator):

Fasting glucose: _____

A1C: _____

MY STRATEGIES

To reach these goals, I agree to:

1. Adopt the plan's strategies for getting more vegetables, fruit, whole grains, lean protein, low-fat dairy products, and good fats into my diet and for cutting back on saturated fat, trans fat, and refined carbohydrates.

2. Follow the Plate Approach at every meal to control portion sizes and calories.

3. Walk most days of the week and build up to performing the Sugar Buster Routine twice a week.

4. Practice a stress-relief technique every day.

5. Track my progress using the 12-Week Planner.

6. Plan my meals in advance using the 12-Week Planner.

7. Note my successes as well as my failures at the end of each week; I promise to cheer myself on every step of the way.

MY MOTIVATION

Here's why I want to do all I can to control my diabetes:

1. _____

_____

_____

_____

_____

2. _____

_____

_____

_____

_____

_____

3. _____

_____

_____

_____

_____

Signed:_____

Date:_____

Witness (optional):_____

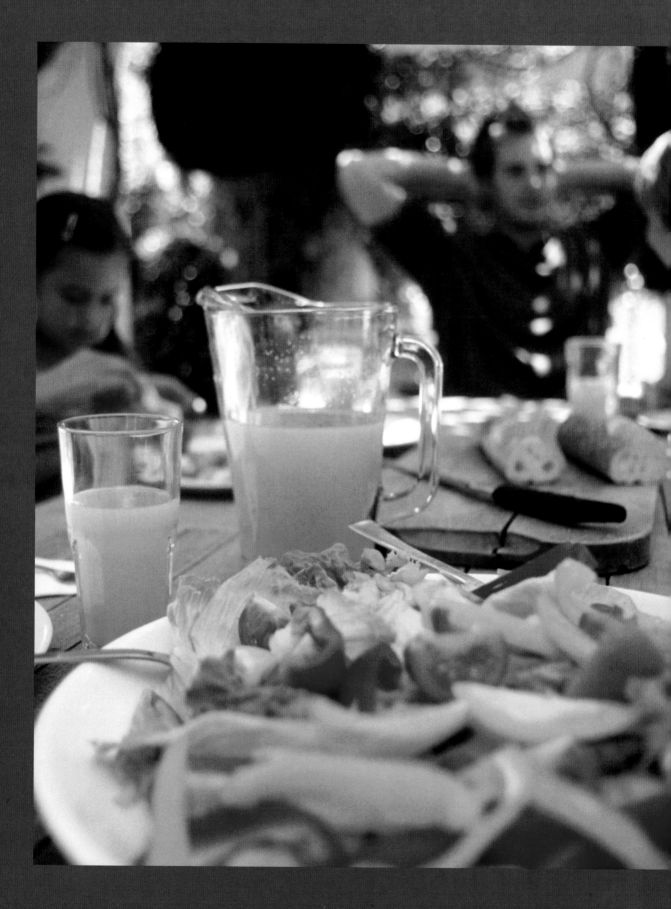

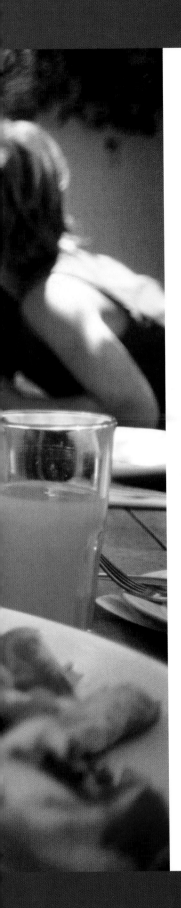

1

EAT
to reverse diabetes

- Delicious Foods
- Satisfying Meals
- Perfect Portions

- Better Health

the plan

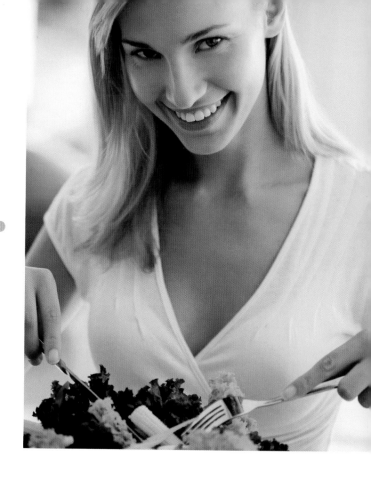

Eating to beat diabetes can seem awfully complicated and, well, intimidating. We've solved that problem by boiling down the best research-proven eating advice for people with diabetes into seven clear goals, each one designed to help you make important changes to your current eating habits without a lot of hassle.

what to do

GOAL 1
Eat five+ servings of vegetables a day

The reason couldn't be simpler or clearer: People who eat more vegetables weigh less, have better blood sugar control, and slash their risk for diabetes-related diseases. Plenty of good reasons to make lunch a lavish salad, bite into baby carrots smeared with peanut butter for a snack, and invite two or even three vegetables over for dinner tonight.

GOAL 2
Cut your refined carbohydrates by half

It's carbohydrate foods that make blood sugar rise. Of course, they are also your body's main source of fuel. The solution: Choose your carbs carefully. Slash your intake of processed grains such as white rice and starchy vegetables like mashed potatoes, and focus on foods that give you a big nutrition bang for your carb buck without sending your sugar soaring.

GOAL 3
Eat three servings of fruit a day

Fruits have almost all the health advantages that vegetables bring, and they taste so good! Yes, fruit contains sugar. But it's chock-full of fiber and disease-fighting nutrients and doesn't contain a lot of calories, so it's perfect for helping you shed a few extra pounds. Nothing's off-limits; just check your blood sugar to find the fruits that work best for you...then enjoy.

GOAL 4
Include lean protein at every meal

Protein has the unique ability to keep your stomach satisfied. Eating lean protein at every meal—think fish, beans, eggs, lean meat and poultry, and low-fat dairy—helps keep blood sugar low, cuts between-meal cravings, and even helps preserve calorie-burning muscle while you're losing weight. We'll help you avoid protein pitfalls and fit this important nutrient into difficult meals like breakfast.

what to record

1. YOUR INTAKE OF KEY FOODS

Every day for the next 12 weeks we want you to use the Planner section to record how well you did against the seven eating goals. Also, for just one week we want you to keep a food diary so that you can begin to understand your dietary strengths and weaknesses. You'll find instructions on page 29 and a blank template on page 246.

2. THE NUMBER OF TIMES PER DAY YOU EAT IN RESPONSE TO STRESS, BOREDOM, OR HABIT

Emotional eating and "mindless" eating are major sources of excess calories, fat, and sugar, packing on pounds and making blood sugar difficult to control. In the Planner section you'll record every day how many times you ate not because you were hungry but in response to a mood or simply because there was food in front of you. Gaining awareness of this type of eating is the key to overcoming it.

3. A MEAL PLAN FOR EVERY WEEK

Sit down once a week and fill out the weekly meal planners in the Planner section. This is a great time to pull out the calendar and look ahead for challenges: Will you have to eat on the run one night as you rush from work to an event? A good plan is all about adjusting for real life so that you stay on track.

---

before you begin

1 Take the quiz on page 26

It will help you assess your current eating habits and the state of your pantry, refrigerator, and freezer. Answer as honestly as you can—the info will help you find strengths as well as obstacles you may not have realized are standing in the way of better diabetes control.

2 Determine how many calories you need per day.

See page 27. Keeping calories in check does wonders for helping you manage diabetes. While the Eat plan isn't about obsessive calorie counting, we ask you to keep a food diary during your first week and compare your total calories to the number you actually need in a day.

3 Stock up on foods in the shopping list on page 252.

Does your pantry need an upgrade? Is your freezer packed with ice cream and Popsicles, but a little short on frozen vegetables and boneless chicken breasts? By stocking up on our recommended foods, you'll be ready to put a healthy meal on the table in a snap.

GOAL 5

Trade good fat for bad

The fat in hamburger meat, chicken skin, and full-fat cheese is not only bad for your heart, it's bad for your diabetes. The same goes for trans fat, found in processed foods that contain hydrogenated oil. But that doesn't mean that all fat is bad. On the Eat plan you'll enjoy plenty of it in the form of sugar-controlling "good" fats found in nuts, avocados, olive and canola oil, flaxseed, and fish.

GOAL 6

Use the Plate Approach for perfect portions

Could your dinner plate hold the key to right-sizing your portions? Yes! With our Plate Approach you won't have to measure or weigh foods at home to avoid portion distortion and overeating. This simple, proven method helps people with diabetes lose more weight and gain better blood sugar control. It's that easy and that effective.

GOAL 7

Plan your meals

If you know ahead of time what's for dinner, you'll be less tempted to turn to takeout or meals from a box. And planning and cooking meals at home gives you your best opportunity to follow the six other goals. You'll also know exactly what you need at the grocery store, so you'll be less tempted by snack foods, sweets, processed foods, and high-fat items.

the quiz

Do you pile your plate with vegetables or with fatty meat and mashed potatoes? Is your kitchen stocked with foods that spell success for people with diabetes or with tempting snacks, high-fat foods, and processed items that will thwart your best efforts to eat three healthy meals a day? This quiz will help uncover your strengths and weaknesses in two areas: your current eating habits and the foods you stock in your kitchen.

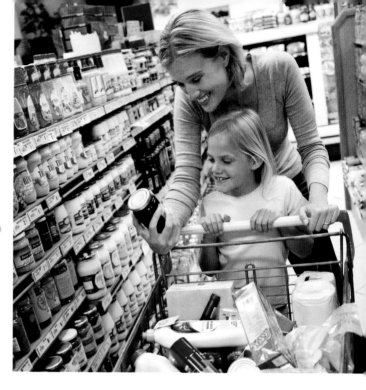

part one your diet

1. **What's the star of most of your lunches and dinners?**
   a. Meat
   b. Starch (pasta, potatoes, bread, rice, or corn)
   c. Vegetables (except potatoes or corn)

2. **Not counting potatoes and corn, how much room do vegetables usually occupy on your plate?**
   a. No room—I eat only potatoes and corn
   b. About a quarter of the plate
   c. Half of the plate or more

3. **What is your usual choice when eating bread?**
   a. White bread
   b. "Wheat" bread made mostly of white flour
   c. 100% whole-grain bread

4. **When it comes to vegetables I:**
   a. Eat mashed potatoes, corn, or French fries, period
   b. Force myself and my family to eat one green, red, or orange veggie at dinner
   c. Love 'em and have no problem eating a rainbow of different colors

5. **How often do you eat salads?**
   a. Salads are boring or too complicated to prepare, so I rarely eat them
   b. Only when I go to a restaurant
   c. Several times per week

6. **Which of these fats do you usually use or cook with?**
   a. Butter or margarine containing hydrogenated oil
   b. Margarine without hydrogenated oil, or corn oil
   c. Olive or canola oil

7. **How often do you consume low-fat milk, cheese, or yogurt?**
   a. Rarely or never
   b. Once a day
   c. Two or three times a day

8. **On average, how many soft drinks do you have each day?**
   a. Three or more
   b. One or two
   c. None

your score

Give yourself 1 point for every "a", 2 points for every "b", and 3 points for every "c". Add your points together.

20-24 points

Congratulations!

You're already following the type of eating plan that helps control blood sugar, keeps your weight in check, and lowers your odds for diabetes complications. The Eat plan will give you new ways to enjoy the foods you already love. We've also got smart strategies for dealing with your next challenge: sticking with the same strategies when you eat out.

16-20 points

Good start, with room for improvement.

You probably need to invite more fruits, vegetables, and whole grains over to your dinner plate and choose higher-calorie foods and refined carbohydrates less often. Start this week and you'll be amazed how fast you see results in your blood sugar and on the scale. Finding smart, easy ways to add a variety of healthy foods—cooked in healthy ways—to your plate can transform this from a boring job into a pleasure. We'll show you how.

9-15 points

It's time for a change.

Your diet relies heavily on processed foods, refined carbohydrates, meats, and the empty calories in soft drinks—all of which get in the way of easy blood sugar control and maintaining a healthy body weight. Give yourself a big pat on the back for picking up this book, and get ready for delicious, healthy eating that will help you keep your blood sugar and weight under control.

8-10 points

Start the Eat plan today!

We suspect your diet is contributing to high blood sugar, stubborn extra pounds, and perhaps even early signs of diabetes complications such as high blood pressure, high cholesterol, and other problems. Pay special attention to the proven healthy-eating advice in this chapter, and talk with your doctor about arranging an appointment with a registered dietitian or certified diabetes educator to help you incorporate healthy eating strategies into your day.

How Many Calories Do You Need?

You don't have to count calories on the Eat plan if you use the Plate Approach (described on page 73). For most foods and most people, it's all you need to keep portion sizes in check and make sure you eat a healthy, calorie-controlled balance of vegetables, grains and starches, protein, and fats. But it's still smart to have a handle on your daily calorie needs.

Step 1

Multiply your current weight by 10. For example, if you weigh 175 pounds, you get 1,750 calories. This is approximately how many calories your body needs to function when it's idle.

$$\underline{\hspace{3cm}} \textbf{ x 10} = \underline{\hspace{3cm}}$$
(your weight in pounds) (calories you need when idle)

Step 2

To fill in roughly how many calories you're burning through physical activity, rate yourself on the following scale:

- If you're totally sedentary, give yourself a 300.
- If you're moderately active, give yourself a 500.
- If you're very active, give yourself a 700.

Step 3

Add the result of step 2 to the number from step 1. For example, if your step 1 number is 1,750 calories and you're sedentary, add 300 to 1,750 to get a total of 2,050 calories per day. This is the number of calories you need to stay at your current weight.

$$\underline{\hspace{2.5cm}} \textbf{ + } \underline{\hspace{2.5cm}} = \underline{\hspace{2.5cm}}$$
(result of step 2) (result of step 1) (calories you need to maintain your weight)

Step 4

Want to lose a pound a week? Aim to subtract 500 calories from that number every day.

part two your kitchen

1. **What are the first three things you see when you open your refrigerator door?**

   △ Full-fat or 2% milk
   ○ Nonfat or 1% milk and/or nonfat yogurt
   △ Full-fat cheese
   ○ 100% fruit juice
   ○ Fresh vegetables and fruits
   ○ Meats like extra-lean ground beef, ground skinless chicken or turkey, pork tenderloins
   △ Meats like ground beef, T-bone steak, sausage, chicken thighs
   ○ Chicken breasts
   △ Soda (including diet soda), sweetened tea, or other sweetened drinks
   △ Regular mayonnaise and creamy salad dressings

2. **What are the first three things you see when you open the freezer?**

   ○ Frozen prepared meals in a box or bag (Weight Watchers, etc.)
   △ Frozen prepared meals in a box or bag (non-diet)
   △ Frozen pizza and/or French fries or deep-fried potatoes
   △ Frozen fish, breaded
   ○ Frozen fish fillets, not breaded, no sauce
   △ Ice cream
   ○ Frozen vegetables and/or fruits

3. **Do you have fresh fruit in your house right now?**

   ○ Yes
   △ No

4. **How many different packaged snack foods (chips, crackers, cookies, pretzels, etc.) do you have in your pantry right now?**

   ○ None
   ○ One or two
   △ Three or more

5. **Which of these are in your pantry right now?**

   ○ Canned beans
   ○ Low-sodium canned soups and broths
   △ White rice, white pasta, white noodles
   ○ Brown rice and other whole grains like barley or whole-wheat couscous
   ○ Whole-grain pasta or noodles
   △ Fruit canned in heavy syrup
   ○ Fruit canned in juice or extra-light syrup
   △ Peanut butter (or another nut butter) or unsalted nuts

your score

Add up the number of green circles you chose. The more circles, the closer your kitchen is to being ready for you to begin the plan.

11-16

Gold star kitchen!
Your cupboards, refrigerator, and freezer contain mostly diabetes-friendly foods like whole grains, beans, fruit, vegetables, lean meat, fish, and low-fat or fat-free dairy products. We'll show you how to use even more of them in fast, delicious ways.

5-10

Your kitchen's sending mixed messages.
Too often, your kitchen sabotages your efforts to control your blood sugar and maintain a healthy weight. There are healthy foods here (give yourself a pat on the back!) but you may find yourself choosing unhealthy options because they're so tempting. Follow our kitchen makeover on page 250 for advice on what to keep and what to toss.

0-4

Your kitchen is hazardous to your health.
The foods in your house are contributing to your diabetes and dangerous belly fat around your middle. Turn to page 250 to make over your kitchen, and use the shopping list on page 252 to restock with foods that will help you follow the Eat plan with ease.

How to Keep a Food Diary

The better you understand the way you're really eating right now—and why—the better you'll be able to identify your strengths, downfalls, and biggest opportunities for improvement. Track what you're eating for the next week using the template on page 246. Write down:

• Everything you eat and drink and how much.

• The time you eat it, as well as the circumstances (such as "dinner at home," "popcorn at the movies," or "I was tired and cranky this morning so I gave in to the doughnuts at work."

• Estimated calories per item.

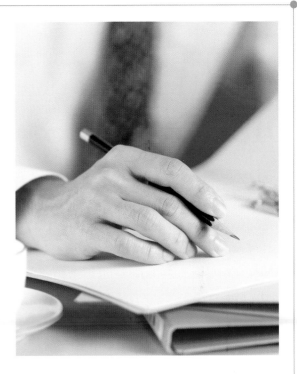

To estimate calories you'll need to do a little sleuthing. For any packaged foods, check the nutrition label, and remember that if it says the package contains two servings and you eat the whole thing, multiply the calories per serving by two. If you've consumed any food or drink from a fast-food outlet, you can usually find the calories for that item online. For other items, refer to the Calorie, Carbs, and Fat counter starting on page 256, or look them up online at sites such as www.caloriecontrol.org. At the end of the week, look over your diary for patterns. You may find that you consume more calories than you ever imagined in the form of midday or late-night snacks, or beverages such as juice, soda, lattes, or beer. Also look critically at your diary to see how well your eating habits match up with the Eat goals, and figure out where they fall short. Are your breakfasts full of carbs but no protein? Are you getting anywhere near five servings of veggies a day? It's amazing what you'll learn when you look at your diet in black and white.

DAY 3	WHAT I ATE/DRANK	ESTIMATED PORTION SIZE	CALORIES	NOTES
Breakfast	Coffee with 2 sugars	1 cup	35	Not enough sleep!
	Cornflakes w/	2 cups	300	
	2% milk	1 cup	120	
Lunch	Ham and cheese sandwich	1	360	Ate at meeting
	Chips - single serving	1 oz	160	
	Diet Cola	12 oz	0	

why the plan works

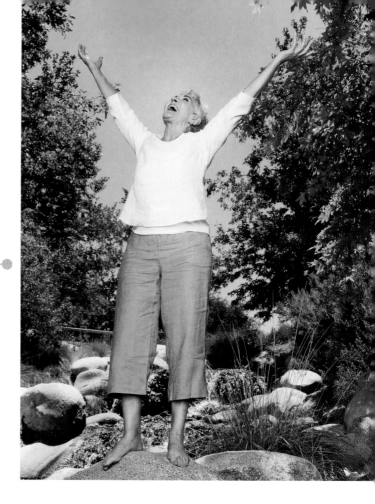

If you have diabetes, your primary goal is simple: to bring your blood sugar under control. There's just no way to better protect yourself from the ravages of the disease. On the Eat plan you'll also lose weight and reduce your risk for all of the serious complications that come with diabetes, from heart attack and stroke to blindness, kidney failure, and even amputation. It's a big promise—one that the plan delivers on, all the while filling your plate to the brim with delicious, satisfying meals. Here's why it works.

It's Easy on Your Blood Sugar

At the heart of the Eat plan are what we think of as "wonder foods"—green vegetables, protein foods like lean chicken and fish, whole grains, low-fat dairy products, and even "luxuries" like olive oil, nuts, and avocado. These foods help keep blood sugar low in a variety of ways.

Slower digestion of meals. At every meal you'll eat right-sized portions of lean protein as well as good fats, such as those in fish, olive oil, nuts, avocado, and flaxseed. These slow-digesting foods blunt the rise in your blood sugar caused by the carbs in your meal simply by expanding the time it takes for your body to digest them. Plus, protein and fat don't raise blood sugar, as carbohydrates do, so including both at each meal instead of filling your whole plate with, say, pasta, automatically helps you avoid sugar spikes. What's more, some of the compounds our bodies make from protein help regulate blood sugar, so including protein in a meal also means your body will process the carbohydrates in that meal more efficiently.

Improved response to insulin. Dairy products and "good fats" (such as nuts, olive oil, and fatty fish like salmon) help reduce insulin resistance, an underlying cause of type 2 diabetes that occurs when your body stops heeding signals from insulin, the hormone that tells cells to absorb blood sugar. Emerging research also suggests that good fats go further, helping your body release the right amount of insulin promptly after eating so that blood sugar doesn't spike after a meal. These fats even seem to help insulin-producing cells in your pancreas live longer.

Fewer sugar spikes. When it comes to carbohydrate foods—the foods that raise blood sugar the most—the plan has you covered. Instead of foods like white rice and starchy potatoes, you'll focus on carbs that have less impact on your blood sugar, including green vegetables and grains such as barley. Researchers have created a system for measuring the blood-sugar impact of carbohydrate foods. It's called the glycemic load or GL for short. High-glycemic foods such as white rice, white bread, and fruit juice are extremely easy for your body to digest, so your blood sugar rises like a hot temper after you eat them. Low-glycemic foods, like non-starchy vegetables, many whole grains, and most beans take a lot more work to break down, so blood sugar levels simmer rather than explode.

On the Eat plan, you'll focus on low-glycemic carbs that go easy on your blood sugar. In fact, the plan devotes three-fourths of the space on your plate to them in the form of non-starchy vegetables, low-glycemic whole grains, and fruit.

It Reduces Your Risk for Diabetes-Related Complications

By getting better control of your blood sugar, you'll help stave off diabetes-related complications, such as serious eye and kidney problems; reduce your risk of heart disease (did you know that people with diabetes have two to four times the usual risk of heart disease and stroke?); and most likely live longer.

The power of plant foods. Our ancestors filled their bellies with wild produce; today, researchers suspect that our bodies evolved to expect big daily doses of the antioxidants, cholesterol-lowering plant compounds called phytosterols, and soluble

Big Bonus Benefits

The Eat, Move, Choose plan helps you lose weight, which may help relieve or prevent a multitude of secondary health problems, including:

- ▶ High blood pressure
- ▶ Heart disease
- ▶ Stroke
- ▶ Gallbladder disease
- ▶ Joint pain
- ▶ Sleep apnea
- ▶ Arthritis
- ▶ Breast cancer
- ▶ Colon cancer
- ▶ Prostate cancer
- ▶ Kidney cancer

fiber found in fruits and vegetables. Without enough of them—and most of us get four produce servings a day or less—heart risk rises. We'll show you how to hunt and gather at least eight servings of produce a day.

The power of a low-glycemic diet. By changing the carbohydrates you eat, you'll garner more protection against heart disease as well as other serious health conditions. When scientists looked at the glycemic load of typical diets in different populations, they found that the higher the GL, the greater the incidence of obesity, diabetes, heart disease, and cancer. In one study, men who ate the most sugar-boosting foods were 40 percent more likely to develop diabetes. And in the landmark Nurses' Health Study, a Harvard School of Public Health research project that's tracked the health and diets of tens of thousands of women for nearly two decades, women were twice as likely to develop heart disease over 10 years if they ate more sugar-boosting foods. The converse is also true: The lower the GL of your diet, the more likely you are to keep your weight under control and stay free of chronic disease.

The power of good fats. The Eat plan goes further, providing your body with good fats that cool chronic inflammation in the body. This kind of inflammation is linked to insulin resistance, which makes it harder for the body to control its blood sugar levels. Inflammation also raises your risk for the medical condition that kills more people with diabetes than any other: heart disease. This plan pampers your heart by giving it the anti-inflammatory fats—in olive and canola oil, avocados, nuts, and fish—and the antioxidants (from fruits and veggies) it needs to stay healthy, and by helping you cut back on the fats that hurt your heart. In fact, eating just a handful of nuts a few times a week can slash your risk of getting heart disease by as much as 25 percent.

It Helps You Lose Weight

You can lose weight on any diet that cuts calories—*if* you can stick with it. And that big *if* is the reason there are thousands of failed diets out there. Too many weight-loss plans unnecessarily restrict healthy foods like whole grains and good fats, or put too much emphasis on blood-sugar-raising carbs. They—and you—miss out on the research-proven staying power of the delicious, high-satisfaction, blood-sugar-friendly meals you'll enjoy on the Eat plan. The plan makes weight loss easier in several ways.

It cuts food cravings. Eating protein at every meal, choosing low-glycemic carbs, and including a healthy amount of good fats in your diet cuts blood sugar swings and therefore food cravings, so you consume fewer empty calories out of a desperate need to eat something—anything—now. Out of 16 studies, 15 found that meals that raise blood sugar quickly resulted in feeling hungrier before the next meal—and eating about 150 extra calories.

It readjusts hunger hormones. Low-glycemic meals also increase levels of leptin, a hormone that decreases hunger (and boosts fat burning), and lower levels of ghrelin, a hormone that increases hunger.

It keeps you full longer. We ask that you eat protein at every meal. One reason: Protein has a special ability to put a damper on hunger, expanding the time between when you eat and when your stomach starts rumbling again. It makes you feel full longer than carbohydrates do—remarkable because protein has the same number of calories (4 per gram) as carbohydrates. Protein also has the advantage of being digested more slowly than carbohydrates, so it slows the rise in blood sugar after a meal.

It keeps your metabolism running on high. In diet studies, people on moderately high-protein diets lost more body fat and less muscle—good news because muscle is your body's metabolic motor, burning calories around the clock whether you're walking or asleep.

It makes meals more satisfying. Fat may seem like a high-calorie splurge, but the truth is, a bit of fat makes meals more satisfying, which can make it easier to stick to a healthy eating plan. Try to go too low-fat, and you'll most likely throw in the towel at some point, probably sooner rather than later. In one study of overweight men and women, those on a moderate-fat diet lost about 9 pounds over 18 months, while those on a low-fat diet actually wound up gaining more than 6 pounds. One key reason was dieting fatigue: Only 20 percent of those on the low-fat diet were still actively participating by the end of the study, while 54 percent of those on the moderate-fat diet were still at it.

It helps you eat fewer calories throughout the day. On the Eat plan we ask you to eat breakfast every day. This not only helps keep your blood sugar levels stable, it also helps you eat fewer calories throughout the day, according to several studies. One report presented to the American Heart Association found that rates of obesity and metabolic problems such as insulin resistance were 35 to 50 percent lower in people who ate breakfast. We also ask you to pile your plate with non-starchy vegetables and fruits. These "high-volume" foods are packed with fiber and water. They take up a lot of room in your stomach, triggering signals that tell your brain that you're full. It's small wonder that researchers find that when people eat lots of vegetables, their calorie consumption goes down— and they lose weight.

It Keeps Portions in Check

We want you to put every type of blood sugar–friendly, health-protecting food on your plate, including higher-calorie "good fats" and whole-grain carbohydrates. But any food, if overeaten, can pack on pounds. That's why right-sized portions are another backbone of our plan. We've devised an innovative Plate Approach that helps you develop an intuitive sense of portion control while giving you plenty of foods that go easy on your weight and blood sugar. With the Plate Approach, you'll become a whiz at no-math, no-measuring perfect portions—a no-worries way to right-size your meals.

It Makes You Feel Better

Modest weight loss—the type you'll experience on the Eat, Move, Choose plan—and the corresponding drop in blood sugar will make you feel better almost immediately by getting rid of the jittery feelings that blood sugar swings can cause and giving you more energy. Just as important, losing weight typically brings down cholesterol levels, blood pressure, and overall risk of heart disease.

Should You Supplement?

You're eating right, you're exercising—is there more you can do to protect your health? You bet! These three supplements can help protect your heart, guard against brittle bones and high blood pressure, and plug the occasional nutritional deficit. You'll notice that we're not suggesting any high-dose, single-vitamin or single-mineral supplements (with the exception of calcium). A growing stack of research suggests that approach is ineffective—or even downright dangerous—for protecting health.

1. Multivitamin A multi can't make up for a poor diet, but it may help fill in nutritional gaps—especially for nutrients that become more difficult to absorb as we age. For people with diabetes, multivitamins can provide critical nutrients, such as magnesium, which many diabetics are deficient in, and chromium, which may help improve blood sugar and cholesterol levels, as well as B vitamins, which help protect the heart and nerves.

What to Take If you're a man or a postmenopausal woman, choose a multivitamin without iron. Make sure it contains 400 mg of folic acid and 400 IU of vitamin D, as well as no more than 100 percent to 150 percent of the recommended daily value for other vitamins and minerals.

Note: Take with meals for best absorption.

2. Calcium Calcium protects the bones and helps keep blood pressure in check.

What to Take The recommended dosage is 600 mg twice a day. Calcium citrate is easier than other forms for people over 65 to digest.

3. Fish oil capsules People with diabetes have an elevated risk of heart disease. Fish oil guards against off-rhythm heartbeats, slows blood clotting, and keeps arteries supple.

What to Take Take 1,000 mg of EPA plus DHA once or twice a day.

Note: Talk to your doctor before taking it, especially if you're on a blood-thinning drug such as Coumadin.

GOAL 1

Eat five+ servings of vegetables a day

RIGHT OFF THE BAT, we know you're probably thinking, "Wow, that sounds like a lot of vegetables." So before we go any further, we want to clear up the confusion over what exactly a "serving" is. It's probably less than you think. See "What's in a Veggie Serving" on page 37. If you're really not used to eating vegetables at all, start with a modest goal of just three servings a day and gradually work your way up to five. Once you get used to eating five servings a day, look for ways to bump that up to seven. There's new evidence that getting seven vegetable servings a day is even better for your health.

From juicy red peppers to sweet little green peas, from meaty portobello mushrooms to crunchy broccoli, vegetables are the ideal food for people with diabetes. Low in fat and calories, they're packed with fiber, vitamins, minerals, and other powerful nutrients that fight disease, pamper your blood sugar, and help you maintain a healthy weight. And let's face it, if you're eating more vegetables, you're eating less of everything else, including fatty meat, carbohydrate foods, and junk food. Now you know why this goal is number 1 on the Eat plan.

Over and over again, researchers have found that eating more vegetables is a key strategy for losing weight and keeping it off. Vegetables make you feel full and satisfied, for very few calories. The simple truth: The more vegetables you eat, the less you'll weigh. In one study at Pennsylvania State University, women who started a meal with a low-calorie salad and then ate a pasta dish ate about 12 percent fewer calories in total than women who skipped the salad and started right in on the pasta. In another study, adding about 6 ounces of vegetables (in this case, carrots and spinach) to dinner helped people feel fuller on fewer calories.

STEP ONE
Shop with Intent

No veggies in the fridge? Then you'll be forced to eat a dinner that's virtually veggie-free or go for chips, cookies, candy, cheese, or whatever else is on hand when you're hungry and need a snack. The first rule of eating more vegetables, then, is to make sure they're ready and waiting, in the most user-friendly forms possible.

Take advantage of prepared produce. We usually don't recommend prepared foods. They're

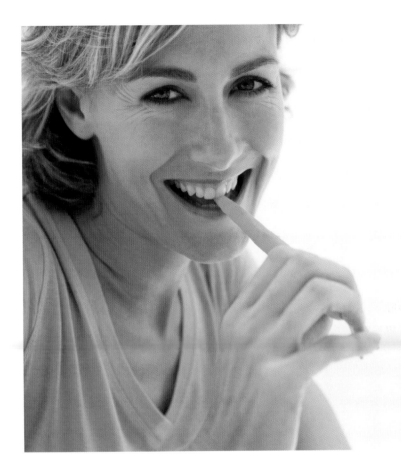

Eating more vegetables is a key strategy for losing weight and keeping it off—they make you feel full for very few calories.

more expensive and often high in artificial flavorings, sugars, and sodium. But when it comes to prepared veggies—bagged salads, prewashed spinach, peeled and diced butternut squash, washed and chopped kale—we're all for it. Numerous consumer studies find that we're more likely to use bagged salads and other produce than produce that requires more preparation.

Buy "now" and "later" fresh vegetables. When you grocery shop, choose just a few vegetables from the produce section that you can use up over the next four or five days, such as lettuce, spinach, and tomatoes. Invest the rest of your fresh-veggie budget in types that keep well, such as carrots, celery, cabbage, onions, winter squash, sweet potatoes, and

garlic. That way, vegetables won't languish in your fridge, and you'll always have produce on hand even when it's tough to get to the store for more perishable items.

Stock your pantry and freezer with canned and frozen vegetables. They can be as nutritious as fresh veggies because they're picked at their peak, when they are the most nutrient-rich. Frozen vegetables are flash-frozen, which seals in the nutrients until the veggies are thawed. Don't worry about losing nutrients that leach into water in cans: The amounts are small, and you lose nothing if you use the water in dishes such as soup. Just be sure to choose naked veggies—those without sauce or cheese.

STEP TWO
Aim for Variety

We have a tendency to lump all vegetables together as if they were a single food. But vegetables can be sweet, bitter, or bland; big or small; and green, orange, yellow, red, brown, and every shade and flavor in between. Given the sheer bounty of natural foods at your disposal, how do you decide which to eat?

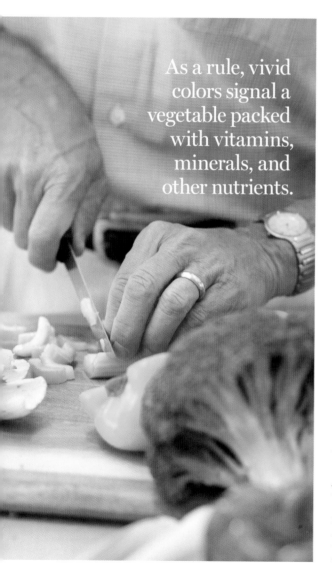

As a rule, vivid colors signal a vegetable packed with vitamins, minerals, and other nutrients.

The first thing to do is to vote with your taste buds and eat produce you like. If you tend to eat only one veggie, such as frozen green beans, try to vary your routine. This will help ensure that you get all the nutrients you need. A serving of broccoli may have dozens of powerhouse nutrients—but not necessarily the same ones as a serving of asparagus.

Getting the variety of nutrients found in a variety of vegetables is important for controlling blood sugar and cutting your risk for diabetes complications like heart disease and high blood pressure. In one British study, people with the highest blood levels of vitamin C were less likely to have high A1C scores, a long-term indicator of high blood sugar. In another study, people with the highest blood levels of beta-carotene—found in carrots and winter squash—had 32 percent lower insulin levels (suggesting better blood sugar control) than those with the lowest levels. Dark, leafy greens such as spinach, Swiss chard, bok choy, collards, and mustard greens provide zinc, a mineral that protects insulin-producing beta cells in the pancreas. Zinc is lost in the urine when blood sugar is too high, so replacing it is vitally important if you have diabetes.

Ready to munch and crunch?

Start by choosing veggies with star nutritional power. As a rule of thumb, vivid colors—dark greens and bright reds, oranges, yellows, and purples—signal that a vegetable is packed with vitamins, minerals, and other vital nutrients. Often, these nutrients are especially helpful for people with diabetes. We highly recommend these five versatile superstars:

Broccoli. Big on volume and small on calories, broccoli is a great way to bulk up carbohydrate-rich dishes (think pasta, casseroles, and baked potatoes) to blunt their effect on your blood sugar and your waistline. This classic is one of the best food sources of chromium, a mineral required for insulin to function normally (remember, insulin helps the body use up blood sugar so there's less in the bloodstream). One cup of broccoli provides almost half of your daily chromium requirement. Fiber, at a hearty 4 grams per stalk, is also part of broccoli's "benefits package."

Carrots. Don't believe the hype that carrots raise your blood sugar rapidly. Chalk up that myth to a problem with the Glycemic Index, a system that preceded the more accurate Glycemic Load. While the type of sugar carrots contain is transformed into blood sugar very rapidly, the amount of sugar in carrots is extremely low. Thank goodness, because they're one of the richest sources of beta-carotene, which is linked to a lower risk of diabetes. Like most vegetables, carrots are also a good source of beneficial fiber. By the way, carrots won't help you throw away your reading glasses, but they will help protect against two sight-robbing conditions: macular degeneration and cataracts.

Spinach, kale, and other dark, leafy greens. Thanks to rich stores of carotenoids (including beta-carotene and other "carotenes"), these yummy greens are among the most antioxidant-rich vegetables on Earth. Antioxidants are powerful weapons against diabetes-related complications, including heart disease and nerve damage, not to mention cancer. They're also loaded with potassium and magnesium, which help keep blood pressure in check.

Sweet potatoes. Eat a baked sweet potato instead of a baked white potato, and your blood sugar will rise about 30 percent less! A sweet deal indeed, especially because these potatoes are packed with nutrients and disease-fighting fiber, almost 40 percent of which is soluble fiber, the kind that helps lower blood sugar and cholesterol. Sweet potatoes

what's in a veggie serving?

Here's the definition of a serving from the National Cancer Institute. All varieties of fruits and vegetables—fresh, frozen, canned, dried, and 100 percent juice—count. Measure out some of these in your kitchen so you can see how reasonable a serving size is.

- 1/2 cup raw, cooked, canned, or frozen vegetables
- 3/4 cup (6 ounces) 100 percent vegetable juice
- 1/2 cup cooked or canned legumes (beans and peas)
- 1 cup raw, leafy vegetables such as lettuce and spinach

are extraordinarily rich in carotenoids, orange and yellow pigments that play a role in helping the body respond to insulin. They're also full of the natural plant compound chlorogenic acid, which may help reduce insulin resistance.

STEP THREE

Have at Least One Vegetable Side Dish at Dinner

Make it an automatic rule: There will be at least one vegetable on your plate at dinner—and lunch whenever you can. This can be as easy as tossing baby carrots or cherry tomatoes into a zip-close bag. These strategies can help make the most of the great flavors and textures in these amazing foods.

Give veggies a roast. Here is one of the great side dishes—easy to make, delicious to eat, and amazingly healthy. Plus, it tastes surprisingly sweet and lasts well as a leftover, meaning you can make large batches and serve throughout the week. Cut hearty root vegetables like parsnips, turnips, rutabagas, carrots, and onions into inch-thick chunks and arrange in a single layer on a cookie sheet. Drizzle with olive oil and sprinkle with kosher or sea salt, freshly ground pepper, and fresh or dried herbs. Roast in a 450°F oven until soft, about 45 minutes, turning once. That's it!

Throw 'em on the grill. If you only use your grill for meats, you've been missing out! Peppers, zucchini, asparagus, onions, eggplant—even tomatoes—all taste amazingly good when grilled. Generally, all you need to do is coat them with olive oil and throw them on. Turn every few minutes and remove when they start to soften. Or skewer chunks of veggies on a bamboo or metal skewer and turn frequently. You can also buy grilling baskets that keep the veggies from falling through the slats in the grill.

Buy a vegetable steamer. It's one of the healthiest ways to cook vegetables because nutrients aren't lost in the water. Choose a metal or bamboo steamer basket, fill it with veggies, place over a saucepan of rapidly simmering water, cover, and cook for 5 to 10 minutes. It's that simple.

STEP FOUR
Sneak in Veggies at Every Opportunity

The average American is lucky to get two servings of vegetables a day—far less than the five we're suggesting. This gap pretty much captures America's

Vegetable Seasoning Guide

Think beyond butter when it comes to seasoning vegetables. Try these delicious pairings:

VEGETABLE	BEST HERBS, SPICES, AND FLAVORINGS
ASPARAGUS	Lemon, garlic, oregano
BROCCOLI	Garlic, soy sauce, mustard, dark sesame oil
CARROTS	Lemon, orange, curry powder, ginger, dill, raspberry vinegar
CAULIFLOWER	Basil, curry powder
EGGPLANT	Basil, garlic, crushed tomato
GREEN BEANS	Garlic, soy sauce, sesame seeds
MUSHROOMS	Parsley, thyme, green onions, chives, sherry, balsamic vinegar
PEAS	Mint, garlic
SPINACH	Garlic, soy sauce, sea salt, nutmeg, balsamic vinegar
SUMMER SQUASH	Lemon, rosemary, tomato, garlic, basil
TOMATO	Basil, garlic, oregano, balsamic vinegar, Parmesan cheese

health problems in a nutshell. If we ate more vegetables and fewer processed foods, we'd lose weight, clean our arteries, balance our blood sugar, and shut down a large number of hospitals. But getting from two servings a day to five doesn't come without planning or effort. We're here to help. Here's how to sneak more veggies into your daily diet.

Breakfast, Lunch, and Snacks

Sneak vegetables into breakfast. One reason we don't get enough vegetables is that many of us consider them merely a side dish to dinner. But eggs are perfect vegetable vehicles. Make egg scrambles a regular breakfast, using a scrambled egg to hold together lightly sautéed vegetables such as peppers, mushrooms, zucchini, asparagus, or onions.

Build a sandwich that has more lettuce and tomato than meat. Stack the meat filler in the sandwich to no higher than the thickness of a standard slice of bread. Then pile on low-calorie slices of lettuce and tomatoes to the combined height of both slices of bread. Presto: Your sandwich tower has the height of the Empire State Building yet the svelteness of the Eiffel Tower.

Have a veggie burger for lunch once a week. Top it with a sliced tomato and lettuce for even more veggie power. Honestly, it will taste better than you imagine.

Open a can of low-sodium soup and add veggies. Toss in a bag of precut broccoli and carrots, either fresh or frozen, and voilà! You have a superfast and easy lunch or dinner entrée, ready to be flavored with your preferred spices, herbs, or hot sauce. As the soup simmers, it will simultaneously cook the veggies, boosting the nutritional value and fiber.

Eat vegetables like they were fruit. Half a cucumber, a whole tomato, a stalk of celery, or a

five things
to do with broccoli

- Chop spears and add them to stir-fries.
- Steam just long enough for the broccoli to turn brilliant green. Eat the softer-but-crunchy spears as finger food for a taste that's different from that of either raw or fully cooked broccoli.
- Add raw or lightly steamed to a garden salad or a vegetable-and-dip tray.
- Sauté with a little garlic and oil and top with a dusting of Parmesan for a quick, low-calorie side dish.
- Steam, then puree and make soup by adding to chicken broth along with a bit of garlic and some onions. For a creamier version, add fat-free evaporated milk.

long, fresh carrot are as pleasant to munch on as an apple. It may not seem typical, but who cares? A whole vegetable makes a terrific snack.

Dinner and Dessert

Start each dinner with a mixed green salad before you serve the main course. Not only will it help you eat more veggies, but by filling your stomach first with a nutrient-rich, low-calorie salad, there'll be just a bit less room for the higher-calorie items that follow. For an instant, perfectly dressed salad, open a bag of prewashed, precut romaine lettuce or mixed greens, add a tablespoon of olive oil and a splash of lemon juice or balsamic vinegar, and shake.

Put a plate of raw vegetables in the center of the table. Nearly everyone likes carrot sticks, celery sticks, cucumber slices, string beans, cherry tomatoes, and/or green pepper strips. They're healthy, they have virtually no calories, they have a satisfying

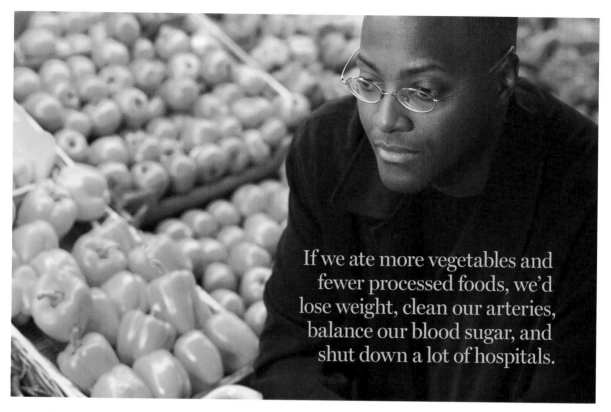

If we ate more vegetables and fewer processed foods, we'd lose weight, clean our arteries, balance our blood sugar, and shut down a lot of hospitals.

crunch, and they can substantially cut your consumption of the more calorie-dense main course.

Once a week, have an entrée salad. A salade niçoise is a good example: mixed greens, steamed green beans, boiled potatoes, sliced hard-boiled egg, and tuna drizzled with vinaigrette. Serve with crusty whole-grain bread. Bon appétit!

Fill your spaghetti sauce with vegetables. Then replace half the pasta you normally eat with more vegetables. We typically take a jar of low-sodium prepared sauce and add in string beans, peas, corn, bell peppers, mushrooms, tomatoes and more. Like it chunky? Cut them in big pieces. Don't want to know they're there? Shred or puree them with a bit of sauce in the blender, then add. And don't stop there. Steamed broccoli or green beans, or baked spaghetti squash (use a fork to remove the spaghetti-like strands), are filling and delicious replacements for the mounds of pasta that often find their way onto our plates.

Order your pizza with extra veggies. Instead of the same old pepperoni and onions, do your blood sugar and digestion a favor and ask for half the cheese, double the sauce and add toppings like artichoke hearts, broccoli, hot peppers, and other exotic vegetables many pizza joints stock these days for their gourmet pies.

Puree cooked veggies into soup. Potatoes, carrots, winter squash, cauliflower, and broccoli— just about any cooked (or leftover) vegetable can be made into a creamy, comforting soup. Here's a simple recipe: In a medium saucepan, sauté 1 cup finely chopped onion in 1 tablespoon vegetable oil until tender. Combine the onion in a blender or food processor with cooked vegetables and puree until smooth. Return puree to saucepan and thin with broth or low-fat milk. Simmer and season to taste.

Go vegetarian one day a week. You can do this by merely substituting the meat serving with a vegetable serving (suggestion: make it a crunchy, strong-flavored vegetable like broccoli). Or you can dabble in the world of vegetarian cooking, in which recipes are developed specifically to make a filling, robust meal out of vegetables and whole grains. For those times, you should get yourself a good vegetarian cookbook.

Use salsa liberally. First, make sure you have a large batch filled with vegetables. One good approach: Add chopped yellow squash and zucchini to store-bought salsa. Then put salsa on everything: baked potatoes, rice, chicken breasts, sandwiches, eggs, steak, even bread. Salsa shouldn't be just for chips. It's too tasty and healthy not to be used all the time.

Throw a bag of pre-shredded carrots and cabbage into your next soup, salad, or casserole. Available in the produce department, these coleslaw ingredients add flavor, color, and lots of vitamins and minerals.

Use vegetables as sauces. How about pureed roasted red peppers seasoned with herbs and a bit of lemon juice, then drizzled over fish? Or puree butternut or acorn squash with carrots, grated ginger, and bit of brown sugar for a yummy topping for chicken or turkey. Cooked vegetables are easily converted into sauces. It just takes a little ingenuity and a blender.

Bake some pumpkin pudding for dessert. It's easy—and delicious! In a bowl, beat together 1/2 cup

Eat Your ABCs

Knowing tasty ways to cook a vegetable makes you all the more likely to eat it. Try these tips.

Asparagus Roast them in the oven with a little olive oil. Delicious! Or make instant asparagus soup by pureeing cooked asparagus, heating it with a little milk, and adding chopped parsley or tarragon.

Broccoli Overcooking can degrade some of broccoli's nutrients, so steam florets lightly, shorten cooking time in the microwave, or quickly stir-fry them in a small amount of olive oil. To eat them almost raw but cooked enough to soften them up, blanch broccoli spears in boiling water for about 3 minutes.

Brussels sprouts The stems are tougher than the leaves, so cut an "X" across the base of each sprout before steaming to allow heat inside the core to soften it. For the mildest taste, choose frozen baby Brussels sprouts. For the best flavor, cook them lightly so they're still a little crisp.

Cauliflower Instead of mashed potatoes, try this tasty cauliflower puree. Boil a head of cauliflower cut into florets, one diced peeled potato, and six peeled garlic cloves until tender. Drain and puree (in batches) in a food processor and thin with enough warm milk to make it velvety. Drizzle olive oil on top and season with salt and pepper.

egg white (or egg substitute), 1 can pumpkin, 2 packets Splenda, 1 teaspoon cinnamon, 1/2 teaspoon nutmeg, and 1/2 cup fat-free evaporated milk. Pour into four 8-ounce custard cups coated with cooking spray. Place on a cookie sheet. Bake uncovered at 400°F for 8 to 10 minutes. Reduce heat to 300°F and bake for another 30 minutes until a knife inserted comes out clean. Serve warm or cold. Yum!

Top 20 Foods for Diabetes

Just about any good-for-you food fits into the Eat plan, including every fresh fruit and green (and red, orange, and yellow) vegetable under the sun. But these 20 foods have properties that make them extra-appealing for people with diabetes.

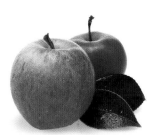

1 Apples This year-round favorite fruit is loaded with soluble fiber—number one for blunting blood sugar swings. A medium apple dishes up an impressive 4 grams of fiber, mostly pectin, which is also known for its ability to lower cholesterol. Go for whole, unpeeled fruit.

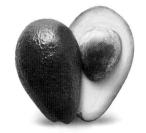

2 Avocado Rich, creamy, and packed with good fat, avocado slows digestion to help keep blood sugar from spiking after a meal. A diet high in the fat it contains may even help reverse insulin resistance, which translates to steadier blood sugar over the long term.

3 Barley Barley may just be the perfect substitute for rice. Soluble fiber and other compounds in barley slow the digestion and absorption of blood sugar dramatically. And unlike rice (either white or brown), barley has minimal impact on blood sugar. Choosing this grain instead of a refined grain like white rice can reduce the rise in blood sugar after a meal by almost 70 percent—and can keep your blood sugar lower and steadier for hours.

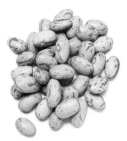

4 Beans The soluble fiber in all types of beans puts a lid on high blood sugar. And because they're rich in protein, beans can stand in for meat in salads and even main dishes. Best of all, all you have to do is open a can.

5 Beef Yes, beef is a diabetes-friendly food, as long as you choose the leanest cuts and keep portions to one-fourth of your plate. Getting enough protein in your meals helps keep you full and satisfied, and it helps you maintain muscle mass when you're losing weight, so that your metabolism keeps burning on "high."

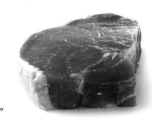

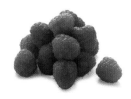

7 Broccoli Filling, fibrous, and full of antioxidants (including a day's worth of vitamin C in one serving), broccoli is also rich in chromium, which plays an important role in long-term blood sugar control.

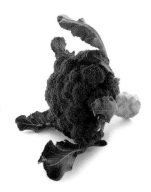

6 Berries Full of fiber and especially rich in all-important antioxidants, berries are a low-calorie, low-sugar way to satisfy a sweet tooth.

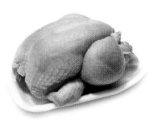

8 Carrots They're one of nature's richest sources of beta-carotene, which is linked to a lower risk of diabetes. And raw carrots (dipped in a little peanut butter or hummus) make perfect snacks.

10 Eggs Eggs are an excellent, inexpensive source of high-quality protein—so high, in fact, that egg protein is the gold standard nutritionists use to rank all other proteins. An egg or two won't raise your blood sugar (or cholesterol in most people) and can keep you feeling full and satisfied for hours after a meal.

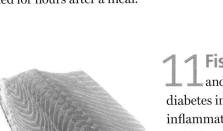

9 Chicken and turkey White meat chicken is one of the leanest, lowest-calorie protein sources money can buy. Turkey breast is even lower in calories. Ground skinless turkey breast is a smart substitute for ground beef.

11 Fish Serve up salmon for dinner and you'll be managing your diabetes in several ways—by fighting inflammation in your body, and getting good fats, which help steady blood sugar. You'll also slash your risk of heart disease, the most deadly diabetes complication.

continued >>>

12 **Flaxseed** These brown shiny seeds hit the diabetes trifecta: They are rich in protein, fiber, and good fats similar to the kind found in fish. They're also a good source of magnesium, a mineral that's key to good blood sugar control because it helps cells use insulin.

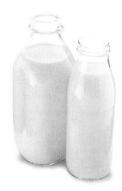

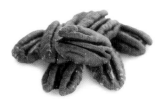

13 **Milk and yogurt** These are rich in protein and calcium, which studies show may help people lose weight. And diets that include plenty of dairy may fight insulin resistance, a core problem behind diabetes. Go low-fat or fat-free when you eat or drink dairy.

14 **Nuts** Where else can you get a protein-rich, fiber-heavy snack that's also loaded with good fat? Nuts couldn't be any friendlier to your blood sugar. Just stick with a small handful per day.

15 **Oatmeal** Thanks to its soluble fiber, it's even better for your blood sugar than starting the day with a whole-grain cereal. And it's extraordinarily kind to your heart.

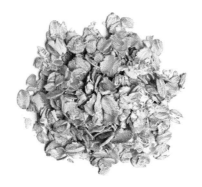

16 **Olive oil** Unlike butter, the good fat in olive oil won't increase insulin resistance and may even help reverse it, helping your body steady its own blood sugar. A touch of olive oil also slows the emptying of the stomach, so your meal is less likely to spike your blood sugar. And of course the oil is heart-friendly.

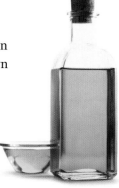

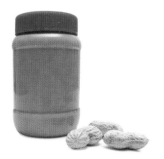

17 Peanut butter
A study at Purdue University found that eating peanut butter can dampen appetite for up to 2 hours longer than a low-fiber, high-carb snack, making this childhood favorite a grown-up weight-loss ally. Monounsaturated fats in PB also help control blood sugar.

18 Seeds
Like nuts, seeds of all types—pumpkin, sunflower, sesame and beyond—are filled with good fats, protein, and fiber that work together to keep blood sugar low and to stave off heart disease. They also are a natural source of cholesterol-lowering sterols, the same compounds added to some cholesterol-lowering margarines.

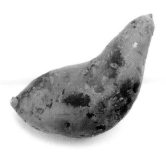

19 Sweet potatoes
Choose a baked sweet potato instead of a baked white potato, and your blood sugar will rise about 30 percent less. Sweet potatoes are packed with nutrients and disease-fighting fiber—almost 40 percent of which is soluble fiber, the kind that helps lower blood sugar and cholesterol.

20 Whole-wheat bread
White bread is one of the five foods in our diets that raise blood sugar the most. Switch to whole wheat and you may improve your sensitivity to insulin, the hormone that manages blood sugar. In one study of 978 men and women, the higher their intake of whole grains, the greater their insulin sensitivity, which translates into better blood sugar control.

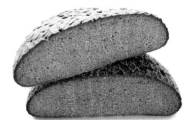

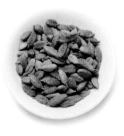

GOAL 2

Cut your refined carbohydrates by half

SIMPLY PUT, MOST AMERICANS eat way too many carbohydrate foods—yet not nearly enough whole grains. Most of the carb foods we eat are the kind that send blood sugar soaring. We munch lots of potatoes, mostly fried. We consume enormous quantities of bread in all forms, most of it made with refined white flour that has little or no fiber. We eat a lot of rice, most of it white. We breakfast on pastries and muffins and snack on bags of potato chips and pretzels (it's true pretzels are low in fat, but they're more or less just empty carbs). And we wash it all down with sugar-sweetened sodas and fruit drinks. In fact, of all the extra daily calories we've taken to consuming over the past decade or two, nearly all come from one source: refined carbohydrates.

It's time to dial down the carbohydrate mania, the smart way.

Let's be clear. We're not talking about a "just say no" approach to carbohydrates. Your body needs the energy and nutrients found in grains, vegetables, dried beans, fruits, and milk (yes, all of these foods count, at least in part, as carbohydrates because they contain starches and/or sugars). Instead, we ask you to make a conscious effort to choose more whole grains and fewer refined grain products; eat smaller portions of grain-based carbs; and spend much more of your "carb budget" on vegetables and fresh fruit.

STEP ONE
Say "Less" to Refined Carbs

Reducing or eliminating just a few foods that spike blood sugar can make a huge difference when it comes to managing your diabetes. In a major study of middle-aged women, five foods emerged as the biggest high-blood-sugar culprits. Together they were responsible for 30 percent of the total effect the women's daily diets had on their blood sugar. See "Smart Substitutions" to learn the five foods and discover lower-GL replacements. Pay special attention to making these switches first. Then move on to these tips.

Skip the dinner rolls. Bread isn't bad for you, especially if it's whole grain. But if you had a sandwich at lunch or toast with your eggs at breakfast, that's probably all the bread you need for the day.

Nix the tortilla for a lettuce leaf wrap. A 13-inch tortilla can contain as many as 330 calories, not to mention 55 grams of carbs. Instead, try wrapping a lettuce leaf around canned tuna or salmon, shredded carrots, diced celery, and pepper slices.

Eat less rice, and choose carefully. Stick with one serving, or 1/2 cup, per meal. Your best choice when it comes to your blood sugar? Converted white rice or brown rice. Avoid jasmine rice, arborio rice (the kind used to make risotto), sticky rice, and long-grain quick-cooking rice. Of all rices, these raise blood sugar the most.

Cut your pasta in half. Even white pasta has a lower GL than bread because of the way the starch molecules are interwoven with protein molecules, making the starch in pasta harder to break down. That means pasta is fairly friendly to your blood sugar, as far as grain foods go. (Cook it al dente instead of well done, and it will have even less impact on your blood sugar.) Still, it's a good idea to avoid making pasta the dominant food on your plate. Serve yourself half of a cup of pasta instead of a whole cup and bulk it up with sautéed peppers, mushrooms, spinach, or other vegetables.

Indulge in parsnip and carrot "fries." Cut down the length of parsnips and carrots to make long, thin strips of the vegetables. Place on a baking sheet, drizzle with olive oil, sprinkle with salt and pepper, and roast in a 400°F oven for about 40 minutes.

Say so long to soda. Want an instant, easy way to eliminate empty carbohydrate calories and gain better blood sugar control? Take aim at sodas. These beverages have zero nutritional value, but each 12-ounce serving of regular soda contains about 150 calories—virtually all of it sugar. (That's equivalent to nine packets of sugar!) And studies

Smart Substitutions

Each substitution raises blood sugar just half as much as the food it replaces.

FOOD	SUBSTITUTION
Cooked potatoes	Whole-grain pasta
Sugary breakfast cereal	High-fiber breakfast cereal
White bread	Coarse 100% whole-grain bread
Muffin	Apple
White rice	Pearled barley

show that soda calories don't fill you up the way food does, so you end up consuming more calories throughout the day than you would if you got those 150 calories from something you could sink your teeth into. What else is there to drink? Plenty.

Water. It has zero calories and quenches thirst better than sugary drinks. Drink it liberally, since dehydration can raise blood sugar. Add a squeeze of lemon or lime juice to make it more interesting.

Sparkling water. Choose plain water or sugar-free, fruit-flavored varieties.

Iced tea. Make your own by steeping two tea bags in a tall glass of cold water. If you drink bottled iced tea, check to be sure it's sugar-free and calorie-free.

Lemonade. Making your own with fresh lemon juice and sweetening it with a sugar substitute cuts out the calories, saving more than 100 calories compared with store-bought lemonade.

STEP TWO

Have Three to Six Servings of Whole Grains Every Day

The total number of grain-based carb servings you should aim for every day will depend on your own personal blood sugar patterns and the dietary advice you get from your doctor, registered dietitian, or certified diabetes educator. But almost certainly you should be eating more whole grains than you do now. A serving is small—one slice of 100 percent whole-grain bread or 1/2 cup of cooked pasta or grains. Even so, most of us eat less than one serving a day.

The Not-So-Sweet Truth about "Diabetic" Treats

Can you eat "sugar-free," "low-carb," and "diabetic" candies, cookies, and desserts to your heart's content? The surprising answer is no. You'd think sugar-free foods like candy and soft drinks would have less impact on blood-glucose levels and waistlines than regular candy or soft drinks. But it's not that simple.

The sweeteners they contain—called sugar alcohols—have half the calories of sugar. Under food-labeling laws, products containing sugar alcohols are permitted to call themselves sugar-free. But in fact sweeteners like maltitol, mannitol, sorbitol, and xylitol may not be sucrose (the technical name for regular sugar), but they do contain carbohydrates, each gram of which can raise blood glucose just as much as sugar does. They can also cause intestinal distress—from bloating and gassy rumbling to diarrhea. The products they're in often have just as many calories as regular treats. Our advice: Pay no attention to "sugar-free" claims on the packaging. Look instead at a product's total carbohydrate count and calories. Then go enjoy a piece of fresh fruit!

Why should you go whole? It's simple. Eating more whole grains has been shown to cut heart disease risk by 25 percent in women and 18 percent in men (again, heart disease is the number one killer of people with diabetes). It also helps keep blood sugar steady. In one study of 978 men and women, the more whole grains people ate, the greater their insulin sensitivity, which translates into better blood-sugar control.

And consider the weight loss benefits: The famous Nurses' Health Study from the Harvard School of Public Health looked at more than 74,000 women and found that those who ate the most whole grains were a whopping 49 percent less likely to gain weight over a 12-year period than those who ate the least.

Whole grains contain all the parts of the grain—not just the starchy low-fiber center, but also the nutrient-rich germ layer and the fiber-rich bran layer on the outside. The result: You get antioxidants, vitamins, minerals, and a wide range of plant compounds that protect against chronic disease in many ways.

Many Americans just aren't used to eating whole grains and may not know where to begin. Fortunately, it's easy to do.

Start your day with a high-fiber cereal. There's really no better way to get one of your daily servings of whole grains than starting your day with a whole-grain cereal. Look for a brand with the word "whole" in the first ingredient and at least 3 grams of fiber per serving. It's also important to look for cereals with low sugar content. That way, you'll control calories and stay off the blood-sugar roller coaster that leads to midmorning hunger pangs and food cravings. (A British study found recently that eating sugary cereal actually led to overeating at lunch.) Top your cereal with berries to squeeze in a fruit serving.

For protein, pour on some fat-free milk and maybe some ground flaxseeds (you'll read more about these soon), and you've got the perfect Eat to Reverse Diabetes breakfast.

Buy bread and rolls with the word "whole" in the first ingredient. This is the simplest way to shift the balance from refined to whole-grain carbs in your diet. Don't be fooled by the marketing terms on the front of the label. For example, coloring a loaf of bread brown and calling it wheat bread doesn't make it whole wheat. Or saying a product is "made with wheat flour" could be true of both whole-wheat bread and angel food cake. If a product is truly whole grain, the label will list whole wheat, whole oats, or some other whole grain as the first ingredient on the label.

Switch pastas. Whole-wheat pasta is widely available, and it tastes better than ever. Also look for whole-wheat couscous, a type of pasta that cooks in five minutes. For pasta that's even friendlier to your blood sugar, go with one of the many new high-fiber, high-protein options that have popped up on supermarket shelves. Some are multigrain pastas, made from grains such as oats, spelt, and barley in addition to durum wheat. Since these are higher in soluble fiber, they have less impact on your blood sugar than regular or even whole-wheat pasta. Some contain flaxseed as a source of heart-healthy omega-3 fatty acids. Some have added protein—40 or 50 percent more than regular pasta—from sources like soy flour, milk solids, or egg whites. This also makes them more blood sugar friendly.

Bake with the whole stuff. Give a boost to homemade baked goods by replacing one-third of the white flour with whole-wheat flour.

Use fibrous fixings. Bran cereal, oat bran, and wheat germ make good condiments when

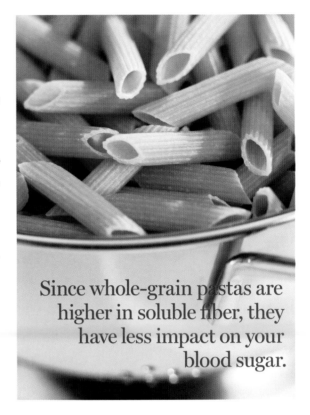

Since whole-grain pastas are higher in soluble fiber, they have less impact on your blood sugar.

sprinkled over oatmeal, applesauce, cottage cheese, or yogurt. In recipes that call for bread crumbs, try oatmeal or whole-grain bread—toasted, then reduced to crumbs in your food processor.

Set a brown rice rule at home and when eating out. With six times more fiber than white rice, brown rice is packed with vitamins, minerals, and natural plant compounds made by nature to protect your health. That's just the beginning. It's also rich in the bone-building mineral magnesium, the immune-boosting antioxidant selenium, and manganese, a mineral important for keeping up the body's natural defenses. Brown rice takes about 45 minutes to cook at home, so start early or make a big batch and freeze meal-size portions. Many restaurants also offer it, if you ask. Just be sure to keep your portion size to 1/2 cup. While it's much better for you than white rice, even brown rice raises blood sugar quite a bit.

Keep bran on hand. Think of bran as the heavy "overcoat" worn by kernels of whole-grain oats, wheat, or rice. It contains the highest concentration of fiber of any part of the grain (12 grams per 1/2 cup for wheat and rice bran; 7 grams per 1/2 cup for oat bran). As you know, fiber helps you feel fuller on fewer calories, smoothing the way for weight loss.

Bran also helps tame wild blood sugar surges after meals. When researchers gave obese children either a sugar solution or a sugar solution plus 15 grams (about 4 tablespoons) of wheat bran, the kids' blood sugar levels were much lower when they ate the bran. If you add bran to your diet regularly, you could really lower your blood sugar over the long term—by as much as 22 percent, research shows. More ways to use bran:

Mix into meat loaf. Use oat bran or another bran as a binder in meat loaf instead of bread. It will help blunt the effect of the mashed potatoes you eat with it by lowering your blood sugar response to the entire meal.

Sprinkle bran flakes on casseroles. You'll hardly know they're there, but the fiber will still work to keep blood sugar lower.

Replace half the flour in muffin recipes with bran. The result is a muffin high in fiber and loaded with nutrients. If you don't have bran flour on hand, try using bran cereal. Some brands have muffin recipes right on the box. Add fruit and nuts for even more fiber.

Try delicious, easy-to-cook bulgur. Also known as kasha, bulgur is wheat grain that's been partially cooked by boiling or steaming, then dried and cracked. That means you're getting a whole grain that cooks in about 15 minutes—great for a week-night dinner.

sugar buster quiz

Q: Raisin Bran or All-Bran cereal?
A: All-Bran

All-Bran cereal has a glycemic load (a measure of how much it raises your blood sugar) of 9; Raisin Bran's GL is 12.

You'll find bulgur in different textures. Coarse bulgur is used for pilaf and rice dishes, medium is used as breakfast cereal, and fine is used for tabbouleh (a Middle Eastern salad made with bulgur, chopped parsley, cucumbers, tomatoes, olive oil, and lemon juice). The finer the grain, the quicker bulgur cooks up.

Serve bulgur pilaf as a side dish. There are a million different recipes, some including dried fruit and some with vegetables and/or herbs. Grab a good cookbook and take your pick. You can also enjoy bulgur in cold salads.

Stuff zucchini with extra-lean beef or pork mixed with bulgur.

Throw together some tabbouleh as an excellent, portable summertime lunch salad or side dish. Toss in chopped vegetables from your garden, such as tomatoes and cucumbers, and add some goat or feta cheese or chicken for extra protein.

Cook up hot bulgur cereal in salted water as you would oatmeal. Top with fresh fruit or with chopped walnuts, dried cranberries, cinnamon, and a drizzle of honey. Some manufacturers make bulgur cereals with extra ingredients, such as soy, which adds extra protein.

The Eat, Move, Choose Carb Pyramid

Because of their extra fiber and nutrients, whole-grain foods (like whole-wheat bread) are a huge improvement over refined grain foods (like white bread). But even among whole-grain foods, some are better for your blood sugar than others. Choosing low-glycemic carbs can make a big difference in your blood sugar numbers. Use this pyramid as your guide.

High-GL Choices

potatoes
French fries
white bread
overcooked pasta
udon noodles
white rice
sticky rice
rice-based cereal

cornflakes
millet
instant Cream of Wheat
most baked goods
non-diet soda
sweetened fruit drinks
dried dates
raisins

Moderate-GL Choices

wild rice, brown rice
wheatberries
pasta cooked al dente
whole-wheat pasta
rye crispbread
chocolate milk
apple juice
pineapple juice

dried figs
bananas
sweet potatoes
black-eyed peas
whole-grain cereals
low-sugar cereals
regular Cream of Wheat
whole-grain and sourdough bread

Lower-GL Choices

most fresh fruits
most vegetables (except potatoes)
coarse barley bread
whole-grain pumpernickel
pearled barley
oatmeal
bran cereal
muesli
lima beans
split peas

milk
soy milk
tomato juice
dried prunes
dried apricots
popcorn
yogurt
lentils
all dried beans
(except black-eyed peas)

STEP THREE
Eat at Least One Food Rich in Soluble Fiber a Day

There are two types of fiber: soluble and insoluble. Most whole grains are rich in insoluble fiber, which passes through you undigested. Soluble fiber is the kind that dissolves in water. It's found in oats, barley, beans, and some fruits and vegetables. Both are very good for you, but only soluble fiber will help you lower your blood sugar in a big way.

Researchers tested the two top grain sources of soluble fiber—oatmeal and barley—on overweight middle-aged women. On days when they ate oatmeal for breakfast, their blood sugar levels over the next three hours were about 30 percent lower than when they ate a sugar-laden pudding. On days they ate barley cereal, it was about 60 percent lower.

How does soluble fiber help control blood sugar? When it mixes with water it forms a gum. Think of oatmeal. You can pick out the grains or flakes when it's dry, but once you cook it, it's one big mush. This gum forms a barrier between the digestive enzymes in your stomach and the starch molecules in the food—not just the oatmeal, but even in the toast you ate it with. So it takes longer for your body to convert the whole meal into blood sugar, and a slower rise in blood sugar is a good thing for your health.

that's easy! ⟵

Simply eating the right breakfast cereal can jump-start weight loss. When 60 women and men had high-fiber oatmeal for breakfast instead of low-fiber cornflakes, they ate 30 percent fewer calories at lunch, reported researchers from the New York Obesity Research Center at St. Luke's–Roosevelt Hospital. The appetite-control factor seems to be all that satisfying fiber, which helps you stay full.

Not coincidentally, barley has a much, much lower GL than either white or brown rice, so go ahead and embrace it as a rice substitute. It's very easy to like. Oatmeal has a lower GL than cold cereal—even whole-grain cereal.

Eating more foods rich in soluble fiber is a key strategy for lowering your blood sugar after meals. It will also improve your health in other ways. Oatmeal is famous for lowering cholesterol; it may also lower high levels of triglycerides as well as high blood pressure. There's even a health claim allowed on oatmeal: "Eating three grams of soluble fiber from oatmeal in a diet low in saturated fat and cholesterol may reduce the risk of heart disease."

To get more soluble fiber into your diet, start with these easy strategies.

Have oatmeal for breakfast. Oats are slow-digesting carbs that are great for your blood sugar if you keep the portion size reasonable. Stick with about a cup, and fill up the rest of your bowl with fresh fruit and a sprinkling of nuts. A steaming bowl of oatmeal—sprinkled with sugar-lowering cinnamon—is more than comfort food. Studies show that oats can reduce post-meal blood sugar and insulin levels in people with diabetes. Oats are also an excellent source of the mineral manganese, which plays a role in blood sugar metabolism.

Add oats while cooking. Make a batch of oat bran muffins and keep them on hand for tasty breakfast treats. And next time you make pancakes or waffles, replace up to one-third of the flour in the batter with oatmeal ground to a fine powder in the blender. Just don't substitute instant oats in a recipe that calls for quick-cooking or old-fashioned oats. The texture is different, and instant oats usually have other flavors added.

Make a crunchy topping for fresh fruit. For dessert, serve oat-rich fruit crisps and cobblers.

Just watch the butter content. It's better to use a good-for-you brand of margarine such as Smart Balance, or canola oil, instead.

Thicken with oats. Use oat flour or even a sprinkle of dry oat bran to stews, casseroles, and soups as a fiber-rich thickener.

Buy a bag of quick-cooking barley. Add it to soups, use it instead of arborio rice (the worst rice offender of all in terms of your blood sugar) in risotto, and serve it as a nutty, flavorful side dish. The possibilities are endless. Pearled, hulled, or quick cooking, all varieties of barley are rich in cholesterol-lowering soluble fiber as well as compounds called beta-glucans that the human body converts into blood sugar extremely slowly. There's new evidence that eating barley at breakfast can keep you feeling fuller and more satisfied at lunch and even at dinner, so that you have fewer cravings and can make healthier choices at those meals.

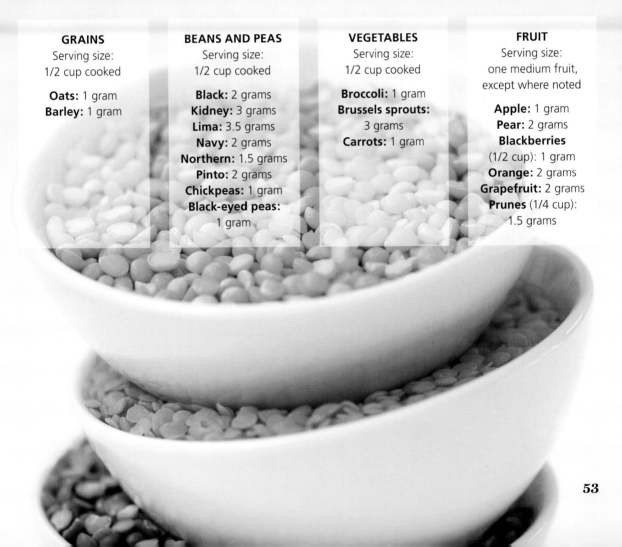

Best Foods for Soluble Fiber

For healthier blood sugar levels, aim to fit as many of these foods as possible into your daily diet.

GRAINS
Serving size:
1/2 cup cooked

Oats: 1 gram
Barley: 1 gram

BEANS AND PEAS
Serving size:
1/2 cup cooked

Black: 2 grams
Kidney: 3 grams
Lima: 3.5 grams
Navy: 2 grams
Northern: 1.5 grams
Pinto: 2 grams
Chickpeas: 1 gram
Black-eyed peas:
1 gram

VEGETABLES
Serving size:
1/2 cup cooked

Broccoli: 1 gram
Brussels sprouts:
3 grams
Carrots: 1 gram

FRUIT
Serving size:
one medium fruit,
except where noted

Apple: 1 gram
Pear: 2 grams
Blackberries
(1/2 cup): 1 gram
Orange: 2 grams
Grapefruit: 2 grams
Prunes (1/4 cup):
1.5 grams

GOAL 3

Eat three servings of fruit a day

EATING MORE VEGETABLES is Goal #1 on the Eat plan, but fruit deserves a place on your plate, too. Surprised? Don't be. Some people get the impression that the natural sugar in fruit makes this sweet treat off-limits for people with diabetes, but that just isn't the case.

Fructose, the kind of sugar naturally found in fruit, isn't absorbed by your body as quickly as sucrose, the kind in table sugar, so it's less likely to cause blood sugar spikes. What's more, fruit is mostly water and fiber, so the amount of fructose it contains is fairly small. Meanwhile, fruits have almost all the advantages that vegetables do. They're brimming with nutrients, they're low in fat, they're high in fiber, and they're relatively low in calories. What it means: This is one sweet treat you can probably eat, in moderation of course, without worrying that your blood sugar will soar. (Dried fruits, especially raisins and dates, are another story.)

With a few exceptions, you can forget any "rules" you've heard about not eating *particular* fruits due to their effect on blood sugar. Truth is, it's personal. We recommend following your doctor's advice about blood-sugar testing after meals and snacks to see how particular foods affect your blood sugar. You may find that certain fruits raise it more than others, which will influence your choices.

STEP ONE
Start the Day with Fruit

Most of us don't eat vegetables at breakfast, so a piece of fruit is the perfect way to get fiber and important nutrients first thing in the morning. Here's how to add fruit to your break-of-day routine.

what's in a fruit serving?

Sprinkle a good handful of blueberries on morning cereal and voila—you've just given yourself one of your three daily fruit servings. What exactly constitutes a serving?

- 1 medium piece of fruit
- 1/2 cup chopped, cooked, or canned fruit
- 3/4 cup (6 ounces) of 100 percent juice
- 1/4 cup dried fruit

Make it a rule: Every breakfast includes a piece of fruit. Cantaloupe, an orange, berries—all are perfect with whole-wheat toast, cereal, or an egg. Or try sliced banana on wheat toast with a tablespoon of peanut butter or sliced apple with almond butter on a toasted whole-wheat English muffin.

Concoct a quick "baked" apple. Wash and chop an apple (leave the skin on for more fiber and nutrients), pile in a small bowl, sprinkle with cinnamon and cover with a microwave-safe paper towel. Microwave until soft, about 4 minutes. Enjoy with yogurt and oat bran sprinkles, or serve over oatmeal for a tummy-warming start on a cold morning.

Shred (yes, shred!) fresh fruit over yogurt. Choose plain, nonfat yogurt and dress it up with grated fresh fruit like apples or pears (use the side of the box grater with the biggest holes for best results). Top with all-bran cereal for a fancy breakfast parfait.

Every Monday, start your week with a fruit smoothie. Add 1/2 cup fresh fruit, 1/2 cup plain nonfat yogurt, and one cup ice to a blender and liquefy. That's a serving of fruit before 8 a.m.!

Whole fruit is almost always a good snack choice—far better than anything (except nuts) that you'd get from a bag.

STEP TWO
Make Fruit Ultra-Convenient for Snacking

Whole fruit is almost always a good snack choice—far better for your blood sugar and your waistline than anything (with the exception of nuts) that you'd get from a bag or a vending machine. A 2-ounce serving of corn chips, for example, has a glycemic load three times higher than that of a medium peach or plum. And you get twice as much food—and zero bad-for-you fat—from one piece of fruit as from that tiny handful of chips.

And let's be honest: Who can stop at a handful? Here's how to keep fruit ready at snack time, any time, any place.

Keep a fruit bowl filled wherever you spend the most time. This could be at work, near your home computer, or even in the television room. And keep it filled at all times with fruit such as bananas, oranges, apples, grapes, or plums. Most fruit is fine left at room temperature for three or four days. But if it's out and staring at you, it's not likely to last that long.

Bring fruit with you anytime you plan on driving for more than an hour. Once you are on the highway and cruising along, an apple or a nectarine tastes great and helps break the tedium. (Don't forget the napkins!)

Make a natural Popsicle. Freeze banana slices or grapes for a delightfully refreshing summer treat.

Tuck an apple in your pocket whenever you go for long walks. It will be your reward for getting to the midpoint of your walk.

Keep cut-up melon in a clear container at the front of the fridge. Use as a first course before dinner; mix with low-fat cottage cheese for breakfast; have a small bowl for a snack; even consider pureeing for a quick sauce over fish.

Have raisins every time you crave a candy bar. Buy kid-sized miniature boxes of raisins—and keep them for yourself. Every time you want a candy, have one box. Raisins are naturally sweet and healthy, and mini boxes are just the right amount to satisfy a yen for a sweet treat. Just be sure to stop at one mini box, because while raisins are infinitely better for you than candy, they have a fairly high glycemic load.

sugar buster quiz

Q: 100 percent juice or whole fruit?

A: Whole fruit

Many of the nutrients and a lot of the fiber found in the skin, flesh, and seeds of fruit are eliminated during juicing, and the calories and blood sugar–raising carbs are concentrated in juice, so you get more than you would if you ate the fruit.

that's easy!

When you drink fruit juice, use a real juice glass, the kind your grandmother had. It holds just 4 or 6 ounces—a right-sized serving.

STEP THREE
Have Fruit at Lunch or Dinner Every Day

Fruit's a natural for snacking, and that apple in the afternoon counts as one of your three daily fruit servings. So did the fruit you had with breakfast. How to fit in one more serving? Plan on having some fruit at lunch...or dinner...or both.

Sweeten your sandwich and add crunch. Add diced kiwi, sliced grapes, or chopped apple to chicken, tuna, and turkey salads.

Throw pineapples or peaches on the barbecue. Brush thick slices of pineapple or peaches with a little olive oil so they don't stick, then grill. Heat brings out the natural sweetness in the fruit.

Mix fruits in with your salad. A sprinkle of raisins, some cut-up strawberries, a diced apple, a small handful of grapes, or some sliced kiwi all make great additions to the typical tossed salad.

Top chicken or fish with fruit salsa. Spice up store-bought salsas with fruit, or make your own fruit-based salsas with pineapple, mango, or papayas. Mix with onions, ginger, a bit of garlic, some mint and/or cilantro, sprinkle on a few hot pepper flakes for fire, and chill.

Finish up with fruit. A slice of watermelon, a peach, a bowl of blueberries or raspberries topped with a dollop of yogurt—they're the perfect ending to a meal, and are so much healthier than cookies or cake.

Dress up fruit for a fancier dessert. A half-cup of strawberries drizzled with balsamic vinegar or soaked in white wine is a sweet, indulgent ending to your meal—and delivers 75 percent of your daily vitamin C requirement. (Recall that antioxidants help protect your body from the ravages of high blood sugar.) Or try roasted plums. Simply mix 1 teaspoon orange zest or ginger, 1/4 cup orange juice, and 3 tablespoons brown sugar and simmer in a saucepan. Add 2 teaspoons of butter or trans-fat-free margarine and stir until melted. Place 8 plum halves, cut side up, in a baking dish, top with the mixture, cover with foil, and bake 20 to 25 minutes at 400°F.

STEP FOUR
Go for Variety

Aim not only to eat more fruit but more *types* of fruit. If you only munch on apples or green grapes or strawberries, you're missing out on important, health-protecting nutrients that people with diabetes need—nutrients you'll get if you eat many different sorts of fruit. So that produce doesn't go bad, buy a combination of long-keeping fruits (such as apples and oranges), a small supply of more delicate fruits (such as berries and peaches) to eat in the first two days after you've gone shopping, and a back-up stash of frozen, no-sugar-added fruits like berries and peaches in the freezer.

Start with these easy-to-find favorites. They are often tastiest and most affordable when purchased in season at a local farm stand or in the supermarket.

Apples. Researchers have discovered that women who eat at least one apple a day are 28 percent less likely to develop type 2 diabetes than those who don't eat apples. That's probably because apples, from tart Granny Smiths to sweet, juicy Pink Ladies, are loaded with soluble fiber—number one for blunting blood sugar swings. A medium apple dishes up an impressive 4 grams of fiber, mostly pectin, which is also known for its ability to lower cholesterol. Looking to trim your tummy? (News flash: Belly fat is bad for blood sugar.) Try eating three small apples a day.

Berries. From ruby red strawberries to midnight-blue blueberries, berries are candy for your taste buds—and powerful blood sugar controllers. Their sweetness is deceptive. Fructose, the natural sugar found in most fruits, is sweeter than what's in your sugar bowl (sucrose), so it takes much less, with fewer calories, to get that sweet taste. Berries are full of fiber, disease-fighting antioxidants, and

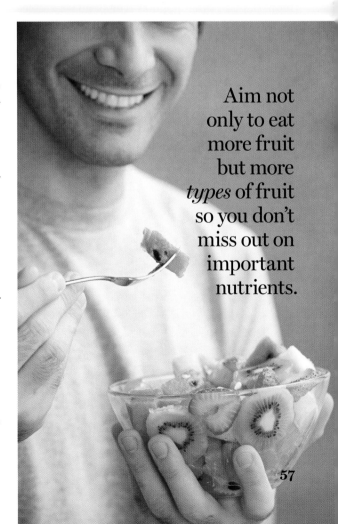

Aim not only to eat more fruit but more *types* of fruit so you don't miss out on important nutrients.

red-blue natural plant compounds called antho-cyanins that may help keep your blood sugar in check. Scientists believe anthocyanins, also found in cherries, may help lower blood sugar by boost-ing insulin production.

Peaches, plums, and apricots. These make perfect low-calorie snacks or sweet additions to entrées and desserts. They're easy on your blood sugar because, like most fruits, they have a high water content, plus a stash of blood sugar–taming, cholesterol-busting soluble fiber. Peaches boast the most fiber of the three. Apricots, which are close cousins to peaches, are richest in beta-carotene, linked with protection from heart disease and cancer. Plums are chock-full of several disease-fighting antioxidants, and dried plums outrank more than 20 other popular fruits and vegetables in antioxidant power.

Be adventurous. Every month, buy one exotic fruit you've never tried. It could be something as relatively common as a mango or as unique as a lychee. You need look no farther than your local supermarket. Today's produce section is definitely not your grandmother's fruit stand. Here are some tips on what these fruits are and how to enjoy them.

Asian pear. Also called an Oriental, Chinese, salad, or apple pear, this firm pear is meant to be eaten immediately—when it's still hard. It's sweet, crunchy, and amazingly juicy.

Guava. It's sweet and fragrant with bright pink, white, yellow, or red flesh. Buy when it is just soft enough to press, and refrigerate for up to a week in a plastic or paper bag. To use, cut in half and scoop out the flesh for salads, or peel and slice. Try cooking and pureeing slightly under-ripe guava as a sauce for meat or fish.

Power Fruits

Of the hundreds of fruits out there, which ones give you the biggest nutritional bang for your buck? We bet on the ones with the most antioxidant power. Antioxidants neutralize free radicals—destructive molecules that damage cells. People with diabetes may have more free-radical damage than people without diabetes, raising risk for heart disease and other health problems. Which fruits pack the greatest antioxidant punch? The good people at the USDA figured it out. Here are the top 10.

1. Blueberries
2. Cranberries
3. Blackberries
4. Prune
5. Raspberries
6. Strawberries
7. Red delicious apple
8. Granny Smith apple
9. Sweet cherries
10. Plum

Kiwi. This fruit never took off until they changed the name from Chinese gooseberry to kiwifruit. Now it's one of the most popular of the exotics. With a flavor that's a cross between strawberries and melon, kiwis are ready to eat when they're slightly soft to the touch. Peel and chop, or cut in half and scoop out the flesh with a grapefruit spoon.

Lychee. Once, lychee trees were found only in southern China, but the popularity of this tropi-cal fruit has caused its spread (it is now widely raised in Florida). The lychee fruit is about 1 1/2 inches in size, oval, with a bumpy red skin. Peel off the inedible skin and you get a white, translucent flesh similar to a grape, but sweeter, surrounding a cherry-like pit. Eat 'em like large grapes. They're available only for a few months a year, but buy a pound next spring and discover why Asians call lychees the king of fruits.

Mango. This is one of the most commonly eaten fruits in the world, along with bananas. The flavor is a combination of peach and pineapple, but spicier and more fragrant (it is sometimes called the tropical peach).

Papaya. With soft, juicy, and silky-smooth flesh, papaya has a delicate, sweet flavor. The center of the papaya is filled with small, round, black, peppery-tasting seeds, which can be eaten but usually aren't. Peel, then slice into wedges or cut into chunks, or slice in half, remove seeds, and scoop out the flesh with a spoon. Unripe papayas can be peeled, seeded, and cooked as a vegetable, and you can grind the seeds like pepper for adding to sauces or salads.

Passion fruit. Passion fruit has golden flesh with tiny, edible black seeds and a sweet-tart taste. When ripe, it has wrinkled, dimpled, deep purple skin. To serve, cut in half and scoop out the pulp with a spoon.

Persimmon. Delicate in flavor and firm in texture, persimmons can be eaten like an apple, sliced and peeled, and are great in salads.

sugar buster quiz

Q: Fresh peach or canned peaches?
A: Fresh peach

Fruit you bite into wins hands-down over fruit you spoon from a can. A peach contains only 35 calories, whereas a cup of peaches canned in heavy syrup has 190. If you buy canned, go for peaches packed in their own juice (110 calories per cup).

Pomegranate. It's the seeds of this crimson fall fruit that you eat. Each tiny, edible seed is surrounded by translucent, brilliant red pulp that has a sparkling sweet-tart flavor. Choose fruit that feels heavy for its size with bright color and blemish-free skin. They can be refrigerated up to a month, while the seeds can be frozen for three months. To serve, cut the fruit in half and pry out the seeds. Use them to top ice cream, sprinkle into salads, or simply as a snack.

Star fruit. Although they look exotic, most star fruits today come from south Florida. Slice them crosswise for perfect five-pointed star-shaped sections as a garnish or for fruit salads. Star fruit's flavor combines the best of plums, pineapples, and lemons.

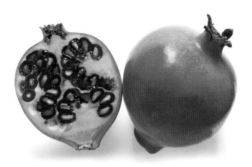

GOAL 4

Include lean protein at every meal

WANT TO CONTROL YOUR BLOOD SUGAR and your weight? Get enough protein in your diet. Studies prove that protein helps keep hunger at bay between meals, and if you're trying to lose weight, taking in enough protein will also help your body hold on to its calorie-burning muscle tissue while you drop pounds.

But the benefits don't end there. Unlike carbohydrates, protein has little or no effect on your blood sugar. Eat a grilled chicken breast or a hardboiled egg and your levels will barely budge. It stands to reason, then, that if you substitute calories from protein for some of the calories you get from carbohydrates, your meals will have less impact on your blood sugar. And because your body breaks down protein slowly, including some turkey sausage or beans with your pasta means that it will take longer for your body to digest the whole meal, resulting in a slower, gentler rise in blood sugar.

Just how important protein is for blood sugar control emerged from a fascinating study. Researchers at the University of Minnesota tested two diets, one high in protein and one with only half as much. The fat content was the same in both diets, but the carbohydrate content varied—volunteers ate fewer carbs on the high-protein diet, more carbs on the low-protein program. In the group that followed the high-protein diet, blood sugar levels were reduced by as much as if the participants had taken pills prescribed to lower blood sugar.

Does that mean that you should sit down to a 12-ounce T-bone steak or fried chicken tonight? No. Fatty cuts of beef, poultry with skin, and some cuts of pork, as well as bacon and some lunch meats, pack lots of heart-threatening saturated fat, which raises levels of "bad" cholesterol. This "bad" fat has also been linked with increased insulin resistance, which contributes to higher blood sugar levels.

On the Eat plan, it's important to focus on *lean* protein foods, so that you get the blood-sugar and

that's easy! ←

Put meat and poultry in the freezer for 20 minutes before you get to work trimming away excess fat. This will firm it up for easier cutting (the meat will become harder than the fat, making a closer "shave" possible) and make marbled fat more visible so you can locate and remove it.

weight-loss benefits of this important macronutrient without the health risks. By cutting back on saturated fat in fatty protein foods like hamburgers and fried chicken, you'll leave room in your diet for eating more blood sugar–friendly "good fats," which is Goal #5.

> Lean beef doesn't just taste good, it's great for helping you achieve and maintain a healthy weight, thanks to its protein.

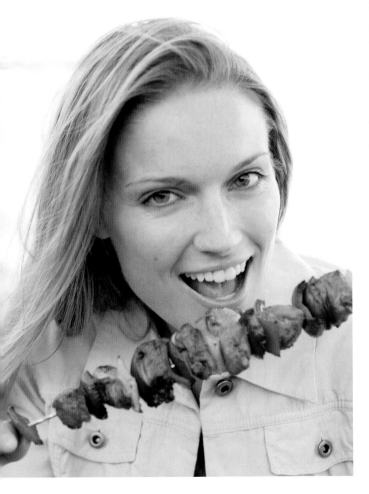

Have Lean Meat Up to Twice a Week

Yes, beef can still be for dinner—or, more accurately, *part of* dinner. Lean beef doesn't just taste good, it's great for helping you achieve and maintain a healthy weight, thanks to its protein. That doesn't mean that sitting down to a giant T-bone or eating mega-cheeseburgers with enough calories and fat for breakfast, lunch, and dinner combined is suddenly okay. It isn't. But it's more than okay to fill one-quarter of your plate with a lean choice like tenderloin. Here's how to get the leanest, most flavorful red meats on your plate.

Pair beef strips with veggies. Stir-fry strips of beef with lots of veggies for an easy way to have your beef and get your vegetables, too. Or throw together fajitas made with flank steak and generous amounts of bell peppers and onions for a quick weeknight meal. Or for a refreshingly delicious Asian-inspired salad, toss hot grilled beef with crisp lettuce, lime juice, and chopped onion.

Remake meat loaf. Create healthier meat loaf by combining finely chopped spinach and onions and grated carrots with extra-lean ground beef. Use oats as a binder.

When company comes, serve up roast beef tenderloin. Don't forget to serve a salad beforehand and at least one veggie side dish.

Turn up the tenderness. Make any cut of beef a standout by marinating it in balsamic vinegar, olive oil, basil, Dijon mustard, and garlic. Or use any marinade that contains vinegar, wine, or citrus juice. The acid softens the tissues of the meat, making it tenderer.

Use half the beef; get all the flavor. In chili, tacos, spaghetti sauce, and casseroles that call

"Skinny" Beef

The following have 10 grams or less of total fat and 4.5 grams or less of saturated fat per serving. We've ranked them from the leanest to the least lean.

▸ Eye round roast
▸ Top round roast
▸ Mock tender steak
▸ Bottom round roast
▸ Top sirloin steak
▸ Round tip roast
▸ 95-percent lean ground beef
▸ Flat half of brisket
▸ Shank crosscuts
▸ Chuck shoulder roast
▸ Arm pot roast
▸ Shoulder steak
▸ Top loin steak (such as strip or New York steak)
▸ Flank steak
▸ Rib-eye steak
▸ Rib steak
▸ Tri-tip roast
▸ Tenderloin steak
▸ T-bone steak

for ground beef use half extra-lean ground beef and half ground, skinless turkey or chicken breast. You'll cut the fat content but still get the assertive, satisfying flavor of beef.

Take another look at pork. Pork loin is a very lean and affordable cut of meat that's flavorful and satisfying, like beef. Among its charms: It cooks quickly in the oven or on the grill and tastes great with a wide variety of marinades and spices (we love garlic and oregano or low-sodium soy sauce and grated fresh ginger). Pork loin's perfect when company's coming for dinner. Or throw a couple of chops on the grill (try garlic-lime marinade or a rub made of chili and garlic powders).

STEP TWO

Turn to Chicken

Chicken and turkey can be high-fat disasters or perfect *Reverse Diabetes* fare. It all depends on the cut and how it's prepared. Breast meat is lower in fat than dark meat such as thighs and drumsticks. And in fact, a 3-ounce serving of skinless chicken breast has 95 percent less saturated fat—the stuff that clogs arteries and blunts insulin sensitivity—than an equal serving of beef tenderloin. It also has 40 percent fewer calories, making it a practically perfect protein food. Just remember that even breast meat loses its health appeal when it's fried (especially in the oils used at many fast-food joints, which essentially turn chicken into a heart attack in a bucket). The skin, meanwhile, with all its saturated fat, is just about the worst thing you can eat. Be sure to remove it either before or after cooking.

Fortunately, lean poultry is incredibly versatile, as well as convenient. Here are easy ways to take advantage.

Enjoy a fast dinner of supermarket rotisserie chicken. Instead of the fast-food drive-through tonight, run into the supermarket for a bag of salad greens and a rotisserie chicken. At home, enjoy a big salad and a slice of breast meat. To keep it lean, skip the skin and don't eat the greasy drippings.

Order turkey or chicken breast at the deli counter. Roll up a few slices and add to salads to pump up their protein content, or eat them in sandwiches on whole-wheat bread topped with mustard, tomato, and plenty of lettuce or even baby spinach. Have two slices or 1.5 ounces per sandwich.

Roast some turkey even when it's not Thanksgiving. Turkey breast is actually lower in fat and cholesterol and higher in protein than chicken breast. You can now buy just the turkey breast in many grocery stores.

Try this instead of fried chicken. Brush boneless, skinless chicken thighs with olive oil and sprinkle with rosemary, salt, and pepper. Bake or grill until juices run clear, about 45 minutes. Chill overnight—this is great lunch or picnic fare. For another option that's just as finger-lickin' messy as the real thing, mix the juice of 1 lemon with 1 tablespoon Dijon mustard, 1/4 cup honey, a pinch of curry powder, and a pinch of salt. Roll skinless chicken drumsticks in the mixture to coat well and bake until done, 45-60 minutes.

Use ground chicken or turkey breast in place of ground beef. Make sure it's ground *breast* meat; if it includes dark meat it will be much higher in fat. This lean meat makes good burgers and tastes great in meat loaf, meatballs, chili, tacos, and lasagna.

STEP THREE
Have Fish Twice a Week

The fattiest protein on your plate should be oily cold-water fish like salmon and mackerel (and to a lesser extent, tuna and other fish). These fish contain diabetes-fighting, heart-protecting omega-3 fatty acids—a fat you almost certainly need to get more of into your diet. A study at the Harvard School of Public Health found that women with diabetes who ate fish just once a week had a 40 percent lower risk of dying from heart disease than did women with diabetes who ate fish less than once a month.

The fats in fish do even more than guard against heart disease. They also cool chronic inflammation in the body, a major contributor to numerous chronic diseases, including insulin resistance and diabetes. Inflammation may even play a role in brain diseases such as Alzheimer's as well as certain cancers.

that's easy!

Keep chicken tenderloins in the freezer for fast meals. Two tenderloins are about 3 ounces, a perfect portion. These skinless, boneless cuts thaw quickly in the fridge overnight or in a bowl of cold water (seal in a zip-close bag first).

Any fish is a great source of protein, and we encourage you to eat it twice a week when you might otherwise have chicken or beef. Shellfish counts, too, so go ahead and indulge in grilled shrimp, lobster, and mussels. They don't contain as much omega-3s as salmon, but they're still low in saturated fat and calories and rich in protein. Worried about your cholesterol? You don't need to avoid shrimp. It does contain cholesterol, but for most of us, shrimp should still get the green light. In a definitive Rockefeller University study, eating large servings of shrimp every single day raised "bad" LDL cholesterol by 7 percent, but it also boosted "good" HDL cholesterol 12 percent—a net benefit.

Here's how to fit in two servings of fish or seafood a week.

Keep frozen fish fillets in the freezer. Vacuum-packed sole, cod, or salmon fillets are the next best thing to fresh. You'll have dinner on the table in a flash—even if you have to spend a few minutes defrosting it first—because fish is done before you know it, making it a perfect weeknight meal.

Fire up the grill. Almost any type of fish tastes fabulous grilled, especially salmon. Brush it with a little olive oil to keep it from sticking. Throw some zucchini strips on the grill, too, and you have a blood sugar–friendly meal. Or, try wrapping trout in foil with lemon slices, dill, thyme, salt, and pepper and bake. Serve over quinoa.

No-Worries Salmon

Recent analysis involving a handful of researchers from different institutions came to this bottom line: Whenever you can, choose wild Pacific salmon instead of farmed salmon, which is typically higher in several chemical contaminants. If you do buy farmed salmon, which has higher levels of omega-3s and is usually cheaper, opt for farmed salmon from Chile. It's the healthiest and safest by far.

No matter which fish you choose, you're better off eating than not eating it. A pair of Harvard University researchers combed through stacks of studies, government reports, and other scientific literature on fish and human health and published their findings in the *Journal of the American Medical Association* in 2006. Their bottom line: Eating fish far outweighs any accompanying risks from contaminants.

Don't overlook salmon in cans and pouches. This is usually wild salmon—same as the pricey, sometimes hard-to-find stuff from the fish counter. Use it to make salmon salad or salmon croquettes and use in quiches and pasta dishes.

Stuff a tomato with tuna or salmon salad. Make the tuna or salmon salad with low-fat mayonnaise or plain yogurt, hard-boiled eggs, chopped apples, celery, and onion. Serve with whole-wheat crackers.

Think sushi for supermarket takeout. Many larger supermarkets have their very own sushi chefs on staff. If you need a quick, prepackaged meal, this is the place to stop. Sushi delivers protein and is generally low in calories. Since some types of sushi—especially bluefin tuna—may be contaminated with mercury, it's best to limit sushi to once a week.

Order grilled salmon when you dine out. You'll avoid temptations packed with saturated fat (like cream sauces and deep-fried goodies) and ensure that you get a serving of healthy omega-3 fatty acids.

Keep a bag of frozen shrimp in the freezer. Thaw them according to the package directions and you have the makings of a fast, high-protein meal or appetizer. Serve boiled shrimp with shrimp sauce as a party hors d'oeuvres. Leftovers? Chop some cooked shrimp and sprinkle over your salad to add low-fat protein. Use a lemony dressing. Or place a shrimp, small chunks of avocado and tomato, and a bit of salsa onto a lettuce leaf. Roll it up and eat! In stir-fries, use shrimp instead of chicken or beef. Add in the last 5 minutes to avoid overcooking. Also try shrimp in your tacos instead of beef.

Have lobster for lower blood sugar. Indulge in this fancy feast—without the melted butter. The upper crust of the crustacean kingdom happens to be a particularly rich source of a little-known mineral called vanadium, which studies suggest enhances insulin's effect in the body, helping to keep an anchor on blood sugar.

STEP FOUR

Enjoy "Bean Cuisine" at Least Three Times a Week

From black beans to chickpeas, cannelini to kidney beans, these slow-digesting little nuggets are rich in soluble fiber—and therefore fantastic for your blood sugar. In a recent study, men and women who ate a meal that included about 6 ounces of chickpeas had 40 percent lower blood sugar an hour after eating than those who ate an equal amount of white bread with jam.

The fiber in beans leads to a slow, steady blood sugar rise rather than a spike after a meal. Beans also pack loads of protein. Are they the perfect food for people with diabetes? Perhaps. Just stick with 1/2 cup or so per meal, since beans do contain carbohydrates.

If you're trying to lose weight, eat beans! Not only are they incredibly filling, they also pack a heap of nutrition in a relatively low-calorie package. Better still, some of the starch in beans is a type called resistant starch that the body can't even digest, so the calories don't count. Beans are also full of folate, a B vitamin that may help reduce some of the nasty consequences of diabetes by helping to keep arteries clean.

The only black mark for beans is the sodium content of canned beans. Cut it in half by rinsing them in cold water before using. What next? Here are a handful of great ways to enjoy beans.

Put them to bed—on a bed of salad greens. Add chickpeas or kidney beans to a salad for a filling fix of protein. They're delicious with chopped red pepper, corn, and tomatoes.

Pour canned beans into soup or chili. Experiment with different combinations of colors, sizes, and flavors. We like the assertive taste of red and black beans mixed together, and the sweetness of white beans.

Spruce up tomato sauce. Add some kidney beans to pasta sauce along with chunks of vegetables for a hearty pasta topping.

Give them a starring role at your next picnic. Make a tasty salad by combining black beans with red onions, tomato, lime juice, cilantro, and shredded spinach.

Use in place of beef in Mexican foods. Mash kidney beans or black beans and use them on tortillas instead of beef or refried beans.

Serve edamame as a side dish. These young green soybeans are wonderful snacks. You can buy them frozen; just steam and serve. They're also a perfect addition to soups and salads. Soy has more protein, ounce for ounce, than beef and almost none of the saturated fat.

Create a high-fiber dip. Serve bean dip or hummus with a whole-wheat pita cut into wedges.

Cook up hearty chili. Cook up a big pot of black bean chili on the weekend and freeze the leftovers. Go meatless, or use ground skinless turkey or chicken breast in place of ground beef to keep saturated fat content low.

Bake chickpeas for a terrific snack. Whether the beans are canned or cooked dried, drain and pat dry. Toss about 2 cups beans with one beaten egg white and a mix of spices. Go for cumin, chili powder, and cayenne pepper for a spicy treat or cinnamon, ground ginger, and nutmeg for a sweet snack. Bake, stirring occasionally, at 400°F until golden and crisp, about 15 minutes.

that's easy!

To get more beans into your diet, invest in a pressure cooker, which lets you cook them—and other foods—in drastically less time than it would normally take. They look like regular pots, but with more elaborate lids that clamp shut, trapping steam and heat inside. Soaked beans cook in just 10 or 15 minutes. Scared of pressure cookers? Don't be. Today's models are much safer and easier to use than the kind your grandmother had.

STEP FIVE
Don't Forget Eggs

Eggs have been much maligned in recent years but the fact is, they're an excellent and inexpensive source of protein, and the most nutritionally complete of all protein sources. One large hardboiled egg has 7 grams of protein to keep you full, and just 2 grams of saturated fat. In studies, people who ate eggs and toast for breakfast stayed fuller longer and ate significantly fewer calories for the rest of the day than people who started the day with a bagel and cream cheese. Because they're all protein and fat, eggs have virtually no impact on your blood sugar, making them a much better breakfast choice than, say, a stack of white-flour pancakes.

Eggs do contain cholesterol, but dozens of studies show that it's saturated fat, not dietary cholesterol, that raises people's cholesterol the most. For people with elevated cholesterol or those who are especially sensitive to the cholesterol in foods (for some people, cholesterol levels do rise after eating a cholesterol-rich meal), experts recommend eating no more than three or four egg yolks a week. Egg whites, which contain no cholesterol, don't count.

If you have an egg tray in your refrigerator door, ignore it. Eggs stay fresh best if you keep them in their original container, pointed ends down.

Keep hard-boiled eggs in the fridge for a protein-rich snack. It's hard to find snack foods rich in protein, but a hardboiled egg is the perfect solution. It's portable, too—but you do have to keep it cold.

Serve a frittata for dinner. Think of it as Italian egg pie. You can add almost anything to your frittata, such as lean ham, diced tomato, spinach, and goat cheese. Use 1 to 2 cups of filling for every four or five eggs.

Make It Milk

On the subject of protein, dairy deserves special mention. Foods such as fat-free milk and yogurt and low-fat cheese are high in both protein and calcium. Why is calcium important? Studies find that making sure you get adequate amounts can help you lose weight. The reason: A lack of adequate calcium triggers the release of a hormone called calcitriol, which prompts the body to store fat. Eating two or three servings of calcium-rich dairy foods per day helps keep calcitriol levels low so your body burns more fat and stores less. Taking calcium supplements doesn't seem to produce the same effect, which leads researchers to conclude that dairy foods may have some other, as-yet-undiscovered weight-loss advantage as well.

But there's more. A mysterious factor in milk seems to help directly protect against insulin resistance. Two Harvard studies found that people who made dairy foods part of their daily diets were 21 percent less likely to develop insulin resistance and 9 percent less likely to develop type 2 diabetes for each daily serving of dairy they had. Pretty impressive!

Not everyone tolerates the lactose in milk well, but if you're bothered by symptoms such as bloating and gas, you can ease dairy into your diet by having small amounts with meals, which slows the rate at which lactose enters your system. You can also forgo milk in favor of dairy foods that are naturally lower in lactose, such as low-fat cheese and yogurt.

Dress up egg salad sandwiches. Add veggies such as grated carrots, chopped leeks, finely chopped shallots, red onion, pea shoots, or plain old lettuce. Mix with a combination of low-fat mayo and plain yogurt. Sprinkle in a classic "egg salad" herb such as tarragon or dill. Or throw in some canned tuna to up your fish quotient for the day.

GOAL 5

Trade good fat for bad

FAT IS USUALLY SEEN as a dietary evil…but is it? Of course butter, cheese, lard, and certain other fatty foods are dense in calories and known to contribute to heart disease. But fat also has important roles to play in the body, helping to form cell membranes, distributing fat-soluble vitamins, and insulating the body against heat loss. And there's an upside to fat for diabetics: It slows the digestion process after a meal or snack, which means that glucose converted from the carbohydrates you've eaten enters the blood more gradually. As a result, fat should play a bigger role in your diet than you might assume—making up as much as 25 to 30 percent of total calories.

But not any old fat will do. As you've already seen, choosing the right fats can actually help your body process blood sugar better. Choosing the *wrong* fats contributes to insulin resistance, which makes blood sugar more difficult to control and raises your risk for heart disease, the number-one killer of people with diabetes. The fats to avoid? Saturated fats in fatty meats, poultry with the skin, and full-fat diary products like whole milk, full-fat yogurt, and cheese. Also avoid the trans fats that still lurk in some margarines, commercial baked goods and snack foods, and processed foods and fast foods.

The right fats? These include monounsaturated fat found in nuts, nut butters, seeds, avocados, and olive and canola oil, as well as omega-3 fatty acids found in fatty fish, walnuts and hazelnuts, and to a lesser extent, flaxseed and flaxseed oil. Unlike saturated fat, which contributes to insulin resistance, these fats may even help reverse it.

that's easy!

Grill time? Instead of burgers, here are some healthier options: salmon burgers, lentil burgers, veggie burgers, and ground chicken burgers. And instead of hot dogs, consider turkey kielbasa or apple chicken sausages.

The health benefits of these good fats are one reason that low-fat, high-carbohydrate diets are no longer seen as the healthiest eating strategy for people with diabetes. It's great knowing you can enjoy healthy fats without guilt or fear, and that you can harness these high-satisfaction, delicious foods to help you stay on track as you lose weight. We'll be honest. When it comes to fat—any fat—you still have to watch how much you eat. At 9 calories per gram, even "good" fat can pack on the pounds. That's why you don't want to simply add good fats; you want to eat them *in place of* saturated fats and trans fats.

Here's how to enjoy good-fat foods without overindulging.

STEP ONE
Cut Way Back on "Bad" Fats

Your first step is to cut out, or significantly cut back on, the leading "bad fat" foods—see The Sat Fat Hit List below. Take special aim at full-fat cheese and fatty cuts of meat (think hamburgers, ribs, and bacon). If you avoid fast food and packaged treats (all too often made with oils full of saturated fat) and cook most of your meals at home, this shouldn't be all that hard to do, once you commit to doing it. Pick one food this week to cut back on, then next week, pick another. Don't worry—your meals will still taste great!

In Goal #4, you discovered smart ways to include lean meat and poultry in your meals. Now follow these additional tips to remove even more saturated and trans fats from your diet. Then read on for clever and flavorful ways to fill the gap with healthy good fats.

The Sat Fat Hit List

Americans get more "bad" fats from these 10 foods than from any others. Often, you can make substitutes: low-fat cheese for full-fat hard cheeses, lean beef for high-fat cuts or burgers, nonfat milk for whole milk, olive or canola oil for soybean-based vegetable oil, fruit sorbet for full-fat ice cream. What will you substitute today?

1. Cheese
2. Beef
3. Milk
4. Oils
5. Ice cream/sherbet/frozen yogurt
6. Cakes/cookies/quick breads/doughnuts
7. Butter
8. Shortening, lard, other animal fats
9. Salad dressings/mayonnaise
10. Poultry (skin, dark meat, fried chicken)

Slash saturated fat in meats. Follow all of our advice in Goal #4 to reduce saturated fat in the meats you eat. Choose leaner cuts of beef, never eat the skin on chicken or turkey, and switch to ground skinless poultry instead of ground beef. Saturated fat from meats and poultry is a major source of this killer fat in the American diet.

Switch to nonfat milk. The fat in milk is the number three source of saturated fat in our diets, so it's time to go nonfat. You can even find fat-free half-and-half for your coffee. If you don't like the taste of nonfat milk, we have two suggestions. First, try ultra-pasteurized nonfat milk, which is thicker and creamier than regular nonfat milk. Or keep two cartons of milk in your fridge: one that's 2 percent and one that's nonfat. Blend them together, progressively adding more nonfat milk as you get used to it.

Say "cheese," only smarter. As a calcium-rich protein food, cheese has a (small) place in your diet. Unfortunately, most cheese is high in saturated fat. That means you'll want to use it sparingly. Make a little go a longer way by choosing a strong-flavored type like Parmesan, Romano, or feta; you'll be able to use less and still get the taste you want. Also, look to lower-fat cheeses when possible. These include part-skim mozzarella, feta, and soft goat cheese.

Experiment with soy crumbles. Chili on the menu? Meatless soy crumbles provide all the protein of ground turkey and the mouth feel of ground meat. Try them for a change of pace to cut cholesterol and saturated fat. You'll be amazed at what a good stand-in they are.

Retire the fryer. Put away the fry bucket and vow to stop frying in your skillet. Broiling, grilling, baking, and sautéing in canola or olive oil are far healthier ways to prepare meals.

Chill out. When preparing soups or stocks, chill broth overnight and skim off congealed fat.

Modernize your margarine. Instead of butter or a margarine that contains trans fats (check the nutrition facts label for trans fat content and examine the ingredients list for small quantities of "hidden" trans fats listed as hydrogenated or partially hydrogenated fats or oils), use a spread with no saturated fat or trans fats.

Repair the recipe. When baking foods like breads, cakes, muffins, and brownies, try using half the amount of oil and replace the rest with an equal amount of applesauce or pureed fruit such as prunes.

Take advantage of nonstick cookware. Why use butter or margarine to keep food from adhering to frying pans when nonstick pans will work. If you want to coat the pan, use a dab of olive oil or a quick spritz of cooking spray.

STEP TWO

Make Olive and Canola Oils Your Oil Staples

Using olive or canola oil (when you need a neutral-tasting oil) most of the time instead of other oils or butter is important. Unlike butter, these oils contain mostly unsaturated fats, which don't increase insulin resistance and may even help reverse it, helping your body steady its blood sugar. Why olive and canola and not corn or safflower? The latter two are thought to promote low-grade

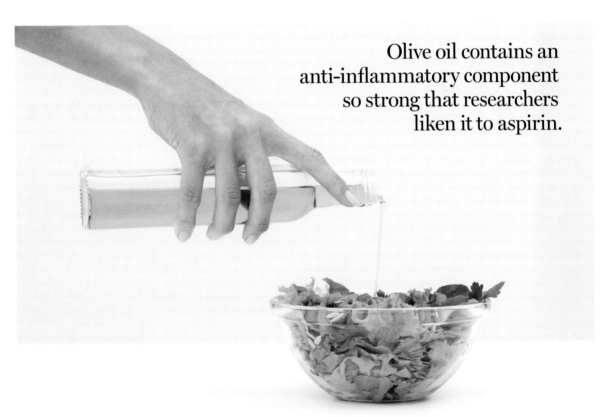

Olive oil contains an anti-inflammatory component so strong that researchers liken it to aspirin.

69

inflammation in the body, which contributes to diabetes, heart disease, and other health problems.

Like all fats, olive oil also slows digestion so that the bread or pasta you eat it with takes longer to break down into blood sugar. In an Australian study that compared the effects of consuming olive oil, or water, or a mixture of water and oil before a high-carb meal, researchers discovered that it took almost three times as long for study volunteers' stomachs to begin emptying—significantly delaying the subsequent rise in blood sugar—when they had the olive oil. Slower rises in blood sugar also equal feeling full longer, which in turn equals weight loss!

Olive oil is like liquid gold because it contains an anti-inflammatory component so strong that researchers liken it to aspirin. This may be one reason that people who follow the Mediterranean diet—a traditional way of eating that emphasizes olive oil along with produce, whole grains, and lean meat—have such low rates of heart disease and diabetes, both of which are linked with inflammation. Here's how to make the most of these oils.

Cholesterol-Friendly Margarine

One reason to limit your use of butter or margarine made with hydrogenated oil is that the kinds of fats they contain raise your cholesterol—definitely a bad thing if you have diabetes. But there is a way to have margarine and lower your cholesterol. Spreads such as Benecol and Take Control contain additives called sterols or stanols, plant chemicals that block the absorption of dietary cholesterol. Studies find that using a total of 1 to 2 tablespoons of this type of spread a day can cut cholesterol by as much as 10 percent.

Dress your salads with the good stuff. Spring for a very nice extra-virgin olive oil for salad dressings. You'll taste the difference, and your salad will be that much more satisfying.

Cook with olive oil in place of butter or margarine. Great cooks use olive oil in just about everything. Use it whenever you can in place of other vegetable oils, margarine, or butter. In recipes that call for butter or margarine, use 3/4 teaspoon olive oil in place of 1 teaspoon butter or margarine. Note, however, that olive oil has a relatively low "smoke point." Extra-virgin oil will start to break down—read burn—at about 375°F; virgin oil will start to burn at 420°F. When cooking at high temperatures, use canola oil instead.

Try a new topping for your potatoes. First of all, make that a baked potato, not a mashed potato. A baked potato with the skin will have less impact on your blood sugar. Then, try using a little olive oil mixed with roasted garlic instead of butter.

Dress up pasta with olive oil instead of butter or cheese. Add a teaspoonful to pasta, chopped tomatoes, crumbled feta cheese, chopped fresh basil, and capers for a fast and oh-so-simple supper.

Turn to canola oil for a "neutral" flavor. Versatile and low in saturated fat, canola oil is a good substitute for butter in baked-goods recipes and in delicate stir-fries when you don't want the more assertive flavor of olive oil.

STEP THREE
Have a Small Serving of Nuts or Seeds Five Times a Week

Thanks to their mix of good fat, fiber, and protein, nuts and seeds are "slow-burning" foods that are friendly to your blood sugar. In fact, Harvard researchers discovered that women who regularly ate nuts (about a handful five times a week) were 20 percent less likely to develop type 2 diabetes than those who didn't eat them as often. Believe it or not, people who include nuts in their diets also tend to weigh less.

Yes, nuts and seeds are high in fat, but it's about 85 percent "good" fat, the kind that may reduce insulin resistance. Good fats, of course, also improve heart health, even boosting levels of "good" HDL cholesterol. In studies, people who ate as few as 5 ounces of nuts a week as part of an overall heart-healthy diet lowered their risk of developing heart disease by 35 percent compared to those who ate nuts less than once a month. Here's how to fit nuts and seeds into your diet.

Use nuts to bump up the protein. Stir chopped walnuts or pecans into rice dishes. Mix pine nuts or chopped walnuts into pasta dishes along with olive oil, basil, and sun-dried tomatoes. Or create your own trail mix for snacking with dried fruit, high-fiber cereal, and your favorite nuts.

Give 'em a roast. Top off pumpkin, squash, or tomato soup with chopped roasted nuts. Or sprinkle your favorite chopped nuts and some dried cranberries on green salads. Roasting nuts brings out their flavor. Preheat the oven to 300°F. Place 1/2 cup of shelled nuts on a baking sheet in a single layer and roast for 7 to 10 minutes. Check near the end of the roasting time to make sure they don't burn.

Enjoy peanut butter sandwiches again. Peanut butter and other nut butters—such as almond or cashew butter—make delicious lunchtime sandwiches, especially if you spread them on coarse whole-grain bread and top with fruit instead of jelly. Banana's an obvious choice, but we also love the taste of strawberries, sliced apple,

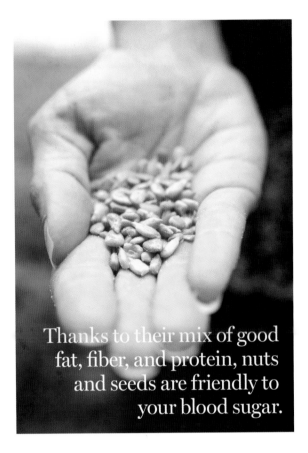

Thanks to their mix of good fat, fiber, and protein, nuts and seeds are friendly to your blood sugar.

peaches, and pears on a nut-butter sandwich with a sprinkle of cinnamon or nutmeg for an added boost of flavor.

Add peanut butter to your snack. Ideally you should be having protein with every meal *and* snack. Sometimes that's hard to do, but not if you remember peanut butter. Portion out one tablespoon and dip baby carrots in it or spread sliced apple wedges or celery sticks with it.

Introduce yourself to flaxseed. Tiny, shiny, and brown, flaxseeds are a godsend to your blood sugar as well as your heart, so if you haven't tried them yet, it's time for a trip to the store. Flaxseed is rich in both protein and fiber (more than 2 grams per tablespoon of ground seeds). It's also a good source of magnesium, a mineral that's key to good blood sugar control because it helps cells use insulin. But what's really unique about these seeds is this: They're incredibly rich in an essential fatty acid called alpha linolenic acid, which the body uses to make the same type of omega-3 fatty acids you get from fish. Ground flaxseed spoils quickly, so buy whole seeds in bulk and grind as needed (warning: eat them whole and they'll come out the same way they went in). Whole seeds will last up to a year stored at room temperature. If you buy ground flaxseed, keep it in the fridge.

Sprinkle ground flax liberally. Once you discover flaxseeds you'll find countless uses for them. They're great on hot or cold cereal or yogurt or low-fat ice cream. You can add them to meat loaf, meatballs, burgers, and casseroles, or add a tablespoon or two to doughs and batters for pancakes, waffles, muffins, and breads. (Just keep an eye on baked goods in the oven; the flaxseed could make them brown quicker than usual.) Also add them to cooked fruit desserts like baked apples or blueberry compote.

Discover the super-seeds. Pumpkin and sunflower seeds (buy unsalted varieties) make great snacks along with a piece of fruit. They're also a tasty replacement for croutons on a salad or sprinkled lightly over steamed green beans or carrots.

that's easy!

To prevent a cut avocado from turning brown in the refrigerator, remove the seed and spray the flesh with cooking spray, then wrap in plastic. Use within three days. If avocados are ripening faster than you can eat them, mash them with 1/2 tablespoon lemon or lime juice per avocado. Place in an airtight container, cover, and freeze. Use within four months.

STEP FOUR
Use Avocado Instead of Butter and Cheese

This rich, creamy fruit is loaded with fat—a whopping 25 to 30 grams each—but most of it "good" monounsaturated fat, the same fat you get in nuts and olive oil. Research suggests that diets rich in this type of fat may help keep blood sugar in check by slowing digestion after a meal. And unlike the saturated fats in butter and meat, monounsaturated fat won't increase insulin resistance. There's even some suggestion that eating more of it could help insulin-producing cells in your pancreas stay healthier. That means avocados are great additions to your diet if you eat them in moderation.

Start with a ripe avocado. Hold the avocado in your hand and press it gently, then roll it to the other side and press again. If it gives just a bit but pressure doesn't leave a permanent dent (an indication that it's too ripe), it's ready to eat.

Eat it as a snack. Instead of a handful of pretzels—practically all carbs—or cheese, cut an avocado into five pieces and eat two of them, drizzled with lemon juice, for a satisfying 110-calorie snack.

Use avocado in place of cheese. Rich in sterols, compounds shown to lower cholesterol, avocado is also a calorie bargain when eaten the smart way. Have one of those slices you cut in the tip above on your sandwich for 55 calories—half the 100 or so calories in an ounce of cheese. Or mash some avocado and spread it on in place of mayonnaise.

Add to salads. Use chunks or slices in place of cheese, or mash avocado and mix with lemon juice for a thick, dressing-like addition. Adding it to salads also increases your body's ability to absorb the good-for-you carotenoids, such as beta-carotene, in salad greens.

GOAL 6

Use the Plate Approach for perfect portions

NOW YOU'RE READY to get down to the nitty-gritty—putting the healthy, tasty foods you've read about in Goals 1 through 5 on your plate. Your assignment: Get a plate and set yourself a place at the table. Learning to fill it with perfect portions of fruit and vegetables, grain- and starch-based carbs, and protein is the key to successful blood sugar control, successful weight loss, and success at lowering your risk for diabetes complications.

The good news: Using the plate approach can make weighing and measuring food for portion control obsolete.

The Plate Approach rebalances your meals to give you the ideal proportions of vegetables, protein, and carbohydrates. Using the Plate Approach *automatically* cuts your calorie intake—the real goal of any weight-loss plan. It also ensures that you won't get too many carbohydrates at one sitting, with no need for you to keep a tally. Best of all, your plate will contain plenty of food, so you'll never feel deprived.

Complicated eating plans, such as the food exchange system that dietitians sometimes recommend for people with diabetes, are supposed to be effective because they make you track every-

thing you eat, theoretically leaving less to chance. But many people find the exchange system too confusing. The Plate Approach accomplishes the same objective (controlling portions and calories) in a simpler way—and it works.

In one study at Emory University School of Medicine in Atlanta, people who used a basic visual guide to make healthy choices lowered

Do You Need a Stricter Approach?

The Plate Approach automatically controls carbs and so helps regulate blood sugar. However, if you use insulin or you're having trouble controlling your blood sugar, you may need a stricter approach, such as carbohydrate counting, a system that helps you keep tight control on carb levels at every meal. Consult a registered dietitian who can customize a plan for you and refer to the carbohydrate counts starting on page 256. You can combine carb-counting with the Plate Approach to achieve better blood sugar control and to reach a healthy weight.

the Plate Approach
at a glance

Using the Plate Approach, the number of calories you save by eating more vegetables and fewer fatty foods can be significant. See for yourself. Because the meal on the bottom also contains fewer starches, it should have much less of an impact on your blood sugar.

TYPICAL AMERICAN MEAL
Calories: 1,358

Protein
8 ounces
fatty steak

Vegetable
1 cup corn

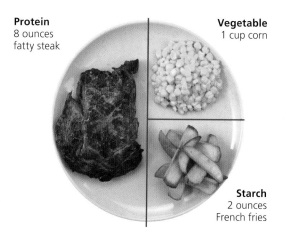

Starch
2 ounces
French fries

PLATE APPROACH MEAL
Calories: 440

Vegetable
1 1/2 cups mixed
vegetables

Starch
1 small
sweet
potato

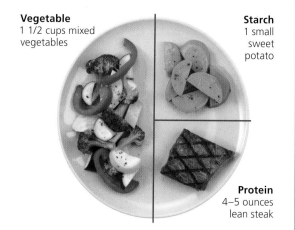

Protein
4–5 ounces
lean steak

their blood sugar, cut calories, and lost weight just as successfully as those who took the trouble to follow a plan that used food exchanges. And in a Canadian study, people with diabetes who followed a similar plate approach lost more weight than those who got conventional weight-loss advice. And they kept using their plate approach even after the study ended.

The biggest change you'll likely see on your plate? That humble helping of vegetables in the typical American meat-and-potatoes diner will become a hearty helping, shrinking the space left over for fatty meat and carbs—the major sources of calories, fat, and blood-sugar-raising starches and sugars.

Use the three main elements of a typical meal—meat, carbs, and vegetables—as your starting point. When you dish them out, your plate in effect becomes divided into three sections. Of course, it's the size of the sections that matters. To picture how your plate should look on the Plate Approach, mentally divide it into left and right halves. Then imagine the right half split into two equal parts. Whenever you eat a meal, keep these sections in mind and fill them in the following way.

STEP ONE
Load the Left Half of Your Plate with Vegetables (and Fruit)

The entire left side of your plate is reserved for produce. This is where you'll put all of your vegetables as well as fruit. Choose anything you like except potatoes and corn, which belong in the starch section. For some meals, you can eat fruit instead of (or in addition to) vegetables.

There's no escaping it: To lose weight, you need to take in fewer calories than you burn. The Plate Approach's solution to cutting calories is remarkably simple: Eat more vegetables and less of everything else. In the Plate Approach, half the real estate on your plate is taken up by vegetables, which are naturally very low in calories, so there's less room for starches and calorie-dense meats.

Vegetables are low in calories yet high in volume because a lot of their weight comes from water. Such "high-volume" foods have the advantage of looking big, so they make your brain expect that you'll be satisfied by eating them. They also take up more room in your stomach, so they trigger a signal in your brain that makes you stop eating sooner. It's small wonder that researchers in weight-loss programs such as that at the University of Alabama in Birmingham find that when people eat lots of vegetables, their calorie consumption goes down—and they lose weight.

Still hungry? You can fill the biggest portion of your plate—the vegetable section—again and again. That's right, there's no limit on the amount of food you can eat from this part of the plate as long as you stop when you feel satisfied. On the right half of the plate, however, stick with one helping of carbohydrate and one helping of protein.

Almost all vegetables are inherently good for you, but beware of transforming low-calorie vegetables into high-calorie ones by frying them in oil or smothering them with toppings, such as cheese sauces, full-fat salad dressings, or butter. By adding just 1 teaspoon of butter, you more than double or triple the calories in a serving of vegetables.

A word about breakfast: We're not going to ask you to fill half your plate with vegetables at this meal, since most of us don't eat vegetables in the morning (although if you're making an omelet, go ahead and pack it with as much produce as possible). Instead, substitute fruit, such as blueberries, strawberries, or bananas.

STEP TWO
Fill the Upper Right-Hand Side with Whole Grains

Grain-based carbohydrates and starchy veggies such as potatoes belong in the upper right-hand side of your plate. This area is reserved for whole-grain pasta, brown rice, barley, noodles, potatoes, or corn. If you're serving starchy beans (legumes such as black beans, pinto beans, kidney beans, or chickpeas) as a side dish, you would put them here.

The benefit? When starches are limited to one-fourth of your plate, you've got automatic carb control, which translates into better blood sugar control.

You already know that carbs aren't dietary disasters and that having three servings of whole grains a day will enhance your health and your blood

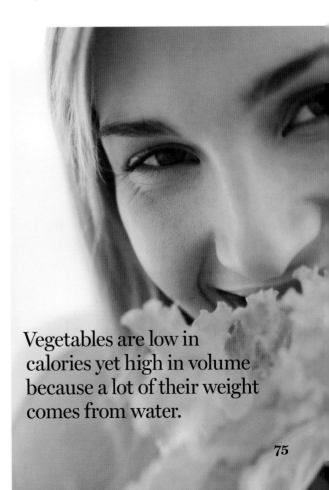

Vegetables are low in calories yet high in volume because a lot of their weight comes from water.

sugar if you have diabetes. But limiting portions is important with both starchy and grain-based carbs. First, they raise blood sugar. Second, some researchers now believe that eating too many carbohydrates make weight control especially hard for people who are already heavy. The reason: Carbs break down easily into glucose, and with enough glucose on hand, the body never has to burn its fat stores for energy.

With the Plate Approach, you'll enjoy a generous yet safe and controlled amount of carbs—no more worries about overeating second helpings of rice or mashed potatoes, no more guilt.

STEP THREE
Put Lean Protein on the Bottom Right-Hand Side of Your Plate

Reserve one-fourth of your plate for satisfying, sugar-controlling protein foods. These include lean red meat, eggs, fish, chicken and turkey, as well as dairy products, such as yogurt or cheese. If legumes are part of your entrée, put them here.

You've already learned that making sure you get protein at every meal is critical. Protein makes you feel full longer than carbohydrates do, and it doesn't raise blood sugar. So why not eat more of it? We're glad you asked. The first reason, of course, is calories. Just about any protein food you eat has more calories than veggies do. The second reason

is fat. As you know now, saturated fats directly impair the body's ability to react to insulin, the hormone that keeps blood sugar in check, and many protein foods contain these fats. Finally, if you fill up on protein at the expense of vegetables or whole grains, your body will be deprived of nutrients that are essential for good health.

STEP FOUR
Internalize the Plate Approach

Not every meal will fit precisely onto different segments of a plate the way we've suggested. For example, a stir-fry might have all the right elements—carbs (brown rice), lean protein (chicken strips), and lots of vegetables (carrots, broccoli, and pea pods)—but the ingredients are mixed together. That's okay. Once you get the basic idea of the Plate Approach down and get used to seeing how much food goes into each section of the plate, you won't need the divisions to guide you. As long as the bulk of the dish is vegetables, with smaller amounts of rice and poultry, a stir-fry is a perfect Plate Approach meal.

You may also have problems using the Plate Approach when you're out to dinner, eating a meal that isn't served on a dinner plate, or eating food that you didn't serve yourself. In these situations, having a sense of what a healthy portion looks like will help you stay on track. See A Visual Guide to Portion Sizes on the opposite page.

A Visual Guide to Portion Sizes

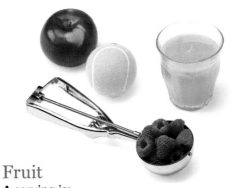

Fruit
A serving is:

1 medium piece of fruit (the size of a tennis ball)

3/4 cup fruit juice

1/2 cup chopped, cooked or canned fruit, or berries (the size of a large ice cream scoop)

Vegetables
A serving is:

3/4 cup vegetable juice

1/2 cup non-leafy vegetables, cooked, chopped, or canned (the size of a large ice cream scoop)

1 cup raw leafy vegetables (the size of a baseball)

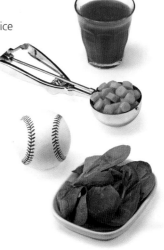

Meat, Poultry, Fish & Beans
A serving is:

3 ounces of cooked lean meat, poultry, or fish (the size of a deck of cards)

1/2 cup of cooked dry beans (the size of a large ice cream scoop)

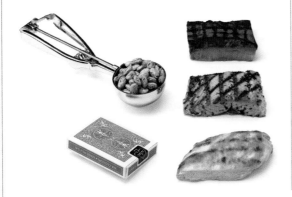

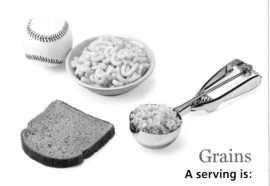

Grains
A serving is:

1/2 cup cereal, rice, bulgur, barley (the size of a large ice cream scoop)

1/2 cup pasta (2 servings equals the size of one baseball)

1 slice of bread

GOAL 7

Plan your meals

SIT DOWN ONCE A WEEK—we suggest setting aside time for this on Saturday or Sunday—to map out your meals for the coming week. In the Planner section you'll find a weekly meal planner to fill out for each of the 12 weeks. You'll restock your kitchen with healthy, low-glycemic staple foods. And you'll shop strategically, so that the foods that end up in your grocery bag are foods recommended by the Eat plan.

Planning your meals—and shopping accordingly (refer to our shopping list on page 252)—sound like no-brainers. But they're actually make-or-break strategies. Studies show that many a good dietary intention falls by the wayside when these steps aren't taken.

If you still have high-fat, high-calorie, high-carbohydrate foods tucked away in your cabinets and refrigerator, and if you don't have a meal plan, it's easy to give in to cravings or to grab the easiest option when you're hungry and there's no time to figure out how to create a healthy meal. If you shop without a list, it's too easy to fall back on processed foods from boxes and packages, to buy those two gallons of double-fudge supreme ice cream because they're on sale, to grab the usual breaded fish sticks, or to be tempted by the eye-catching cookies and crackers that get all the most visible spots in supermarket aisles. (Have you ever noticed that the oatmeal's always stuck on the bottom shelf, or that there are few fancy signs on the fresh produce? Healthy food *whispers* in the grocery store while other foods scream.)

Planning is a powerful way to set yourself up for success. Each time you walk into the kitchen to prepare a meal or into your favorite deli, coffee shop, or restaurant for a meal, you'll already know what you're going to do. Once you've planned what you'll eat, it's a snap to eat what you've planned. You've thrown up a major roadblock to three common dietary downfalls: Giving in to temptation, to hunger, or to old habits.

What's on your menu this week? Consider these meal-by-meal ideas.

STEP ONE
Start with Breakfast

You've heard it before, but we'll say it again: Breakfast is the most important meal of your day. Studies show that breakfast eaters weigh significantly less than people who skip morning meals, and those who skip breakfast eat more later in the day—probably because they become so hungry that overeating is inevitable. Getting breakfast into your system kicks your calorie-burning furnace into gear and keeps it burning hot throughout the morning. Otherwise, it will stay on "low" because your body turns it down while you sleep to conserve energy. And of course breakfast helps prevent dangerous blood sugar lows.

While the foods we usually have at breakfast won't always fit onto a dinner plate, you can still use Plate Approach principles to guide your choices and portion sizes. Just be sure to include some protein, a moderate portion of whole grains, and a serving of fruit or vegetable.

Put eating first. Try to have breakfast shortly after getting out of bed. That way, you'll eat before you remember that you have to take out the trash, walk the dog, pay bills, or do any other distracting tasks that can gobble up your time.

Plan on protein. One challenge with breakfast is getting protein into your meal. When you're not eating eggs (which are rich in protein), look to nonfat milk, yogurt, and peanut butter. Grab a container of fat-free, sugar-free yogurt and top it with 3 to 4 tablespoons of high-fiber cereal or a palmful of ground flax- seeds and sliced fruit. Or one whole-wheat mini-bagel topped with 2 tablespoons peanut butter, served with a medium banana and a cup of black or green tea.

that's easy!

Got a minute? That's about all you need to cook up a hot egg sandwich that you can carry out the door with you. Just crack an egg into a saucer and whisk it with a fork. Microwave on high for 30 seconds, take it out and whisk again to keep the edges from overcooking, then nuke it for another 30 seconds. Serve on coarse whole-grain toast. Note: You'll want to pop the bread into the toaster before starting the egg—otherwise, the egg may be done first.

Top high-fiber cereal with fruit. Look for a whole-grain brand that contains 5 grams or more of fiber per serving. There are plenty of them on the market. Some brands also include a substantial amount of protein. A high-fiber cereal plus fat-free milk counts as your carbohydrate and protein servings. Just top with fruit, and you'll have a perfect Plate Approach meal.

Add veggies when you can. How about a two-egg omelet filled with 1/2 cup vegetables (such as sautéed onions, green peppers, and mushrooms) and topped with 1 ounce shredded fat-free sharp cheddar cheese, served with a slice of whole-wheat

Breakfast on the Go

Even when you're eating on the go, it's possible to have a balanced breakfast that includes protein, carbohydrate, and a fruit or vegetable using these "fast-food" combinations.

PROTEIN	CARBOHYDRATE	FRUIT
1 HARD-BOILED EGG	1 small low-fat bran muffin	1 medium banana
1 OUNCE STRING CHEESE	1 whole-grain English muffin	1 medium apple
1 PINT LOW-FAT MILK	1 whole-grain cereal bar	20 seedless grapes
8 OUNCES LOW-FAT YOGURT	1-ounce box whole-grain cereal	1 orange or peach
1 OUNCE WALNUTS	1 whole-grain cereal bar	1 pear or plum

toast? Or a fried egg between two whole-grain English muffin halves with several slices of tomato and 1 ounce reduced-fat cheddar cheese?

Invent your own "breakfast food." Some people say they just don't like breakfast. In many cases, what they really mean is that they don't like traditional breakfast foods. But who says breakfast has to be eggs, toast, or cereal? As long as your body gets a mix of protein and carbohydrate, it doesn't matter what you eat. It could be some leftover soup, a peanut butter and banana sandwich on whole-grain bread, some turkey on a slice of bread with a small orange on the side, or an egg salad sandwich (made with canola oil mayonnaise) on a whole-grain English muffin—like fast food but with healthier carbs and less fat.

Pack a chicken sandwich on whole wheat and a green salad, and voilà— the pefect lunch.

STEP TWO
Create the Perfect Lunch

What makes an ideal midday meal? Eating it absolutely no more than five hours after breakfast (and preferably sooner) for starters. Otherwise, you'll get too hungry and overeat. You also want a meal that will energize you rather than send you into an afternoon slump. That means one with ample protein but not too much fat or too many carbs.

You probably have a little more time for lunch than for breakfast, so don't rush: Slowly savoring your food will make you feel more satisfied, so you'll be less likely to overeat.

Pair lean protein with whole grains. Protein and whole-grain carbs are a snap at lunch—a lean protein like sliced turkey or chicken on whole-wheat bread, for example, or leftover sliced pork tenderloin and brown rice from last night's dinner. Just add a salad or a handful of carrot sticks to fill your produce quota.

Include fruit. Grab a piece from the fruit bowl on your counter or from your refrigerator before you leave the house. Otherwise it can be rough to get fruit into your lunch if you're eating away from home.

Make sure your salad contains lean protein. Grilled chicken or beans of any kind make the grade. Try a green salad topped with 3 ounces grilled chicken and 1/2 cup grilled vegetables (such as onions, portobello mushrooms, and green and red peppers). Drizzle with 2 teaspoons of a vinaigrette dressing made with olive oil. Serve with a small whole-grain roll.

Sneak in veggies. To make sure you get plenty of vegetables in your lunch, add a salad or load up your sandwich with lettuce and tomato or add other veggies, such as cucumbers, bean sprouts, onions, or roasted red peppers from a jar.

Open up ready-to-eat soup. Your grocery store stocks numerous healthful soups sold in microwavable cartons. According to research conducted at Pennsylvania State University, broth-based soups weigh down your stomach, enabling you to feel full on fewer calories. Toss a bean and vegetable soup along with a cheese stick and a carton of skim milk into your lunch bag. In just a few seconds, you'll have packed all the protein and fiber you need to power your body and brain through the afternoon.

STEP THREE
Create a Dinner You'll Love

Uncomplicated foods fit easily into the Plate Approach—pile veggies on one side, spoon a serving of brown rice or barley into the carbohydrate position, place chicken or another lean protein into the designated spot. Follow suggestions in Goals 1 through 5 to expand your repertoire and mix and match a variety of delicious, easy to prepare dinner foods.

You'll also find handy meal-planning suggestions with every weekly meal planner in the Planner section.

What about combination foods, such as soups, stews, casseroles, and pasta dishes with sauces that may contain vegetables and protein? Take a look at the ingredients and plan accordingly. Pasta with shrimp and broccoli covers all the

---

quick and easy lunches

Second to breakfast, lunch is the easiest meal to throw together. Try these suggestions.

Sandwich, American style. A turkey or chicken breast sandwich on whole wheat with lots of tomatoes, some sprouts if you have them, and lettuce or even baby spinach leaves. Avocado is another nice addition.

Sandwich, Mediterranean style. Hummus stuffed into half of a whole-wheat pita with bean sprouts, diced tomatoes, cucumbers, and shredded carrots.

Bean salad. Rinse and drain a can of black beans and a can of sweet corn. Add 1/2 of an avocado, cubed. Mix with a drizzle of olive oil, 1 tablespoon balsamic vinegar, and a pinch of cumin. Makes several servings.

A veggie wrap. Place 2 cups loosely packed raw spinach leaves in food processor and grind. Mix in 1/2 cup fat-free ricotta and 1 tablespoon Parmesan cheese, and wrap in a whole-wheat tortilla.

Mediterranean tomato salad. Dice fresh tomato and cucumber, mix with a thinly sliced red onion and black olives, add some low-fat feta, and drizzle with a little olive oil, red wine vinegar, salt, and pepper.

A bowl of chili. Make it with beans and ground skinless turkey and serve with a small green salad.

A pita pizza. Start with a whole-grain pita and top with 1/2 cup broccoli, 2 ounces of part-skim mozzarella, and 2 tablespoons tomato sauce. Enjoy with a tossed salad with 1 tablespoon low-fat dressing.

---

bases—just be sure there's lots of broccoli, only a moderate amount of pasta, and enough shrimp to fill a quarter of your plate. You'll probably want to add a side salad to bump up the produce portion of the meal. Serving a hearty vegetable-beef stew or chicken-and-vegetable soup? Just add whole-grain rolls and a colorful fruit salad.

Start with these strategies to help you get a healthy meal on the table, even on busy weeknights.

Have an inventory of recipe standbys. Fewer than 60 percent of Americans know what they're having for dinner come 4 p.m. Planning ahead is the answer. No one expects you to come up with a new meal every night. The trick is to find 8 or 10 healthy recipes you love (you may even want to keep a list on your refrigerator), then rotate them in. Start with three low-fuss, nutritious recipes that you can almost cook in your sleep. For example, you might designate Monday as casserole night, Tuesday as grilled fish night, and Wednesday as roasted chicken night. Include tried-and-true vegetable and whole-grain side dishes as well. This eases the headache of grocery shopping—you'll need many of the same groceries from one week to the next.

Write your grocery list as you fill in your meal planner. When you sit down to plan your meals, think about what's in your freezer and fridge, what your family likes to eat, what your upcoming week entails (are you eating out one night?). Then plan out the week's worth of menus. At the same time, write out your grocery list—then go shopping. Post the list of menus on the kitchen refrigerator or bulletin board so its the first thing you see when you get home. Voilà! No more thinking ahead. Just follow your own instructions.

Use parts of last night's dinner for tonight's meal. This allows you to cook once and eat twice. For example, if you have roasted chicken one night, use the leftovers to serve up chicken fajitas or chicken salad the next. Similarly, if you make grilled fish one night, try fish tacos the next. Prepare all key protein foods—chicken, turkey, fish, and so on—in larger-than-needed amounts so they will last two nights instead of one. Do the same

---

quick and easy
dinners

Some of our favorite diabetes-friendly dinners:

- ■ A stir-fry of shrimp (keep a bag of shelled shrimp in the freezer) and precut veggies, served over 1/2 cup brown rice or barley.
- ■ Barbecued chicken breast, steamed broccoli, strawberries, and an ear of fresh corn.
- ■ Lasagna made with lots of vegetables, ground skinless chicken or turkey, whole-wheat noodles, and fat-free ricotta, served with a tossed salad.
- ■ Baked or grilled fish, sautéed spinach, steamed carrots, and barley.
- ■ Steamed or stir-fried vegetables mixed with 1/2 cup whole-grain pasta, sliced chicken breast, and a dusting of Parmesan cheese. Serve with a tossed salad.
- ■ Pork tenderloin or a center-cut pork chop, steamed green beans with sliced almonds, one-half of a baked sweet potato.

---

with rice and other grain side dishes. Serve it up as a regular side dish one night and use the leftovers to make a casserole, stir-fry, or soup the next.

Make new recipes on the weekends, when you have more time to cook. You'll enjoy the cooking process more when your mind feels rested and unfettered. Once you get the hang of the new recipe, incorporate it into your weeknight repertoire.

Double the recipe. Freeze the leftovers and you have a ready-cooked meal for next week.

Start dinner in the morning. Slow cookers are back in fashion for a reason—they're wonderful! Take any cut of meat or poultry, put it in the pot (even frozen), add a can of diced tomatoes or a can of low-fat, low-sodium creamed soup, and turn on low. You'll come home in the evening to a great-smelling house and a delectable dinner that needs only a whole grain and vegetable to complete.

STEP FOUR
Enjoy Dessert on Occasion

We didn't forget about ending your meal on a sweet note. That's where those three servings a day of fruit come in handy. Deploy them strategically at the close of your meal for a delicious finale. Ripe strawberries with a dollop of yogurt or light whipped cream (make sure it doesn't contain hydrogenated oil), a baked apple dusted with cinnamon, a beautiful fruit salad loaded with ripe summer berries, or sliced citrus in winter are all fabulous, fresh ways to get colorful and tasty fruit onto your dessert plate.

STEP FIVE
Write Down Your Snack Strategy

A healthy diet rises or falls on the quality of foods you eat between meals. Depending on what your blood sugar control plan from your doctor allows, fitting in a nutritious, low-glycemic snack or two every day will help you stay on track by helping you avoid overeating at meals.

Snacks can demand some advance planning if you want to reach for healthy choices; vending machines certainly don't offer a lot of options. In fact, it's not a bad idea to dump the whole concept of

sugar buster quiz

Q: Black coffee or coffee drinks?
A: Black coffee

It has almost no calories, and recent research shows that moderate coffee drinking is actually good for you. If you prefer a cold drink, ask for plain iced coffee (with fat-free milk if you like) and add a teaspoon or two of sugar. Fancy coffee drinks, on the other hand, can be loaded with sugar and a staggering amount of saturated fat. At Starbucks, a Double Chocolate Chip Frappucino Blended Crème with whipped cream, Venti size (24 ounces), has 86 grams of sugar and a whopping 25 grams of fat, more than half of it saturated. That's more fat and saturated fat than you'd get in a McDonald's Quarter Pounder with Cheese.

"snack foods," which typically includes chips, crackers, and candies. What does that leave? Plenty. A small handful of nuts is a perfect snack, rich in protein and good fat. Or try one of these choices:

- 8 ounces of fat-free, sugar-free yogurt
- 1 ounce of fat-free string cheese
- 1 snack-size plastic bag of cherry tomatoes or sliced raw red peppers, carrots, or cucumbers
- 4 cups of air-popped popcorn
- 1 small apple, orange, banana, or other fresh fruit plus a half-ounce of nuts for protein
- 1 tablespoon of peanut butter spread on four whole-grain crackers.

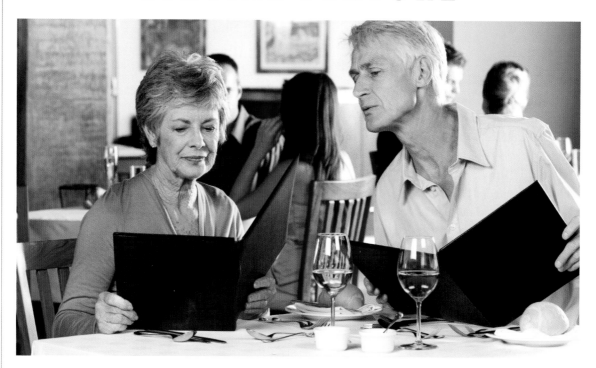

Dining Out Wisely

Who doesn't love dining out—whether it's breakfast at your favorite neighborhood diner, a quick lunch in a delicious deli, or a relaxing dinner. When you eat out, eat smart—following the same eating goals you use at home. Avoid oversized portions, excess fat, and an overload of refined carbohydrates (the bread basket! The mountain of pasta! The desserts!), and the only price you'll pay will be your check, not your health.

Restaurants are in the business of making you feel like a VIP. All the low lighting, soft music, and mouthwatering scents drifting from the kitchen are designed to make you stay longer. Add an indulgent wait staff and a cocktail or glass of wine before your meal, and you're set up to adopt a devil-may-care attitude toward what you order and how much of it you eat. The best way to avoid overindulging is to walk through the door prepared.

Eat Smart While Eating Out

These strategies tip the odds in your favor for getting a blood sugar-friendly meal in any restaurant.

Choose your restaurant with care. Make the challenge of eating out easier by being smart about what kinds of restaurants you patronize. Avoid the temptation of all-you-can-eat places or buffet-style restaurants, where portions are hard to control. Avoid places known for enormous portions, like many chains and most steak houses. And you probably won't find a lot of *Reverse Diabetes* foods on the menu at eateries that specialize in deep-frying an entire breaded onion. Enjoy a meal at one of these on your birthday, sure, but don't do it on a regular basis.

Make friends with the waitperson. Once you're in the right kind of restaurant, get ready to get friendly with the waitperson. Ask them to hold the bread basket so you're not tempted to fill up on usually high-GL carbs while waiting for your meal to arrive. Inquire about how a dish you're considering is prepared (Is it swimming in butter? Are the vegetables present in only token amounts?), and find out how big the portions are. At the same time, ask for a glass of water. Remember to drink plenty of water with your meal.

Order creatively. When you order, be bold: Order soup, salad, and an appetizer (not fried) for your meal rather than an entrée. Split an entrée and share a side order of vegetables to get more veggies into your meal and cut calories. If a main dish comes with a potato, ask if you can get an extra vegetable instead. (Especially if you're a regular customer, you're likely to get your way.) If you plan to order dessert, plan to share it, too. The best situation is when you get to know a restaurant's regular fare, including how big the portions are, and use that knowledge to outsmart the menu.

Draw the line. Ask whether the kitchen can prepare half portions. Many restaurants are more than willing to do so. Some even offer half portions on the menu. If the dish you order turns out to be too big, ask the waiter right then and there to divide the portion and set half aside for you to take home. Don't wait until you've started to nibble, and don't depend on your willpower to eat only half of what's in front of you. If you know in advance that the entrées at a particular restaurant are outsized, ask for a half portion as the meal and request that the other half be brought at the end in a takeout container.

Be colorful. Meat and creamy sauces are usually beige, right? Where do most dishes get their brightest colors? From vegetables and fruit, of course. Choose the most colorful dishes on the menu, and chances are you'll order the healthiest, lowest-calorie selections. Spicy red salsas, deep purple beets, green salads, yellow corn, bright orange and yellow sweet peppers turn your plate into a rainbow of colors. As long as vegetables arrive without added fat, they're yours to eat to your heart's (and your blood sugar's) content.

Dip into the sauce. Ordering salad dressing on the side and drizzling it on sparingly is one of the oldest healthy-eating tricks. Remember that you can order other sauces on the side, too, from gravy to guacamole. Give yourself no more than a tablespoon. And put your fork to good use.

Steer clear of anything breaded, crispy, creamy, or buttery. Choose grilled, baked, steamed, or broiled foods instead. When ordering soups and sauces, stick with those that are broth-based or tomato-based.

Stick to one drink—and have it with your meal. Wine, beer, and liquor add calories to your meal and may encourage overeating.

continued >>>

85

Eating Out Italian

A single slice of pizza with vegetables is a fine choice, especially if it's made with a whole-wheat or thin crust. A cup of pasta with marinara sauce is all right, too. The problem is, few of us stop there.

Ironically, southern Italian food, prepared the traditional way, is among the healthiest in the world. Unfortunately, Italian restaurants are often parlors for the presentation of huge mounds of overcooked pasta and pizza. And even before these arrive, you'll have ample opportunity to eat bread. So unless you want to overload on carbs and send your blood sugar for a wild post-meal ride, tread carefully. Here's how.

If you want pasta, order a dish from the appetizer section of the menu, or share. That's the traditional way—a small first course of pasta followed by simple grilled meat, poultry, or fish and a side of sautéed greens. As for pasta sauces, opt for those based on tomatoes (marinara), vegetables, white wine, and garlic—not cream. Watch out: Pasta primavera is often made with lots of cream.

If it's on the menu, order simple grilled beef, veal, pork, chicken, fish, or shellfish. Add a side order of sautéed spinach or broccoli rabe (a slightly bitter Italian version of broccoli). Finish with a mixed green salad with vinaigrette dressing.

For dessert, ask for fresh berries or fruit ice, if it's available, or a small plate of cookies to share. Stay away from the custards and cheesecake, the cannoli and the tiramisu.

WHAT TO ORDER

■ Appetizers/Sides

Minestrone soup; pasta e fagioli (fagioli means "beans"); green salad; grilled or marinated vegetables; broiled shrimp (no butter); steamed mussels.

■ Entrées

Pasta with marinara or Bolognese sauce; pasta with red clam sauce; chicken cacciatore; chicken or veal marsala; grilled fish; mixed grill; thin-crust cheese or vegetable pizza.

WHAT NOT TO ORDER

■ Appetizers/Sides

Garlic bread; fried mozzarella sticks; antipasto (it's mostly high-fat cheese and high-fat meat); stuffed mushrooms (usually high in fat).

■ Entrées

Pasta with Alfredo (cheese) sauce; penne alla vodka; shrimp scampi (rich in butter or oil); pasta primavera (usually made with cream); fried calamari or anything else that's fried; eggplant parmigiana (eggplant is a sponge for oil); anything stuffed.

Eating Out Mexican

Ordering from a fast-food Mexican place is about as big as a blood sugar challenge can get. Portions are generally huge, the tortillas used for burritos are larger than your head and filled with a cup or more of white rice (blood sugar enemy #1), and the entrées tend to be loaded with cheese—and we don't mean the low-fat variety. Thread your way around these potholes, and you can arrive at a delicious, healthy meal.

Ask the waitperson to take away the tortilla chips. The Mexican equivalent of a big breadbasket is either a bowl of chips or nacho chips covered with cheese. Just say no.

Order a healthy starter instead. Look for ceviches (marinated raw fish or seafood); guacamole, which is full of "good" fats (ask for soft tortillas instead of deep-fried chips to dip, and don't over-eat them); gazpacho, a spicy cold vegetable soup; black bean soup; and tortilla soup (chicken in broth with vegetables and thin fried tortilla chips). Ask for extra salsa for the table and eat it with a spoon rather than on chips.

For an entrée, look to fajitas. These are made with lean beef (or chicken or shrimp) grilled with onions and peppers. Other good choices are grilled chicken or fish dishes.

Order tacos or burritos without high-fat sour cream. Ask for extra salsa instead, or use just a dab of guacamole.

Go for soft tacos and tortillas. Hard tacos are fried, so you're better off with soft tacos. A small tortilla is the equivalent of a slice of bread. If you're not eating rice, two or three soft tacos are fine, but stick to one or two if you are having rice. If you're getting a burrito, ask for no rice and more beans.

As a side dish, go for rice and beans instead of Mexican rice. Thanks to the beans, this dish has a lower GL than rice alone. But check first to be sure the beans aren't refried. Refried beans are likely loaded with fat.

Have dessert at home. Desserts at Mexican restaurants, such as flan and fried ice cream, are usually high in calories and fat, so skip them and eat something healthier elsewhere.

WHAT TO ORDER
■ Appetizers/Sides
Tortilla soup; gazpacho; rice and beans (not refried); soft tortillas with salsa.

■ Entrées
Chicken or steak fajitas; soft chicken tacos (portion: two tacos); chicken or bean burrito; grilled chicken or fish; grilled chicken salad without the taco bowl.

WHAT NOT TO ORDER
■ Appetizers/Sides
Tortilla chips; nachos; quesadillas; refried beans.

■ Entrées
Taco salads; hard-shell tacos; chimichangas; beef or cheese enchiladas; beef burritos; anything "grande."

continued >>>

Eating Out Chinese

The traditional Chinese diet is a healthy one, with lots of vegetables, stir-fries with small chunks of meat or fish, and soy foods. But that's not evident in the typical fare in a Chinese restaurant here, where the meal is likely to be heavy on greasy meats and swimming in sauces with lots and lots of calories. Even the vegetables are usually laden with a fatty sauce. Here's your game plan.

Ask for brown rice. Many restaurants give you the option. Remember, white rice is a blood sugar disaster waiting to happen. And don't eat the whole bowl or container of rice. Spoon a half cup onto your plate and leave the rest. Or do as a Chinese native would: Put a small amount in a small bowl and hold the bowl up, using your chopsticks (or fork) to eat a little rice in between bites of your main dish. Or be bold and don't eat any rice at all.

Start your meal with wonton or egg-drop soup. This will take the edge off your hunger without a lot of calories (avoid soups with coconut milk). If you want a ravioli-type appetizer, order steamed vegetable dumplings, but nothing fried.

When it comes to entrées, order from the "healthy" menu. Here is where you'll find steamed chicken and vegetables with sauce on the side and similar low-fat choices. Another good choice is moo goo gai pan (chicken with mushrooms). If you like stir-fries, ask the waitperson to have yours prepared with less oil and more veggies, and get the sauce on the side.

Make sure you order plenty of vegetables. If you really want to make the meal healthier, order a plate of steamed vegetables and add them to other dishes. Or ask for sautéed vegetables or Szechuan-style string beans.

Take advantage of the bean curd (tofu). Ordering family-style? Include a heart-healthy, low-fat dish like bean curd with sautéed Chinese mixed vegetables (ask for sautéed bean curd, not deep-fried).

Plan to take home leftovers. Portions are often large. Think of about one cup of a dish (without rice) as a serving. Ask for a take-out container right away, so you can store the rest out of sight.

WHAT TO ORDER
■ Appetizers/Sides
Wonton soup; egg-drop soup; steamed dumplings.

■ Entrées
Moo goo gai pan; chicken chow mein; steamed chicken with broccoli, sauce on the side; steamed chicken with mixed vegetables.

WHAT NOT TO ORDER
■ Appetizers/Sides
Hot-and-sour soup; velvet corn chowder; egg rolls; fried wonton; fried dumplings.

■ Entrées
General Tso's chicken; Kung Pao chicken; cashew chicken; moo shu pork; orange beef; spicy eggplant (eggplant soaks up oil).

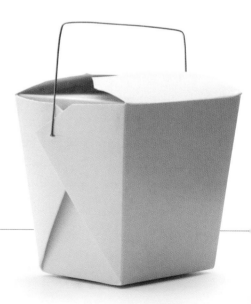

Fast Food Without Fear

An occasional visit to a fast-food joint never killed anyone. Burgers and fries are still the staples on these menus, but the restaurants are now offering a greater selection of healthier fare. True, you'll have trouble locating a decent vegetable, other than salads, but you can keep the fat and calorie damage under control by ordering grilled sandwiches, salads, and even vegetarian burgers, chili, soup, and low-fat dairy desserts. Aim to make your meals "fast" ones less than once a week.

Opt for simple grilled fare, if you can find it. If there's a grilled chicken sandwich and the chicken isn't breaded, that's a good start. Wendy's Ultimate Chicken Grill (320 calories) is a good choice, as is McDonald's Premium Grilled Chicken Classic Sandwich (420 calories). If you can, order it without mayonnaise or creamy sauces. This can save 100 calories or more.

A simple hamburger isn't bad either—if you order the smallest one. At 220 calories, Wendy's Jr. Hamburger is a low-cal burger. (By contrast, a Burger King Double Whopper with Cheese has 1,010 calories.) Another good option is a vegetarian burger. Burger King regularly offers vegetarian burgers (the BK Veggie; 420 calories), and McDonald's has them at some locations.

Order à la carte. A "value" meal that includes fries and a big soft drink is often cheaper, but it's no nutritional bargain—the total calories can top 1,000! Unless you drink diet soda, skip the soft drink and ask for water—or orange juice, hot tea, coffee, or low-fat milk—instead. If it's a special treat, get the fries but buy the smallest size.

Take advantage of the salads. Just skip the cheese, bacon bits, and other add-ons. Ask for vinaigrette dressing. Try a salad as an entrée. Good choices include Burger King's Tendergrill Chicken Garden salad (with vinaigrette) and Wendy's Mandarin Chicken Salad (with Oriental sesame dressing).

Have fruit and yogurt. At Wendy's, you can get mandarin oranges for 80 calories. McDonald's offers Fruit 'n' Yogurt Parfait for 160 calories.

WHAT TO ORDER

■ Appetizers/Sides/Drinks

Garden salad; baked potato; fruit and yogurt parfait; water; low-fat milk; diet soda.

■ Entrées

Grilled chicken sandwich; grilled chicken salad (skip the crispy noodles); junior hamburger; veggie burger; soft chicken taco; soft steak taco.

WHAT NOT TO ORDER

■ Appetizers/Sides/Drinks

French fries (if you must, order the small); hash browns; thick shakes; regular soda; sweetened iced tea.

■ Entrées

Double burgers; burgers with cheese or bacon; fried chicken sandwich; fried fish sandwich.

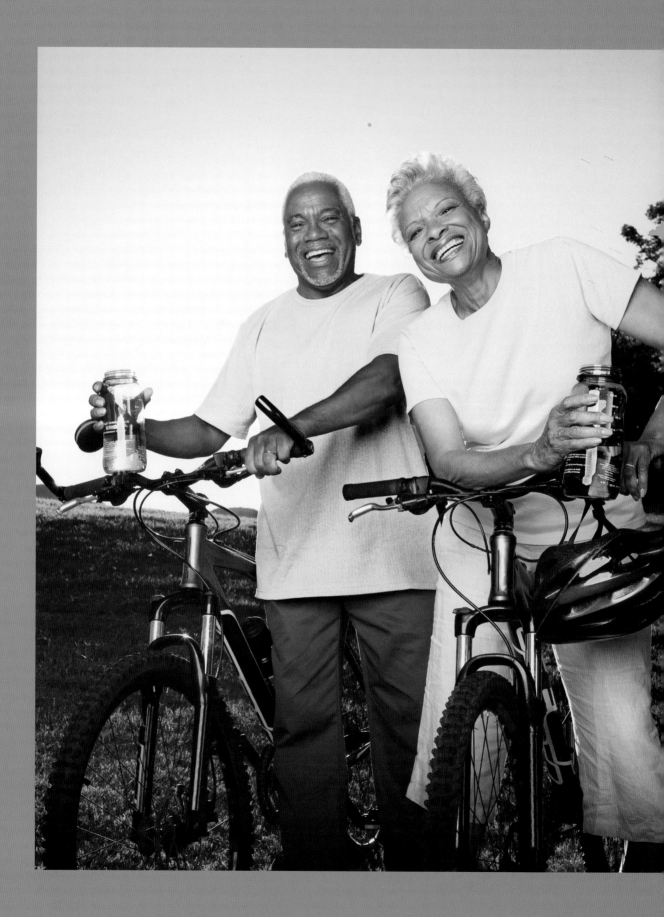

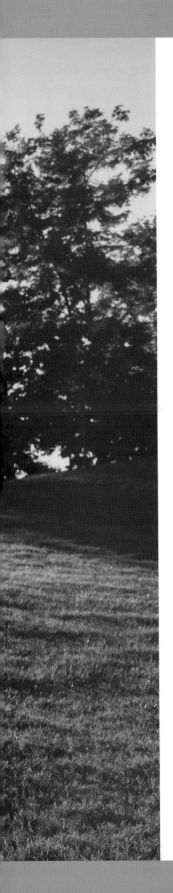

2

MOVE
to reverse diabetes

- Fitness Walking
- Easy Everyday Activity
- Simple Strength Moves

- Better Health

the plan

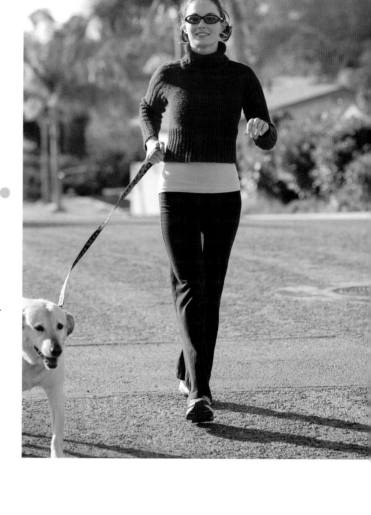

Easy and effective, our research-based Move to Reverse Diabetes plan stacks the deck in favor of better diabetes control. It does naturally what some drugs do: sensitizes cells to insulin so they soak up more glucose. Follow the plan for 12 weeks and you'll almost certainly see lower blood sugar levels. Your body will also burn more calories all day long, which means extra weight will come off more readily.

what to do

GOAL 1
Know how to exercise safely with diabetes

Exercise can make or break your efforts to lose weight and control your blood sugar—but when you have diabetes, you need to make sure you're exercising smartly and safely. It's important to guard against hypoglycemia (blood sugar that dips too low), to protect your feet, and, especially if you take insulin, to time your workouts.

GOAL 2
Walk at least five days a week

The core of the Move plan is a walk in the park… or around the neighborhood…or on a treadmill. Putting one foot in front of the other is a simple yet powerful way to meet *Reverse Diabetes'* twin goals of lower blood sugar and weight loss. Start with just 10 minutes a day and build up to 45-minute walks—energizing, calorie- and fat-burning workouts that feel great.

GOAL 3
Build muscle with the Sugar Buster Routine

Muscle mass is the secret to all-day blood sugar control and to maintaining a healthy weight with ease. Our Sugar Buster moves are safe, easy on your joints, and can be done in small pockets of downtime. You'll ease into the Sugar Buster Routine in Week 4 of our program and build up to performing all nine exercises twice each week.

GOAL 4
Make active choices every day

Equally important on the Move plan, you'll put everyday physical activity back into your life. Studies show that making active choices, from doing lawn work to going bowling, is a no-sweat way to lose weight and reduce your risk for diabetes and other health problems. We'll show you how to energize your life and burn hundreds of extra calories each day.

what to record

1. THE NUMBER OF MINUTES YOU WALK EACH DAY

Use the 12-week Planner section to record this info. How much should you walk? "Your Goals Week by Week," below, outlines your exercise assignments. If you choose to wear a pedometer and count your steps every day, write your steps down, too.

2. WHETHER YOU PERFORMED THE SUGAR BUSTER EXERCISES

Beginning in Week 4 you'll add the Sugar Buster exercises to your weekly routine. Your ultimate goal is to perform the whole series of exercises twice each week. As you'll see in this chapter, you can accomplish your goal in any way that fits your schedule.

3. OTHER EXERCISE YOU GET

Every time you make an active choice instead of an inactive choice during your day, give yourself a pat on the back by writing it down. That includes small stuff, like taking the stairs instead of the elevator, and bigger stuff, like mowing the lawn or playing a game of softball in the backyard. Recording these choices will motivate you to get up and move even more often.

Your Goals Week by Week

New to exercise? Short on time? No worries. The Move plan will ease you into a comfortable exercise routine that won't make you crazy.

WEEK	WALKING TIME	SUGAR BUSTER ROUTINE
1	10 minutes, 5 days a week	None
2	15 minutes, 5 days a week	None
3	20 minutes, 5 days a week	None
4	25 minutes, 5 days a week	Do each sequence once*
5	25 minutes, 5 days a week	Do each sequence once
6	30 minutes, 5 days a week	Do the entire routine twice
7	30 minutes, 5 days a week	Do the entire routine twice
8	35 minutes, 5 days a week	Do the entire routine twice
9	35 minutes, 5 days a week	Do the entire routine twice
10	40 minutes, 5 days a week	Do the entire routine twice
11	40 minutes, 5 days a week	Do the entire routine twice
12	45 minutes, 5 days a week	Do the entire routine twice

*choose a different day for each

before you begin

1 Take the quiz on page 94

It will help you assess your current fitness level, your attitude toward physical activity, and whether you're ready to find ways to fit more fitness into your day. Remember, these questions are for your eyes only. Answer as accurately as you can. You'll uncover valuable information that will help you customize the Move plan to fit your personality, your likes and dislikes, and your schedule.

2 Read the safety information under Goal #1

There you'll find a thorough discussion about exercising safely with diabetes. Read and digest the information before you start the plan.

3 Buy a good pair of walking shoes

High blood sugar and circulation problems mean that people with diabetes are at high risk for slow-healing sores that can lead to dangerous infections. That's why good walking shoes aren't a luxury for people with diabetes—they're a necessity. Turn to page 103 for advice.

93

the quiz

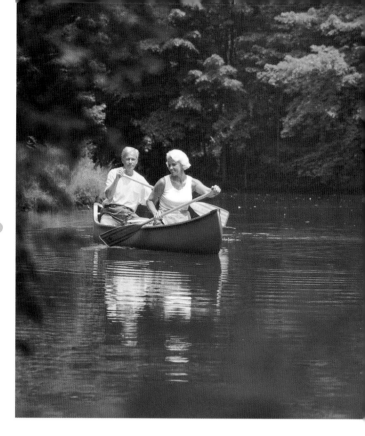

Are you ready to harness the power of movement to beat diabetes? This short quiz will help you understand where you stand—mentally, emotionally, and physically—when it comes to using physical activity to lower your blood sugar, lose weight, and beat stress.

1. **My opinion about walking is:**
   a. It's a slow but cheap mode of transportation. Period.
   b. It's probably good for you, but certainly not serious exercise.
   c. It's a legitimate form of exercise I should do more of.
   d. It's not only great exercise but also a wonderful source of relaxation and pleasure.

2. **If the weather's nice, I might walk for this long:**
   a. 1 minute—the time it takes to get from my car to the supermarket entrance.
   b. 5 minutes—the time it takes to find a nice bench in the park.
   c. 20 minutes—a relaxed stroll in the sun is a rare but pleasant treat.
   d. 30 minutes or more—I jump at every chance to be outside and moving.

3. **My favorite parking spot at the mall is:**
   a. I don't know; I shop online.
   b. Right up front; I'll circle until a primo spot opens.
   c. Relatively near; I don't mind a little extra walking.
   d. The farthest lot; this gives me a chance to get in one more brisk stroll.

4. **If I walked briskly for 15 minutes, I would feel:**
   a. Surprised. I never walk unless it's to get from the house to the car or the car to the office or store.
   b. Like someone knocked the wind out of me.
   c. A little pooped, but still able to hold a conversation.
   d. Invigorated and ready for another lap.

5. **I would rate my strength as:**
   a. Low. When I get out of a chair, I have to push off using the armrests.
   b. Not what it used to be; the grocery bags seem to weigh a ton, and I think twice before picking up small children.
   c. Uneven. Some parts of my body are fairly strong, others are rather weak—even flabby.
   d. Pretty darn good; I could lift a bag of potting soil or carry luggage.

6. **When I think about exercise that builds muscle I:**
   a. Don't think I need it. I'm not a bodybuilder.
   b. Am intimidated by it—I worry that I'll have to go to a gym or lift heavy weights.
   c. Am willing and interested but don't how to do it at home.
   d. Have tried it and seen results—bring it on!

7. **When I think about fitting exercise into my schedule I:**

    a. Feel overwhelmed. I'm too busy already!

    b. Guess I could trade a TV show for some exercise time but would rather not.

    c. Know there are some things in my schedule that I could eliminate or streamline to make exercise a priority.

    d. Have already cleared a dedicated exercise time most days of the week.

8. **On a typical Saturday afternoon, I'm:**

    a. Watching the game on TV or otherwise deepening the depression in my chair.

    b. Watching the kids' soccer or baseball game or driving around to do my errands.

    c. Enjoying life—playing golf, bird-watching, doing something active with the kids or grandchildren.

    d. Working in the yard, doing major housework, home repairs, or washing the car.

9. **I've used exercise to lower my blood sugar in the following way:**

    a. I have to confess that I haven't tried it!

    b. I've noticed that my blood sugar seems lower after I've been active, but I haven't made a conscious effort to use it that way.

    c. I try to get regular exercise because it's good for my blood sugar, but I'm not consistent.

    d. Not only do I exercise regularly to keep my blood sugar lower, I check my blood sugar before and after exercise to make sure it doesn't go too low.

10. **My usual foot-care routine includes:**

    a. I don't pay any attention to my feet—who knows what's going on down there.

    b. I glance at my feet after I bathe.

    c. I try to wear the right shoes and to check my feet regularly.

    d. I trim my toenails regularly, check my feet every day, and insist on wearing shoes that don't rub or pinch.

your score

Give yourself 1 point for each "a," 2 points for each "b," 3 points for every "c," and 4 points for each "d." Add your points together.

30–40 points
Hooray!
You're in gear. You're already living many aspects of the Move lifestyle. Now we'd like to challenge you to work your way up to 45 minutes of walking, five days a week, and to set aside time for our muscle-strengthening Sugar Buster Routine twice a week. Doing these consistently will allow you to reap big rewards.

17–29 points
You're coasting.
You're interested in exercise, but tend to put other commitments—and other people's expectations—first. Now's the time to renew your commitment to yourself and your health. Start by fitting in small bouts of exercise all day long (like taking the stairs instead of the elevator) and setting aside time for fun physical activity, like shooting some hoops or taking the grandkids to the park. Yes, these count as calorie-burning exercise—and they'll get you into the mindset for moving every day.

10–16 points
You're stalled.
Put the book down and take a 10-minute walk now. We want to prove to you that: a) You do have time for exercise; b) It doesn't take a major time commitment to reap the rewards of physical activity; and c) Exercise feels good—and fits into any schedule. Resolve to make time for yourself so that you can fit this important component of the Eat, Move, Choose plan into your life. Remind yourself of the benefits: better blood sugar control, a healthier weight, lower stress, and less risk for serious diabetes complications.

why the plan works

In as little as 30 minutes you can lower your blood sugar today—and put yourself on the path to better blood sugar for months and years to come. At the same time, you'll ease stress, boost feel-good brain chemicals for a happy glow, and give your weight-loss efforts a nudge in the right direction. Yes, exercise can accomplish all that. A growing stack of research shows that the goals of the Move plan—regular walking, easy strength-training, and making every day more active—are key to minimizing and even reversing the problems that underlie diabetes. Here's why the plan works.

It Conquers "Sitting Disease"

Are you sitting down? If you are, you've got plenty of company because you're engaged in the *un*-activity that the typical American now spends an amazing amount of time doing. No one keeps accurate statistics on our cumulative sitting time, but the available data reveal that the average American is seated for 12 to 14 hours each day: behind the wheel of a car (one to two hours); watching television (three hours or more); and parked behind

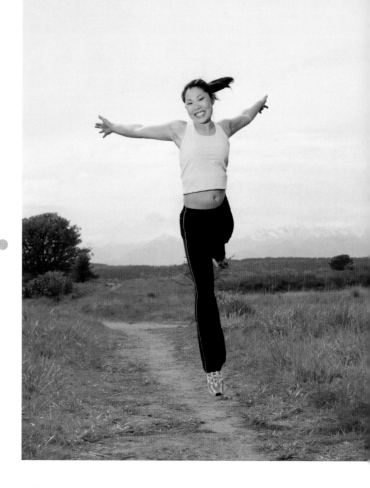

a desk (seven to nine hours). Add an hour of sitting at mealtimes and seven hours of shut-eye, and you're looking at an astonishing 19 to 22 hours of almost complete downtime every single day. What about fun that's physical? National surveys report that one-quarter of adults—and a full one-third of women—do absolutely no leisure-time physical activities. Another third don't do enough for meaningful health benefits.

It's hardly a coincidence that two-thirds of the population now tip their bathroom scales into the danger zone; that millions have diabetes; and millions more have prediabetes or are insulin-resistant, a condition that sets the stage for dangerous high blood sugar.

Getting you up and moving again is an integral part of *Reverse Diabetes*. On the Move plan you'll combat sitting disease in three powerful ways that are proven to work: with regular walking, with our easy Sugar Buster strength-training moves, and by making small but significant active choices throughout the day—everything from throwing yourself into calorie-burning chores to finding fun in motion (bowling, dancing, gardening, playing croquet in the backyard). Studies reveal that fitting in plenty of everyday "lifestyle" exercise is just as effective in maintaining weight loss as formal exercise programs so don't count it out.

It Helps Reverse Your Diabetes

Type 2 diabetes is a condition in which the body's use of insulin is impaired. Because insulin can't do its job of getting glucose (blood sugar) into cells, the glucose builds up in the blood, resulting in high blood sugar. But what if you could improve your body's use of insulin? Wouldn't you essentially be reversing—at least to some degree—your disease? You bet. And that's just what exercise can do for you.

Lower blood sugar. Putting your muscles into action is like hitting your car's accelerator: It instantly boosts the demand for fuel—namely, glucose. First your muscles exhaust their own supply of blood sugar, stashed in muscle cells. Then they clean out the stores in your liver. Finally they draw glucose straight from the bloodstream. The result: lower blood sugar immediately—and lower blood sugar for hours after you've been active. That's because after you've finished exercising your body gives top priority to replenishing glucose stores in the liver and muscles rather than the blood, so your blood sugar will stay lower for hours—perhaps for as long as a couple of days, depending on how hard you worked out. (As you'll discover, that's also one reason you should be careful your blood sugar doesn't dip too low after exercising if you take insulin or oral diabetes medications.)

Greater insulin sensitivity. If you exercise regularly, you can help your body become more sensitive to signals from insulin, the hormone that directs cells to absorb sugar from your bloodstream. Exercise forces muscles to use glucose more efficiently by making cells more receptive to insulin. It's as if getting physical gives your cells a kick in the pants: If they absolutely must have more glucose, they'll work harder to get it. Exercise also boosts the number of insulin receptors on the surface of cells, making those cells more receptive to the hormone. Even if you've been a die-hard couch potato for years, you can ratchet up your insulin sensitivity with exercise in as little as one week.

Some of the best evidence for exercise's effectiveness against diabetes comes from research in people with impaired glucose tolerance, a sign of insulin resistance. These people are at high risk for developing diabetes in just a few years. But in one University of Pennsylvania study, every 2,000 calories they burned per week through exercise dropped their risk of diabetes by 24 percent. What does that mean for someone who already has diabetes? Improving blood sugar through exercise could delay your need for medication if you don't take it now, could help you lower your dose or delay the need for a higher dose (never change a dose

Motionless in America

According to the National Center for Health Statistics report, 70 percent of American adults don't get regular exercise, defined as half an hour of light to moderate activity five times a week, or 20 minutes of vigorous exercise three times a week. Nearly 4 people in 10 get no exercise at all. Not coincidentally, regions of the country that have the most sedentary populations also tend to have the highest rates of diabetes.

on your own), or even allow you to stop taking a medication.

It Turbo-Charges Weight Loss

At least 80 percent of people with type 2 diabetes are overweight. In fact, being overweight is perhaps the single most important contributor to the disease. So if you have diabetes, shedding extra pounds is critical. But it's not necessarily easy.

Let's say you wanted to lose a pound a week, a reasonable goal. To do it without exercise you'd need to cut 500 calories a day—not a small number by any means. (That's two full-size candy bars or an entire large hamburger with the bun.) But if you burned 250 calories a day through exercise, you'd have to cut only 250 calories from your diet. That would make your eating plan seem a whole lot less stringent.

Exercise facilitates weight loss in several ways.

More fat burning. Think of exercising as adding booster rockets to the slow burn of weight loss. After about 30 minutes of sustained exercise, the body runs out of "ready fuel"—it taps out the glucose in the blood. To keep you going, it's forced to turn to the fat for energy, ravaging fat storage sites throughout the body (think flab) and the blood (think "bad" cholesterol and triglycerides). The more active you are, the more energy you use, and the more fat you'll burn.

Faster metabolism. On the Move plan, you won't stop at walking. You'll also deploy another weapon in the exercise arsenal that helps fight diabetes: strength training. This type of exercise builds your muscle mass. That's critical because just like bigger cars, bigger muscles burn more fuel—in this case, glucose—which lowers your blood sugar even further. But there's more. Since muscle tissue burns energy faster than fat tissue—burning about

15 times more calories a day—having more muscle means you'll burn more calories all the time—even when you're watching TV.

A startling fact: Unless you take steps to stoke your metabolism—your body's calorie-burning "engine"—you can lose a third to half of your lean body mass and replace it with twice as much body fat by the time you're 65. That's a double whammy for diabetes, since muscle tissue helps you burn off blood sugar, and excess fat increases insulin resistance. You know what else a slower metabolism means: weight gain. The good news is that if you work every major muscle group just twice a week, as you will on our Sugar Buster program, you can replace 5 to 10 years' worth of lost muscle in just a few months.

It Cuts Your Heart Attack and Stroke Risk

Exercise cuts your chances of having a heart attack or stroke—and that's good news for people with diabetes, whose risk for cardiovascular disease can be two to four times higher than it is for others. In one study, people with diabetes who took part in an aerobic-exercise program lasting only three months saw levels of heart-threatening triglyceride and ticker-protecting HDL cholesterol levels improve by an impressive 20 percent. At the same time, blood pressure levels fell significantly.

It Fights Abdominal Fat

Research on the connection between weight and health has taken a surprising turn: It seems that a large waistline increases risk for both diabetes and heart disease more than simply being overweight does. Why? If your waistline is expansive (especially if it's over 35 inches for women or 40 inches for men), you're likely to be carrying around visceral fat.

Unlike the relatively harmless fat on your buttocks, hips, thighs, and even just below your skin at your waist, visceral wraps around internal organs and churns out dangerous substances. These include inflammatory compounds, which make blood stickier, and fatty acids, which prompt your liver to produce more blood sugar and LDL ("bad") cholesterol and less adiponectin, a hormone that regulates the use of blood sugar and keeps appetite in check.

Surprisingly, not all weight loss programs reduce deadly visceral fat because diet alone is not enough to get the job done. But we've got the solution: a healthy diet *plus exercise*.

Study after study shows that regular walking can help you lose abdominal fat far more effectively than dieting alone. And you don't have to train for the Olympics to see results. Japanese researchers tested obese men before and after they joined a modest walking program for one year. All they did was increase the number of steps they took during their daily activities, such as walking from the car to the grocery store. The result: the amount of fat around their abdomens significantly decreased. Their blood pressure and cholesterol levels also improved—important news for people with diabetes, who face an elevated risk for heart disease.

It Tames Tension

Remember that glow you get after a walk on the beach or down a country lane in autumn? It's no surprise that exercise is an instant stress-reliever and mood-booster. But did you know that this feel-good effect can have a profound impact on your blood sugar? Researchers from Duke University in Durham, North Carolina, have found that releasing tension and calming your mind is an important blood-sugar control strategy. Here's how it works.

Fringe Benefits

Exercise helps control diabetes and reduces the risk of heart attack and stroke. As if that weren't enough, it also:

▶ Helps prevent certain cancers, such as colon cancer.
▶ Improves or maintains blood flow to sex organs, potentially enhancing sexual function and enjoyment.
▶ Preserves cognitive function, including memory.
▶ Retards bone loss that can lead to osteoporosis.
▶ Boosts the ability of immune-system cells to fight invaders.
▶ Slows physical decline that accounts for most impairments associated with aging.
▶ Eases arthritis pain by strengthening and stretching the muscles, tendons, and ligaments that support joints.
▶ Guards against back pain by strengthening muscles that support the spine.
▶ Aids digestion and helps prevent such ailments as irritable bowel syndrome.
▶ Promotes a good night's sleep.

Lower levels of stress hormones. These hormones, including cortisol, raise blood sugar and contribute to weight gain, especially that dangerous visceral fat we just mentioned. Bringing your stress levels down, then, should mean lower blood sugar and less extra weight.

Protection from diabetes burn-out. Living with diabetes is a lifetime job, and sometimes it can feel overwhelming. Exercise helps by producing feel-good chemicals in the brain that can boost your mood, relieve stress, and alleviate the blues. And the feeling of accomplishment you get can do wonders for your confidence and boost your sense of control. If you can do this, you *can* take control of diabetes.

GOAL 1

Know how to exercise safely with diabetes

EXERCISE OFFERS such powerful blood sugar benefits it's almost like taking medicine. But just as you have to use medications judiciously and watch out for any side effects, so you have to use exercise wisely and take steps to avoid problems such as low blood sugar and foot injuries. You'll also want to customize your workout plan to fit your personal needs and circumstances. Here's how.

STEP ONE
Talk with Your Doctor

Check with your doctor before starting any exercise program, especially if you're over age 35, have had diabetes for more than 10 years, or already show signs of heart disease, poor circulation, or nerve damage. Most people should have no problem with the exercises in this chapter, especially if they start gradually. But it's worth at least a quick discussion with your doctor. Here's what your conversation should cover.

Ask if you should take any special precautions. Ask if you have any diabetes-related conditions that would limit or change your routine.

For example, if an exercise stress test indicates heart trouble, you may be advised to walk at a more moderate pace. If you have high blood pressure or eye or kidney damage, you might have to avoid the strain of weight lifting. And if your feet have suffered nerve damage, you may be better off kicking in a pool than pounding the pavement.

Ask about side effects of any medications you take. Some oral diabetes medications can cause muscle ache or fatigue, while others can make you dizzy or nauseated. Be sure you and your doctor are clear about how intensely you intend to exercise and how your medication's side effects may limit your activities.

STEP TWO
Learn How to Time Your Exercise

If you take insulin or oral diabetes drugs, it's important to time your exercise strategically so that blood sugar doesn't fall to dangerously low levels during your walk or workout. If you work out too soon after taking insulin or an oral drug, the glucose-lowering tag team of medication plus movement can be *too much* of a good thing and lower your blood sugar further than you'd like. To ensure your safety, check with your doctor about taking steps like the following.

Avoid peak hours for insulin and oral medications. Try to time your workout so that you're not exercising when the activity of insulin or pills peaks—often within the first hour or two of an injection or taking your diabetes medicines. This may be less of an issue for people who use insulin than it has been in the past. With the increased use of insulin pumps and intensive injection therapy, it's possible for people to exercise any time they can fit it in. Talk to your doctor or diabetes educator for specific advice.

If you're working to cut back on or eliminate your medication use, your doctor may start by having you take less (or none) before your workout. In effect, you may be able to exercise in place of taking your medication if the effects on your blood sugar prove to be similar.

Choose your injection site with care. If you inject insulin into muscles you'll be using, they will absorb it faster and send your blood sugar plummeting. Solution: Unless you're going straight into sit-ups, inject into the softer folds of your midsection. If you're working your abs, wait to exercise until about an hour after your injection to give the insulin a chance to disperse throughout the body.

Exercise after eating. Instead of relying on snacks to head off low blood sugar during your walk, be diligent about planning to exercise after a meal so that you can take advantage of higher, more sustained blood sugar levels.

STEP THREE

Test Your Blood Sugar Before, During, and After Exercise

Grab your blood-sugar meter and a test strip! Before you start to exercise, blood-sugar testing can tell you when it might be better to hold off, at least

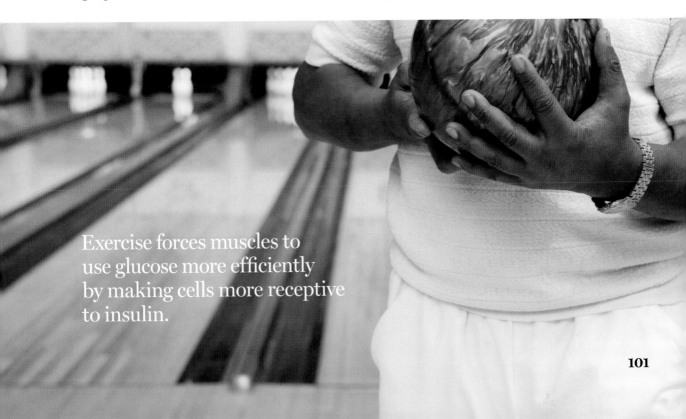

Exercise forces muscles to use glucose more efficiently by making cells more receptive to insulin.

until your glucose levels can meet your muscles' demands. It's wise to test your blood sugar again afterward, too, to see how far it's fallen. This will give you a sense of how exercise affects your blood sugar levels so that you can make adjustments in meals, snacks, and the timing of your exercise.

We've included a log on page 254 where you can record your daily food intake and physical activity to give you a clear picture of how your efforts pay off. Use it as a template (make photocopies), and be sure to examine it and take note of any patterns.

Protect against hypoglycemia. Don't exercise if your blood sugar is below 100 mg/dl. Instead, have a piece of fruit or other snack containing at least 15 grams of carbohydrate, then test again in about 20 minutes. Keep snacking until blood sugar rises above the 100 mg/dl mark.

Protect against hyperglycemia. Test for ketones using a urine ketone test strip if blood sugar before exercise is above 240 mg/dl. If the test detects ketones, don't start exercising until you've taken more insulin to handle glucose uptake during your workout. If ketones are absent, don't exercise if blood sugar is above 400 mg/dl.

Drink plenty of water. Don't wait for thirst to hit before drinking; thirst can be a sign of high blood sugar and could bring your workout to a halt while you check for hyperglycemia. Instead, drink one to two cups 15 minutes before exercising, at least a half cup every 15 minutes during your workout, and another one to two cups afterward.

STEP FOUR
Be Prepared for Low Blood Sugar Emergencies

Exercise works so well at bringing down your blood sugar that you need to make sure it doesn't drop *too* low. Hypoglycemia can happen even if you've planned carefully so it's important to be prepared for this emergency. Here's how.

Know the signs of low blood sugar—and when to stop exercising. Confusion, shaking, lightheadedness, or difficulty speaking all indicate that you should quit exercising *immediately* and take steps to stabilize your glucose level. We can't stress this enough. When you first detect symptoms of hypoglycemia don't wait "just one more minute" or "just awhile longer to see if symptoms improve." True, some symptoms can be confusing: sweating and a rapid heartbeat could just be a natural response to exercise—or signs of hypoglycemia. It's always wise to err on the side of safety.

Carry the right snack with you. A small carbohydrate snack can rapidly bring dropping blood sugar back up in an emergency—but only if you remember to bring one along with you every time you walk. When blood sugar dips too low, you can quickly bring it back up with 10 small jellybeans or

The Blood Sugar Paradox

Why does blood sugar go down sometimes but go up other times after exercise? Muscles use glucose for energy, so as a rule, blood sugar goes down when you're active, as the body moves glucose from the liver and bloodstream into the cells. But that assumes there's enough insulin on hand to help with this transfer. If you take insulin and your dose is too low, glucose can build in the blood during exercise and cause hyperglycemia. That's why it's important to consult your doctor for advice on exercising and to check your blood sugar before and after (and perhaps even during) exercise to understand how physical activity affects you.

the number of glucose tablets your doctor or certified diabetes educator suggests.

Check your blood sugar during long walks. When you're taking a long walk, stop and check your blood sugar after 30 minutes to make sure your blood sugar stays in your target range.

Use the buddy system. It's not always obvious when hypoglycemia is setting in (in fact, denying that anything's wrong can be a classic sign of early hypoglycemia), so it's wise to walk or work out with somebody else or in a place where other people are available if you need help, especially if you're exercising vigorously. Tell your workout partner what to watch for. If you work out at a gym, make sure the gym records indicate that you have diabetes, info that could be important in case your blood sugar dips.

Carry identification. Even if you're just strolling through the neighborhood with a friend, carry ID with your name, address, phone number, contact information for your doctor and a family member, and the names and dosages of your medication or insulin.

Stay alert afterward. Blood sugar can continue to fall long after you've exercised so don't let your guard down for signs of hypoglycemia until 24 hours after your workout.

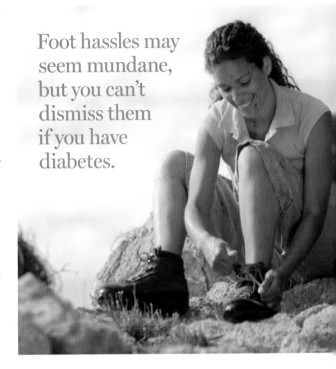

Foot hassles may seem mundane, but you can't dismiss them if you have diabetes.

STEP FIVE
Have a Foot-Protection Plan

The feet can take a beating when you have diabetes. Poor circulation from damaged blood vessels slows healing and makes feet more prone to infection, while nerve damage can dull sensation and leave you oblivious to injuries that can quickly get out of control. In the grand scheme of things, foot hassles may seem almost comically mundane, but you just can't dismiss broken skin, corns, calluses, bunions, or ingrown toenails when you have diabetes. Left untreated for long, such conditions can put you at risk of losing a foot—or even a leg—to gangrene. In fact, about 15 percent of people with diabetes in the United States eventually develop foot problems that threaten a limb, and more than 50,000 must undergo amputations every year. Don't be one of those people.

Buy the right pair of walking shoes. The sole piece of equipment you need on the Move plan is a good pair of walking shoes. They'll help you travel farther and faster with more comfort—and no blisters or injuries.

Shop at a respected athletic-shoe store. A skilled salesperson can size your feet and find the best shoe for your foot shape and size. Tell the

that's easy! ◄—

At doctor's appointments, take off your socks and shoes even if your doctor doesn't tell you to. Your feet should be examined at every visit for signs of skin breakdown, hot spots, cracked heels, or ingrown toenails. Put your glucose log book between your toes. This way you'll be sure that both your feet and your log book will be examined!

salesperson what type of terrain you'll be walking on and how many miles on average you plan to walk a week.

Bring an old pair of walking shoes—and your walking socks—to the store. The salesperson can look at the wear pattern on your shoes to determine what type of shoe you need. For example, if the inner heel is more worn than the outer heel, your foot probably turns in excessively as you walk. In this case, you'll want some extra arch support and a shoe designed for "motion control." Be sure you try on walking shoes while wearing the socks you plan to walk in, not thicker or thinner ones.

Try on your shoes and walk around the store. Make sure the shoe hugs your heel; your heel should not slide up and down as you walk. The shoe should also have a firm arch support, and the forefoot of the shoe should bend with the natural bend in your foot. Most important, the shoes should feel comfortable when you walk.

Do the twist test. A good walking shoe should be flexible enough to accommodate your foot's natural heel-to-toe roll. If you can't twist the sole from side to side, it's too stiff.

Examine your feet daily. If you have nerve damage, you could have sores, cuts, swelling, and infection that you can't feel, so give your feet an exam once a day, perhaps at bedtime. Go over them with both your eyes and your hands. Let your doctor know if you find evidence of any problems. Besides blisters, cuts, bruises, cracking, or peeling, look for areas that are shaded differently (either paler or redder), which could indicate persistent pressure from shoes. Feel for areas of coldness, which could be a sign of poor circulation, or warmth (along with redness), which might be evidence of an infection. If you have trouble seeing the bottoms of your feet, place a mirror on the floor and look at the reflection.

Clean and treat minor scrapes and cuts right away. If you find a small cut or sore on your foot, treat it immediately. Wash your hands with soap and water. Then wash the wound with soap and water, rinse with more water, and pat it dry with a clean towel or tissue paper. Dab some antibiotic ointment onto a cotton swab and smear a thin layer of the ointment onto the wound. (Don't apply the ointment with your finger.) Cover the wound with an adhesive bandage. If the wound doesn't look better within a day, or if you see signs of infection, such as swelling, redness, warmth, or oozing, call your doctor or podiatrist immediately.

Keep your tootsies smooth and dry. Avoid cracked skin and reduce the risk of infection by toweling off your feet thoroughly after bathing, especially between your toes. Rub lotion or cream on the tops and bottoms of your feet to keep them moist, and sprinkle talcum powder or cornstarch between your toes to prevent fungal growth.

Trim your toenails. Do it at least once a week after bathing, cutting straight across the nails and smoothing them with a nail file or emery board. If this is difficult for you, ask your podiatrist to trim your toenails at your next visit.

GOAL 2

Walk at least five days a week

IT'S TIME TO HIT YOUR STRIDE! Starting today we want you to lace up a good pair of sneakers or walking shoes and head out the door. Why walking? It's something almost anyone can so, almost anywhere. And it costs nothing at all. Best of all, it's a great excuse to get outside, something most of us do too infrequently. (Remember that practically any weather is good walking weather as long as you're dressed for it.)

On the Move plan you'll build to 45 minutes of walking five times a week. But for now, the important thing is to get out there—and build a routine you'll love so much you can't live without it. Start as slowly as you like. Gradually you'll pick up the pace and add to the length of your walks, so that by Week 10 you'll be working your heart and muscles enough to really make a difference. Keep track of your walking in the Planner section.

To motivate yourself to walk more, consider buying a pedometer, a small gadget that counts your steps. If you do, log your steps along with your minutes in the Planner pages. Aim for 25,000 steps a week at first (for details, see Make Every Step Count on page 108). Here's how to fit walking in so that it becomes a must-have part of your day.

STEP ONE

Find the Perfect Time and Place

Customizing your walking routine so that it fits your schedule and your unique preferences can make the difference between success and *oops... I didn't fit my walk in again today.* There's no one-size-fits-all solution, no time of day or location that works for everyone—and that's the true beauty of walking. Whatever works for you is the right way to do it, whether you decide to start by fitting in a couple of 10-minute strolls in-between job, home, and other activities; walking on a treadmill during your favorite TV show; or indulging in a long, brisk jaunt in a scenic park. Walking is the centerpiece of the Move plan, and if you make it work for you, you'll be able to stick with it come what may. Here are some strategies for making it happen.

Roll out of bed, get dressed, put on your shoes, and go. It's easy to get caught up in your day-to-day activities and tell yourself that you don't have time for a walk. If you exercise first thing in the morning, however, there will be no

105

need for excuses. Research shows that people who plan to exercise in the morning are more likely to fit in their workouts than people who plan to exercise later in the day. And exercising in the morning may offer a side benefit: You'll sleep better at night. When researchers at the Fred Hutchinson Cancer Research Center in Seattle, Washington, compared morning and evening exercise, people who exercised at least 225 minutes per week in the morning had an easier time falling asleep at night than those who completed the same amount of exercise in the evening.

Or, walk in the evening. That sleep study aside, we still like after-dinner walks. They get you away from the television, they keep you from eating too much at dinner, it's when your neighbors are outside, and it's just a lovely time of day. Don't let unlovely weather stop you either—that's what jackets, boots, and umbrellas were invented for. There's something childlike and fun about a walk in the rain or snow.

Split it up. When you're too busy to go for your usual 30- or 45-minute walk, divide and conquer. Get out there for 5 or 10 minutes at a time. That may be as simple as taking a five-minute walk break around the building after completing a project at work. Such short walking breaks will refresh your mind, so you can return to work with more vigor. In fact, research shows that most of us can only focus at top capacity for 30 minutes at a time. After that, concentration begins to drop off. Your intermittent walk breaks may make you more productive.

Walk in the prettiest area in your town (or the next town over). It just might encourage you to walk more often. When researchers from the University of Wollongong in New South Wales, Australia, surveyed walkers about their walking habits, they found that men who perceived their neighborhoods to be "aesthetic" were more consistent about walking around their neighborhoods. Other research finds that neighborhoods with well-maintained sidewalks and safe and well-lit walking areas encourage walking over neighborhoods that don't have those features. In fact, people who live in so-called walkable neighborhoods walk an average of 70 more minutes each week than people who live in neighborhoods lacking such characteristics, according to a study completed at Cincinnati Children's Hospital Medical Center.

Try a treadmill. If the mail carrier can deliver mail in any weather, you can walk in any weather, as long as you're dressed for it. But if you live in a climate that's often too hot or too cold for comfort, consider investing in a treadmill. A word of advice: Try before you buy. Features to think about include the deck size (a longer walking surface feels less cramped than a short one, but be sure your chosen machine will fit the space available in your home), shock absorption (thicker belts, floating decks, and special shock absorbers decrease the wear and tear on your legs and feet but also raise the price),

sugar buster quiz

Q: Sidewalks or dirt paths?
A: Dirt paths.

If you're over 60, walk on soft surfaces. As you age, the fat padding in your feet deteriorates. The absence of this natural shock absorber can make walking on sidewalks and other hard surfaces feel like foot torture. Flat grass and dirt paths will provide more cushioning for your feet than roads or sidewalks.

and the range of speeds and incline levels. (Most walkers will be fine with a top speed of 5 to 6 miles per hour, but consider a wide incline range so you can vary your walks and add a bigger challenge.)

Go to an indoor track—with cash registers. Many malls open early for walkers. You could also easily walk for 20 minutes in a big warehouse store or at a Walmart or Kmart.

STEP TWO
Set Your Pace

If you already walk for exercise, picking up the pace can help you get fit faster, according to a slew of scientific studies. In an eight-year analysis of 72,488 female nurses ranging in age from 40 to 65, researchers found that those who worked up a sweat for just 90 minutes a week—the equivalent of about 12 minutes a day—lowered their risk for chronic health conditions like diabetes and heart disease by 30 to 40 percent. Similarly, the Harvard Health Professionals study of 44,452 men ages 40 to 79 found that those who ran for an hour or more each week dropped their heart disease risk by 42 percent.

You don't have to (and should not) heave and gasp and hurt to reap these rewards. New exercisers can raise their heart rates into the vigorous zone with little more than brisk walking. When University of Massachusetts researchers asked 84 overweight men and women to walk 1 mile at a pace that was "brisk but comfortable," the vast majority of the volunteers stepped right up to an average 3.2 mph pace, which translates into hard to very hard intensity (70 to 100 percent of their maximum heart rates). The best part? It was easier than people expected, the researchers report.

Here's how to set the right pace, whether you're a beginning fitness walker or a veteran.

five ways to
find more walking time

No time to exercise? We don't buy it! There's no one who can't spare a few minutes for a walk. Remember, exercise helps your cells soak up more glucose so there's less of it in your bloodstream. And once you get going, it feels terrific. Take advantage of these five hidden pockets of downtime to shake a leg.

- **Turn off the TV.** You can fit in a 30-minute walk just by giving up one sitcom. Do you really need to watch reruns or the local evening news (the world can wait until tomorrow)?

- **Use your tube time.** If you watch more than one hour of TV a day, invest in a treadmill and log a couple of miles during your favorite program.

- **Hustle at halftime.** Next time you go to a sporting event—whether it's professional football or your grandson's softball game—don't stay on the bench. Get up and walk around during pregame warmups, halftime, in between quarters, or during time-outs. Just steer clear of the hot dog stand.

- **Use your lunch break.** Eat lunch at your desk, then take a walk around the building or the block. You'll have more energy for the afternoon—and will be more likely to avoid hitting the vending machine for a pick-me-up.

- **Pay your bills online.** Or sign up for automatic bill paying through your credit card company. With the time you save, you can fit in one 30-minute walk. And your bills will never be late!

Beginners: Take it slow and easy. Your top priority is regular walking, not setting new speed records. Be sure you're comfortable with your routine and that it fits into your life, even on busy days. If you're new to walking or haven't hit the pavement for a while, or if your doctor—or your body—tells

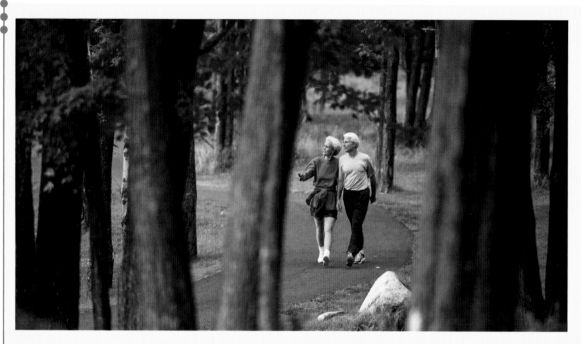

Make Every Step Count

Can a little plastic gadget that costs under $30 help you walk more and lose weight? Count on it. Pedometers are scarcely larger than a book of matches and clip unobtrusively to your belt or waistband. Some can be worn in a pocket. They count each step you take, and some also track miles and calories burned. For many people, simply knowing that the number on the readout is increasing with every step inspires them to take more.

Experts recommend shooting for an ultimate goal of 10,000 steps a day for weight loss and fitness. We recommend a more modest goal of adding 5,000 steps (including those you accumulate on your daily 20-minute walk) to what you're doing now. Those 5,000 steps add up to a real weight-loss advantage, reported researchers in a recent University of Pennsylvania study of 179 women and men. The volunteers all followed a healthy diet, and for 40 weeks, they either went to the gym four times a week, did calisthenics at home, or simply tried to increase their daily steps by 5,000. At the end, the steppers lost as much weight as the others and kept it off just as easily. How to get there:

Establish your baseline. Wear your pedometer on a typical day before you begin the Move walking program. Put it on as soon as you wake up and note how many steps you take. That's your baseline. You'll quickly discover that everyday activities such as taking out the trash use about 100 steps per minute. So does strolling at a lively pace while shopping at the supermarket or mall. Hustling to an appointment tallies about 130 steps per minute.

Start walking. We recommend that you follow the walking plan even if you're also counting steps. It automatically increases your walking time over the 12-week program—and automatically boosts your step count. We estimate that the plan's fitness walk will add about 1,250 steps for every 10 minutes of walking you do.

Go for "extra credit" steps. If your daily activities plus a walk doesn't add up to 5,000 steps, find opportunities to step out throughout the day. Park farther from the supermarket entrance, walk the mall before you begin shopping, or play a little longer with the dog, the kids, or the grandchildren. Every step counts.

you to start slowly, we recommend beginning with baby steps. Walk for just 10 minutes at a comfortable pace and gradually, over the next few weeks, build up to 20 minutes. Then pick up the pace.

Always warm up first. Start every walk with five minutes of easy-paced walking—about the same pace at which you'd do your grocery shopping—to get your body warmed up. Then, cool down at the end of each walk with another five minutes of easy-paced walking. This allows your heart rate to gradually speed up and slow down.

Breathe deeply as you walk to a count of 1-2-3. Many people unintentionally hold their breath when they exercise and then suddenly feel breathless and tired. Oxygen is invigorating, and muscles need oxygen to create the energy for movement. So as you inhale, bring the air to the deepest part of your lungs by expanding your tummy and inhale for a count of three. Then exhale fully either through your nose or mouth, also to the count of three.

Take the talk test. Once you're walking for 20 minutes or more each day, aim for a brisk pace—the speed you'd reach if you were 10 minutes late for an appointment. If you're able to recite the Pledge of Allegiance without hesitating, your exercise level is easy. If you can get it out phrase by phrase with little pauses for breath in between, you're right on target. If you can barely make it to "to the flag" without gasping for air, you're working too hard (that said, if you're in good shape and your heart is healthy, it's okay to exercise in this heart-rate zone, but only for a few minutes at a time).

Walking for 30 minutes or longer? Add in faster bursts. Incorporating brief bursts of faster walking during your walks helps you burn more fat and calories in the same amount of time. Move at your usual speed for three to five minutes, then walk even more briskly for one to two minutes. To pick up the pace, take short, quick steps. (Most people try to walk faster by elongating their strides, but this actually slows you down and can lead to joint and shin injuries.) Bend your arms at 90 degrees and pump them quickly. After your fast-walking interval, settle back into your usual brisk pace for three to four minutes, then pick up the pace again for one to two minutes. Do this several times during your walk. Boosting the intensity intermittently can increase the calorie burn by as much as 60 percent.

Walk faster early in your walk. If you want to increase the amount of fat you burn during your walk, add some bursts of faster walking toward the beginning of your walk. Many walkers wait until the end of the walk to speed up, treating their faster walking as a finishing kick. Yet a study published in the *European Journal of Applied Physiology* found that exercisers burned more fat and felt less fatigued when they inserted their faster segments toward the beginning of a workout. It works because you speed up your heart rate early and keep it elevated for the rest of your walk.

that's easy!

Don't feel like walking? Vow to walk for just 10 minutes, and head out the door. Chances are, once you've warmed up, you'll exercise for longer than you anticipated. Even if you don't, 10 minutes is better than no minutes at all. You'll lower your blood sugar, burn calories, and maintain this important fitness habit.

STEP THREE
Stay Motivated

Once you're up and moving, maintain your momentum. Some people revel in the ritual of walking the same route at the same time every day. But for

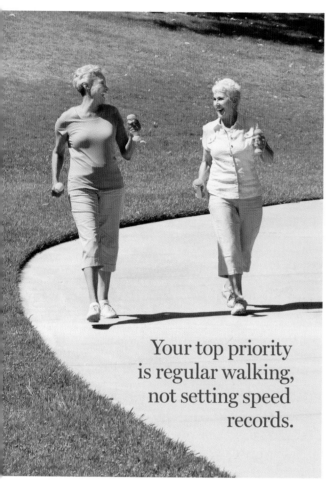

Your top priority is regular walking, not setting speed records.

the United Way—and for the next two weeks, pledge to contribute $1 for every mile you walk. You'll take pride in the fact that you are walking for something beyond yourself, which will motivate you to go longer and faster. After every walk, mark the amount you owe on a chart, and when you reach $50, send a check. Whoever thought exercise could be tax deductible?

Walk for entertainment one day a week. Instead of walking around your neighborhood, walk through the zoo, an art museum, or an upscale shopping mall. First circle the perimeter of your location at your usual brisk pace. Then wander through again more slowly to take in the sights.

Take the entire family on your daily walks. Not only will you be modeling good fitness habits for your children, but you'll also be able to supervise them while you walk rather than getting a sitter. If your children walk too slowly, ask them to ride their bikes or roller-skate alongside you. To keep everyone entertained, play your usual repertoire of long car trip games such as "I Spy." You can also try a scavenger walk, where you start out with a list of items to find during your walk and check off the list as you spot them.

Once a week, complete your errands on foot. If you live within a mile of town, or even a convenience store, start from your house. If you live out in the middle of nowhere, drive to within a mile of your destination, park, and walk the rest of the way there and back. You'll be surprised how much you can accomplish on foot, and even better, how many people you'll meet along the way.

Explore your world. Spy on the new houses going up in the development nearby. Or walk down a street in your own neighborhood that you've never been on (and say hi to the neighbors you've

most of us, variety is the key to staying interested. These steps will keep your foot-powered plan fun and inspiring.

Walk with a friend. If she's expecting you, you're more likely to get out of bed on cold winter mornings or skip the cafeteria in favor of a lunchtime walk. If one of you backs out for any reason, put $5 in a kitty. Hopefully this will never happen, but if you manage to build up any substantial sum, donate it to charity.

Pick a charity. Sign up for a charity walk or choose a cause or nonprofit you believe in—such as breast cancer research, the American Red Cross,

never met). Or check out the hiking trail in a nearby park. Varying your terrain will do more than keep you mentally engaged. It will also help you to target different leg muscles, improving the effectiveness of every outing.

Take a dog with you. Once your dog gets used to your walks, he or she will look forward to them and give you a gentle nudge (or annoying whine) on the days you try to get out of it. There's nothing more effective than a set of puppy dog eyes to extract your butt from the couch and get it out the door. Don't have a dog? Offer to walk an elderly neighbor's dog twice a week. That commitment thing will keep you motivated.

Pump up the volume. Research proves it: Listening to music while walking helps you walk longer, probably because you're distracted by the songs and almost forget that you're exercising. So load up your favorite tunes, especially those with a fast beat, and plug yourself in! Just be sure to keep the volume low enough that you can hear traffic and stay aware of your surroundings.

Posture Perfect

Improving your walking posture will help you burn more fat and calories and help prevent muscle and joint pain. Readjust yourself to the following standards:

▶ Stand tall with your spine elongated and your breastbone lifted. This allows room for your lungs to fully expand.

▶ Keep your head straight with your eyes focused forward and your shoulders relaxed. Avoid slumping your shoulders forward or hunching them toward your ears.

▶ Roll your feet from heel to toe.

▶ As you speed up, take smaller, more frequent steps. This protects your knees and gives your butt a good workout.

▶ Allow your arms to swing freely.

▶ Firm your tummy and flatten your back as you walk to prevent low back pain.

GOAL 3

Build muscle with the Sugar Buster Routine

IMAGINE KEEPING your blood sugar in better control all day long, even when you're sleeping, taking in the latest James Bond movie, or sipping a cup of coffee with a friend. You can accomplish this feat if you invest just a little bit of time in building up your muscles. Remember, using your muscles forces your muscle cells to soak up more glucose. The bonus: You'll look trimmer, have more energy for daily tasks like carrying groceries or grandkids, and even improve your balance.

Building sexy, sugar-sipping muscles is the goal you'll achieve if you follow the plan's Sugar Buster Routine. This set of nine exercises couldn't be simpler: All you need is a pair of sneakers, comfortable clothing, and a few everyday objects—a towel or exercise mat for exercises done while sitting or lying on the floor; a chair, table, or countertop for support for a few moves; and the stairs in your home.

Building sexy, sugar-sipping muscles couldn't be simpler. You'll look trimmer, feel more energetic, and improve your balance!

Once you've mastered the moves and they become easy, you can add light hand weights or ankle weights if you'd like, but right now working against your own body weight is all you need. That also means you can do these exercises anywhere—in a hotel room while you're traveling, behind your office door at work, or in your living room, bedroom, or TV room.

Turn back to Your Goals Week by Week on page 93 to remind yourself how and when to ease into the routine (start in week 3 of the Eat, Move, Choose Plan). When you perform any part of the routine, remember to record it on the Planner pages—give yourself credit where credit is due!

Getting Started

The investment you need to make in order to reap the blood sugar and weight loss benefits of strength training may be smaller than you think. The routine that we've designed can be done in about 20 minutes—roughly the time you'd spend watching commercials during a typical hour-long TV show—so it's easy to do this workout during your favorite program.

The timing. We've broken the workout into three sequences, which take about five to seven minutes each, so that in the beginning weeks, you can do just one sequence on a particular day. You might do the Upper Body sequence on Monday, the Core Body sequence on Wednesday, and the Lower Body sequence on Saturday, for instance. The three moves in each sequence don't even have to be done at the same time. You could spend just a couple of minutes doing one move in the morning, then spend a few more minutes doing the other two moves in the evening. As you get stronger, start doing the whole routine at once, and do it twice a week.

The rules. Both efficient and effective, the Sugar Buster Routine includes basic exercises that will come easily regardless of your past experience or level of strength now. Perform 8 to 12 repetitions of each exercise, then rest for 30 to 60 seconds in between exercises. Once the moves become easy, you can add a second set of repetitions. You'll also find tips for taking many of these moves up a notch once you get strong enough that even two sets of repetitions are easy.

One suggestion: Don't repeat the same exercise two days in a row. Muscles need time to rest and repair themselves between strength-training sessions. You'll get better results if you give each muscle group a day or two off before working it again.

upper body sequence

Wall Push-Up

This is easier than a regular push-up but does the same job.

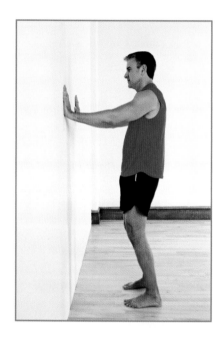

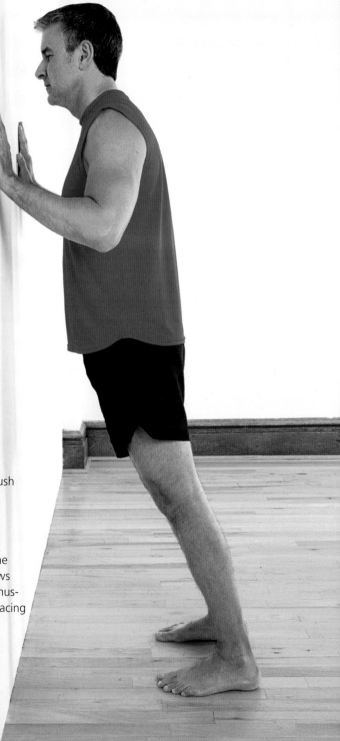

● **ONE** From a standing position about 12 to 18 inches from a wall, put your hands on the wall about shoulder-width apart at chest level, with palms flat and fingers pointed toward the ceiling.

● **TWO** Slowly lower your chin toward the wall. Smoothly push back from the wall to the starting position.

smart tip

As you lower yourself to the wall, keep your elbows out to the side. That works the chest muscles better than keeping elbows close to the body, which shifts the load more to the triceps muscles of the arms. If you feel pain in your hands or wrist, try placing hands farther apart or closer together on the wall.

Armchair Dip

This is an exercise that encourages you to work muscles exactly the way you use them for everyday activities.

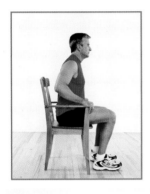 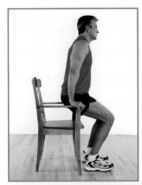

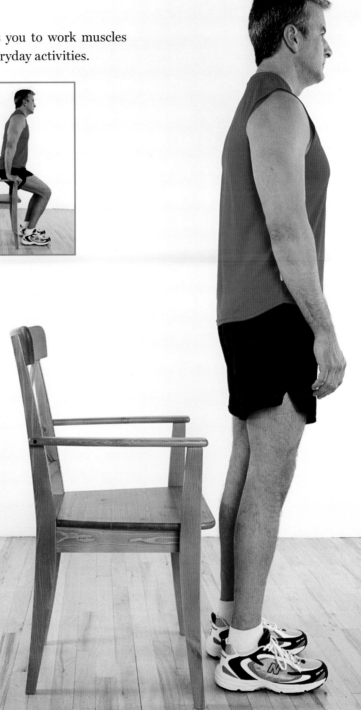

- **ONE** Sit in a sturdy armchair, back straight and feet flat on the floor about hip-width apart. Place your hands on the chair's arms about even with the front of your body.

- **TWO** Using mostly your arms but assisting with your legs, push yourself out of the chair to a full standing position, letting go of the chair as you stand.

- **THREE** Lower yourself back into the chair, putting hands on the arms of the chair as you slowly come down, using your arm muscles to return to the starting position.

smart tip

For a variation, maintain your hold on the arms of the chair until you fully extend your arms, then slowly lower yourself back into the chair.

115

upper body sequence

Seated Biceps Curl

This exercise for the biceps muscles will make hefting suitcases and heavy grocery bags a breeze and build shapely upper arms you won't mind baring in a sleeve-less or short-sleeved shirt.

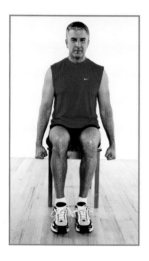

● **ONE** Sit up straight on the front half of an armless chair, feet flat on the floor, with your arms hang-ing down by your side.

● **TWO** Smoothly bend your elbows, keeping them positioned at your side, raising your hands toward your shoulders while rotating your palms a quarter turn so they face your shoulder at the top of the movement. Smoothly return to the starting position.

smart tip

If this exercise becomes too easy, try performing it while holding light dumbbells. Start with 1- or 2-pound weights.

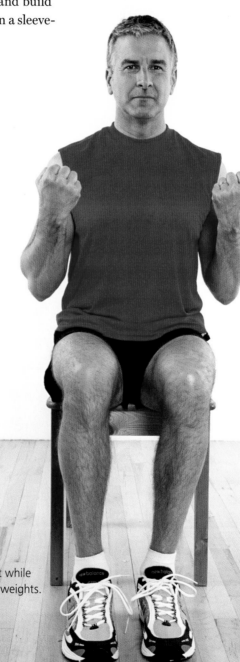

core body sequence

Bird Dog

This move works muscles of the hips, but also the back, chest, shoulders, and arms. The multielement motion improves balance and coordination and helps promote good posture.

● **ONE** Get down on your hands and knees on the floor, a rug, or an exercise mat.

● **TWO** Extend your right leg out behind you, keeping your foot a few inches off the floor as you straighten your knee.

● **THREE** At the same time you extend your right leg, reach out straight in front of you with your left arm. Return to the starting position and repeat with the other leg and arm to complete one repetition.

● **FOUR** Continue alternating legs and arms until you finish a set.

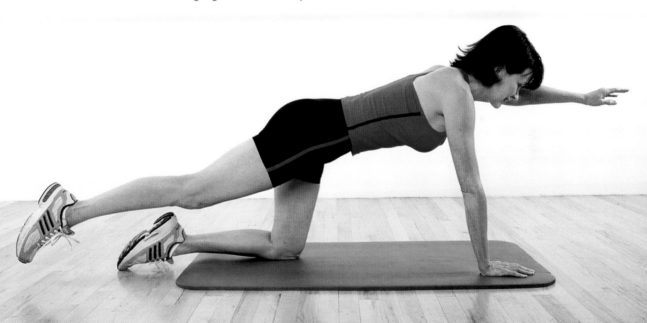

smart tip

Try to keep your back as flat as possible during the movement. If this exercise becomes too easy, try this variation: When you extend your leg behind you, raise it until it's parallel to the floor.

core body sequence

Abdominal Curl

The sit-up is a fundamental part of any well-rounded routine; this version is a little easier and also safer but still effective for strengthening your abdominal muscles.

- **ONE** Lie on your back with feet flat on the floor, knees bent, and arms folded across your chest, each hand touching the opposite shoulder.

- **TWO** Raising your head, use your abdominal muscles to pull your shoulders off the floor so you can look at the top of your knees. Keep enough space to fit a baseball between your chin and chest.

- **THREE** Slowly lower your shoulders back to the floor.

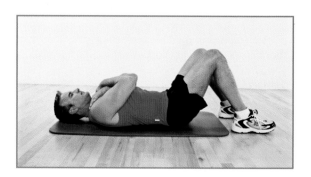

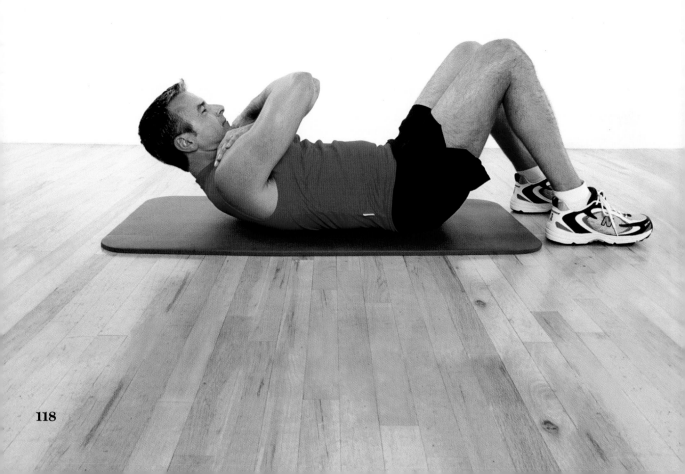

The Bicycle

This exercise is a favorite strength and endurance builder for athletes from football players to figure skaters. It helps tone the muscles along the sides of your abdomen, called the obliques.

- **ONE** Lie flat on your back with your legs straight and your hands behind or lightly touching your ears.

- **TWO** Lift your head off the floor and bring your left knee toward your head, stopping when your knee is about waist level and your thigh is perpendicular to the floor. At the same time, bring your right elbow toward the elevated knee so that your torso twists slightly and your elbow and knee are as close as possible over your abdomen.

- **THREE** Slowly return to the starting position. Rest for one second and repeat with the opposite limbs.

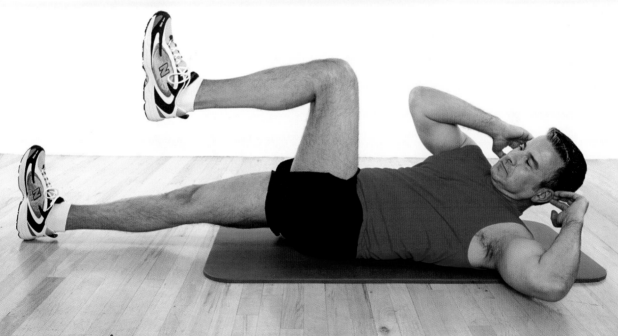

smart tip

This exercise should take about 5 seconds, with 2 seconds to bring knee and elbow close, and 3 seconds to return. As you become stronger, reduce the resting time for a more difficult workout. All motions should be smooth and controlled, which keeps resistance on muscles longer and improves strength and tone more quickly.

lower body sequence

Stair Step-Up

This move helps build strong leg muscles and requires absolutely no equipment. Yes, you can use a special exercise step, but it's not necessary. A regular step in your home is preferable because you can lightly grasp the stair rail for support. To keep track of repetitions, count step-ups on just one foot.

- **ONE** Stand in front of a step with both feet on the floor about hip-width apart.

- **TWO** Place your right foot solidly on the stair and step up. Bring your left foot up and touch it lightly on the step before lowering it back to the floor.

- **THREE** Step down with your right foot.

- **FOUR** Step up with your left foot, bringing your right foot up and touching it lightly on the step, then lowering it back to the floor. Alternate steps in this way, counting one repetition when each foot has stepped up one time.

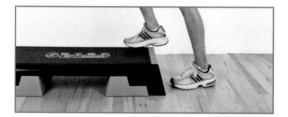

smart tip

Make this exercise more difficult by using only one foot instead of alternating. For example, use the right foot to step up, step down, then step up again rather than alternating with the left foot. When you've finished a set of step-ups with the right foot, do a set with the left.

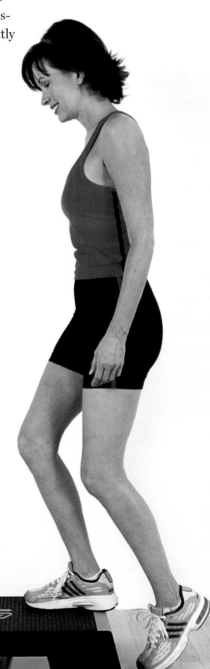

Side Hip Abduction

This exercise works the abductor muscles on the outside of the hip and outer thigh.

- **ONE** Lie on your right side with both legs extended and resting one on top of the other, supporting your head with your right hand.

- **TWO** In a smooth and controlled motion, lift your fully extended left leg straight up as high as you comfortably can. Then lower it back to the starting position. After one set, repeat with the other leg.

smart tip

If you feel unstable in the starting position, try bending the lower leg to provide a wider base of support. If this exercise becomes too easy, try performing it while wearing light ankle weights. Start with half-pound or one-pound weights.

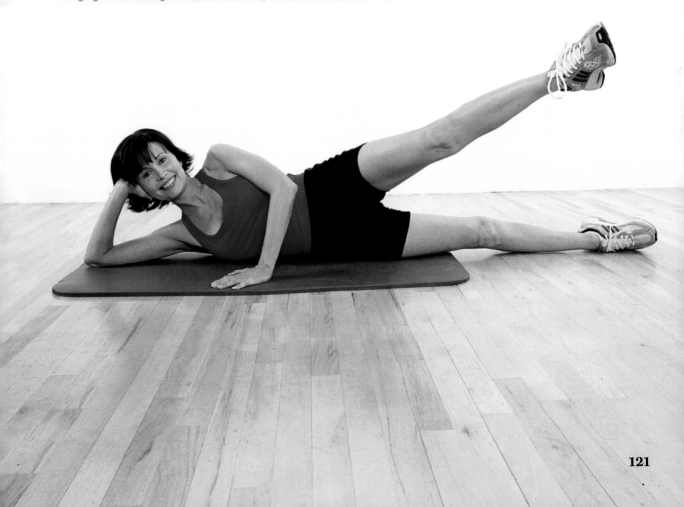

lower body sequence

Standing Hip Extension

Perform this exercise facing a sturdy chair, countertop, or table you can rest your hands on for balance and support. It works your hips, buttocks, hamstrings, and lower back.

ONE Stand with feet about hip-width apart, lightly holding a chair or counter.

TWO Without bending the knee, move your right leg from the hip back behind you. Return slowly to the starting position. After one set, repeat with the other leg.

smart tip

Don't lock the knee of the leg you stand on, but instead keep it slightly bent. While the motion is pendulum-like, you shouldn't let momentum do the work. Perform the move slowly, especially during the return phase. If this exercise becomes too easy, try it with a light ankle weight.

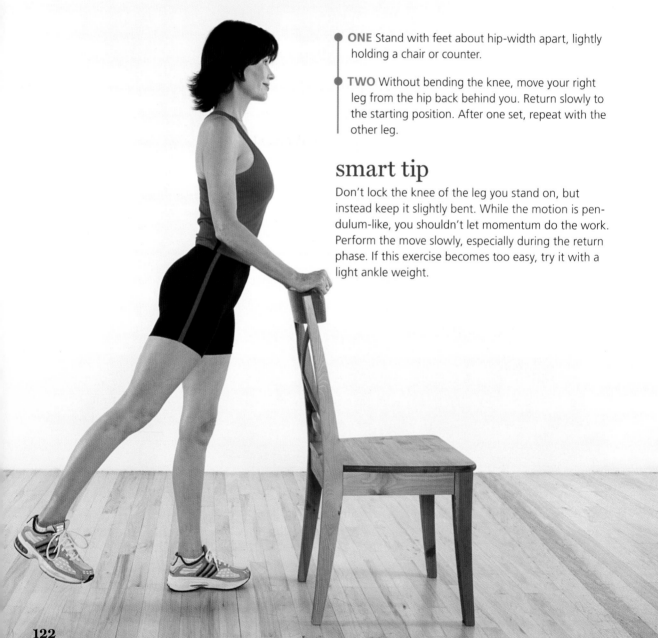

GOAL 4

Make active choices every day

WHAT KIND OF EXERCISE can you do while stuck in a line at the grocery store, when you have to relay information to a coworker, or when it's time to entertain the kids or grandkids? How about small, stealthy, calorie-burning moves that also use up blood sugar and help you lose weight—without taking time out of your day?

Thanks to modern technology we've engineered so many old-fashioned "inconveniences" out of our lives that we're packing on pounds. That's why we've made "living an active life" an essential part of the Move plan. It's just as important as walking and strength training for helping you achieve and maintain a healthy weight and for keeping your blood sugar in check.

Rediscovering the joys of an active lifestyle is fun. We bet you'll find yourself figuring out loads of new ways to fit more activity into your day, whether you play kickball with the kids in the backyard; stand and pace rather than lounging on the couch during phone calls; bound up the stairs rather than taking the elevator; or find yourself volunteering to take the dog out for an extra walk.

This vivacious approach to daily life is also energizing—not energy-sapping, as the typical sedentary lifestyle typically is. The more you sit on the couch or chair, the less you feel like getting up. But when you make active choices, your appetite for movement and activity is whetted, making the rest of the Move plan easier and more enjoyable to follow. Here's how to start living the active life today.

STEP ONE
Seize Opportunities to Move Every Day

At home, at work, and everywhere in between, there are dozens of opportunities to move your body instead of sitting still. We've outlined just a few ideas; feel free to come up with more of your own.

At Work

Get more "face time." Instead of sending e-mails or calling coworkers, stop by their desks to ask a question or figure out a solution to a work issue. Doing this instead of sending just one e-mail a day could save you 11 pounds over 10 years.

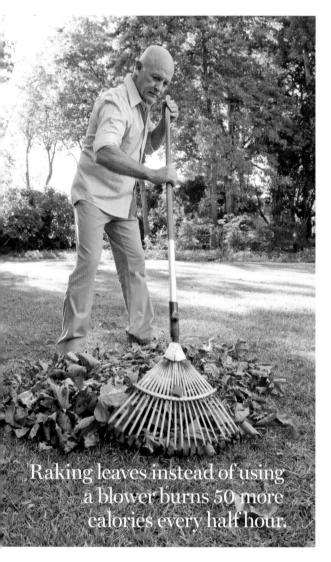

Raking leaves instead of using a blower burns 50 more calories every half hour.

Go the long way. Circle the building before heading to lunch. Use the bathroom or copy machine farthest from your desk. Doesn't it feel good to stretch your legs?

Take the stairs, of course. Just two flights daily could help you melt 6 pounds in a year. In fact, climbing stairs for two minutes five days a week provides the same calorie burn as a 36-minute walk. At home, instead of piling items on stairs so you can take all of them upstairs at once, take them one at a time.

Plan a walking meeting. Need to schedule a small meeting? Suggest a walking meeting instead of a confab in an airless conference room. Take a small notebook and a pen. Chances are, you'll have better ideas and forge a better relationship with your fellow walkers.

At Home

Cook as if it's 1904. Chop veggies by hand instead of in the food processor, whip eggs with a fork or whisk, mix cake batter with a big spoon instead of the mixer, dig out your manual can opener, and, if you have time, wash and dry the dishes by hand. It will all add up to a small workout.

Rake leaves instead of using a leaf blower. You'll burn 50 more calories every half hour.

Scrub your floors more often. Putting some elbow grease into cleaning floors is more intense exercise than vacuuming—and it makes your floors look better to boot.

Spiff up your ride. Wash your car by hand. You'll save money by not going to the car wash and burn up to 280 calories in an hour. Why not vacuum the upholstery and carpeting, wash the plastic trim on the insides of the doors, and do the insides of the windows, too?

Take energy breaks. Every half hour, walk around your office or down the hall for five minutes. Jump up and down in your own office. Do push-ups with your hands resting against your desk. Do 10 leg lifts, then stand up and rise on your toes 10 times. Stretch your arms high 10 times, too.

Get a new rolling "chair." Try sitting on a large exercise ball instead of a desk chair, at least some of the time. You'll use your abdominal and back muscles all day to help you balance.

Trim the old-time way. Leave the electric edger and trimmer in the garage and grab your old hand tools. Comfort hint: Use thick foam or an old carpet square to cushion your knees.

Rehab the push mower. Revive a lovely summer sound: the whisk-whisk-whisk of a muscle-powered push mower. Buy one and consider it an investment in a piece of exercise equipment, or rehabilitate the old one stashed way in the back of the garage. Sharpen the blades, oil the mechanism, and go. Ah! No exhaust fumes, no ugly power-motor noise.

Double-dig. Gardeners know that the best planting beds are double-dug. When you put in a new bed or turn over the soil in your vegetable patch in the spring, leave the power tiller in the shed and get out there with a sharp shovel. Dig each row twice—first to a single shovel's depth, then down one more shovel's worth. Refill the row by putting the first digging's soil in the bottom and the second's on top. You'll have more fertile soil on top and fluffy dirt down deep, so tender roots can grow strong, creating beautiful, healthy plants.

Plant bulbs. Garden catalogs start advertising sales of fall bulbs in midsummer. That's the time to think about daffodils, daylilies, tulips, and a host of other gorgeous spring and summer flowers for next year. Order a bunch and plant them over several fall weekends. Your efforts will be rewarded with a stunning display once winter's gone.

Stop buying weed killer. Be a friend to the earth and to your own muscles: Pull, dig out, and cut back weeds yourself. Your arms and back will get a workout.

Anytime, Anywhere

Take the escalator at the mall or train station, but climb the stairs while you ride. You'll get there faster and use your muscles while you're at it. Just five minutes of stair climbing burns 144 calories.

Don't sit when you can stand. When cooling your heels while waiting in a doctor's office, drugstore, or airport, stay on your feet. Standing burns 36 more calories per hour than sitting.

STEP TWO
Sneak in "Stealth" Exercise Moves

Most of us hate to kill time, but we face countless opportunities during the day to do just that. Opportunities? That's right: From now on, be alert for small moments of downtime during your day and embrace them when they come; they're perfect chances to build some extra exercise into your day.

On the Road to Fitness: Car Moves

Reserve these fast, effective exercises for stoplights and long traffic jams.

Steering wheel lift press. While stopped at a red light, grasp the bottom of the steering wheel with your palms up. Inhale and then, while exhaling, push up on the wheel with your palms as hard as you can. Hold while breathing normally until the light turns green. Works the biceps, the primary load-bearing muscles of the arms.

Ab squeeze. While stopped at a red light or stop sign, take a deep breath through your mouth, dropping your diaphragm so your stomach pushes out. While exhaling, squeeze your abdominal muscles so your back presses into the car seat. (Imagine that a hook around your spine is pulling you back.) Hold for up to 60 seconds while breathing normally. Improves posture and tones the gut to support your back and make you look slimmer.

125

We mean actual exercises—the Stealth Exercises described on page 128. Do them while standing in line at the bank, sitting in traffic, or cooling your heels while waiting at the assigned time and place for friends or family members (who apparently don't know how to tell time). Others you can do in the privacy of your home while you go about everyday activities, such as brushing your teeth or heating a pot of water for tea.

STEP THREE
Make Active Fun Your First Choice

At a neighborhood picnic, are you the person with their hands in the chips and deviled eggs or the one with her hand in a baseball glove, attempting to defend third base? At the park, are you the parent in the thick of the Frisbee game or climbing the monkey bars or the one huddled on the park bench looking bored? We promise: You don't have to be fit, fast, or good at sports to get out there and have some fun.

Play with kids. Impromptu games of basketball, touch football, or tag or just jumping rope or throwing a ball will help you use energy and set a good example of active play for the children. Calories burned: 80 to 137 every 10 minutes.

See exercise as a new social opportunity. Use your desire to get more physical activity as your motivation to sign up for a tango class, biking club, or Pilates lesson—something you've always wanted to try or something you never thought you'd do. Making new friends will be an added bonus—and seeing them will serve as motivation to show up.

Make it a family event. Set up a badminton net or softball diamond in your backyard and get a game going with your family (and neighbors if you need more players). And opt for active family fun such as water parks, sledding hills, playgrounds, pools, and zoos.

Join a sports team. Most communities have soccer, baseball, softball, even basketball teams for, ahem, older athletes. If you want a little less intensity, try coaching a kids' team or even refereeing. It will keep you on your feet.

Go bowling instead of going out for ice cream. You'll burn 100 calories in just a half hour. Haven't bowled in decades? Ask to have the bumpers put up along the sides of the lane; it'll improve your score and make the game more fun.

Join a hiking club or grab a map and a friend and go exploring. If you love wandering in nature, pick a park, mountain, beach, or lake that's close by. Find a map and check if there's an admission fee. Also consider cultivating an interest in birds. Bird-watching is one of America's hottest hobbies, thanks to the wonderful diversity of colors, shapes, songs, and personalities among American birds.

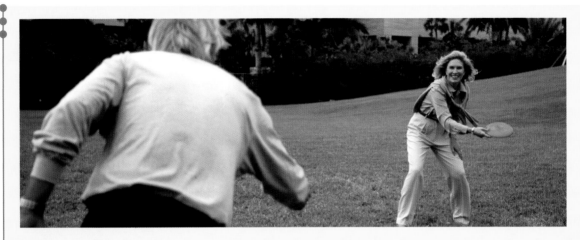

15 Ways to Burn 100 Calories

Whether you're trying to lose weight or maintain a healthy weight, it's important to not get overwhelmed by the big picture—"I have to lose 20 pounds"—but, instead, to focus on the little, everyday things that can make a big difference. For instance, if you burn an extra 100 calories a day, even if you don't change your eating habits at all, you'll lose about 10.5 pounds over the course of a year. What's it take to burn 100 calories? Not much.*

1. **Go roller-skating.** In just 12 minutes (assuming you haven't broken your arm) you've burned off 100 calories.

2. **Go grocery shopping.** A 38-minute grocery shopping trip burns 100 calories; you'll burn another 100 calories carrying the groceries to your car and then into your house.

3. **Play Frisbee.** Half an hour is all it takes—and that assumes you're not doing a lot of running after wild throws.

4. **Put up your Christmas tree.** Forty minutes of stringing lights and hanging ornaments is all that's needed to burn 100 calories and decorate for the holidays.

5. **Usher for your church or synagogue.** After 45 minutes, you'll have not only greeted all the parishioners, but will have burned 100 calories.

6. **Make dinner.** Pick one that requires chopping. If it takes you 35 minutes to get dinner ready, you've just burned your 100.

7. **Jump rope.** Even slow jumping burns 100 calories in 11 minutes; jump faster, and it takes only about 7 minutes.

8. **Clean out your garage.** Put in half an hour of sorting. By then, you'll have cleared at least one small space and burned 100 calories.

9. **Jog in place for 11 minutes.** Do it during the commercials of a 30-minute TV show.

10. **Dance the flamenco.** Just 15 minutes of fast ballroom dancing will do it.

11. **Walk your dog.** In half an hour, you'll have burned 100 calories, and he'll have stretched all fours and sniffed to his heart's content.

12. **Iron your clothes.** And your partner's and your kids'. Do it for 40 minutes.

13. **Hit the driving range for 30 minutes.** You'll improve your golf game and burn 100 calories.

14. **Play golf.** Carry your clubs and walk the course, and you'll burn 100 calories every 20 minutes.

15. **Go fishing.** It's peaceful and stress-free, and 30 minutes of it burns about 100 calories.

*All estimates based on a 150-pound, 42-year-old woman.

The *Reverse Diabetes* Stealth Exercises

Tree Pose

You can do this variation of a yoga move while combing your hair or brushing your teeth.

Stand up straight with your legs together. Slowly raise your right knee to the side, resting the bottom of your right foot against the inner calf of your left leg. Balance there for a count of 15, keeping your left knee unlocked. Pull your stomach in for support and keep your back straight and your chin up. Repeat on the other side.

BENEFIT Strengthens the lower body and core support muscles of the lower back and abdomen.

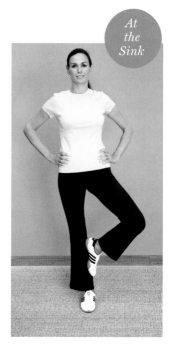

At the Sink

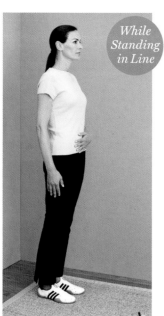

While Standing in Line

Standing Ab Squeeze

Keeping your neck, shoulders, and arms relaxed, pull in and tighten the muscles of your abdomen. (Picture a belt being tightened around your midsection.) Hold for 30 seconds, breathing as normally as possible. Do three times.

BENEFIT Doing this exercise while standing strengthens muscles that support your back against the strain of extra weight in your gut.

Butt Buster

Stand up straight with your feet hip-width apart. Squeeze the muscles of your buttocks together as tightly as you can, hold in your stomach, and move your right leg about 2 inches behind you with your foot off the floor. Hold for 10 seconds, then switch legs.

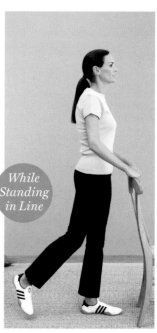

While Standing in Line

BENEFIT Strengthens the humble but powerful muscles in your rear, which are involved in virtually every movement your body makes.

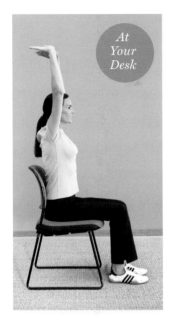

Overhead Press

At Your Desk

Sit up straight with your back firmly against the back of your chair and your feet flat on the floor, about hip-width apart. Raise your arms over your head with your palms flat and your elbows facing to the sides. Inhale and press up as if you were going to push the ceiling with your hands. Hold for 30 seconds, breathing normally. Repeat.

BENEFIT The palm position of this exercise isolates and strengthens the muscles of the shoulders.

Thigh Toner

Sit up straight. While tucking in your stomach muscles, curl your hands into fists and place them between your knees. Squeeze your fists with your thighs and hold for 30 seconds. Repeat.

BENEFIT Strengthens and firms the difficult-to-isolate muscles of the inner thighs.

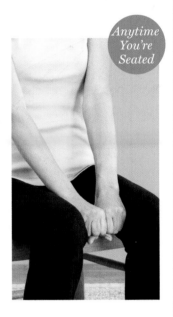

Anytime You're Seated

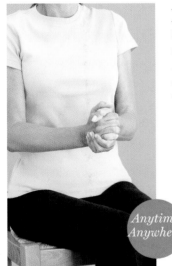

Palm Clasp

Sit up straight and grab one hand with the other. Press your palms together hard for 5 seconds, then release. Do four times. You can also do this one at red lights or while watching TV.

BENEFIT Strengthens the chest and arms.

Anytime, Anywhere

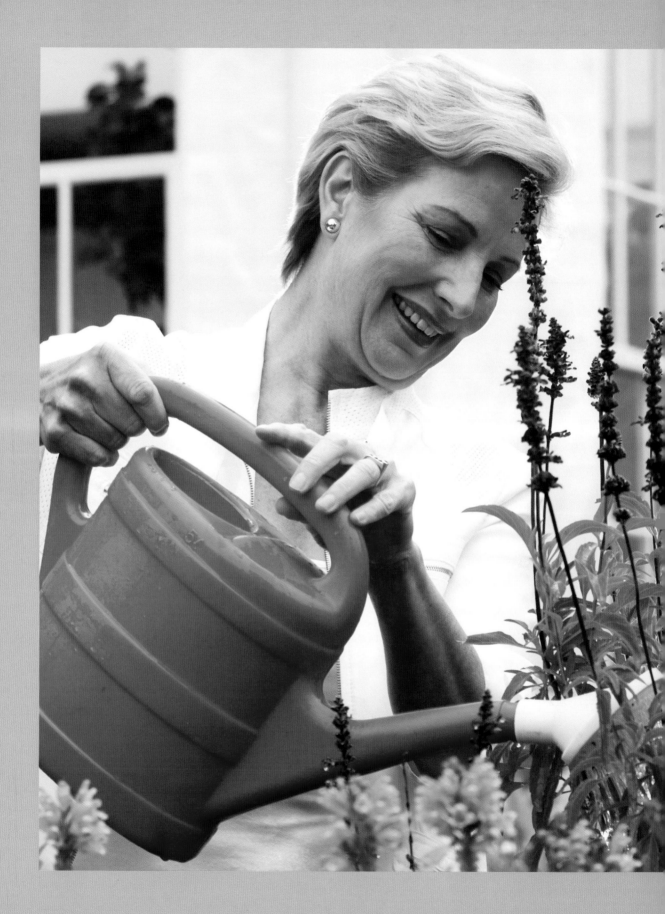

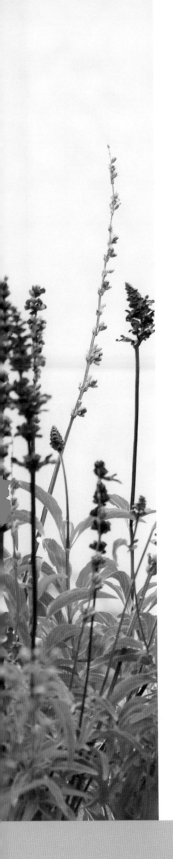

3

CHOOSE

to reverse diabetes

- Deep, Restful Sleep
- Relaxing "Me" Time
- Planning Ahead

- Better Health

the plan

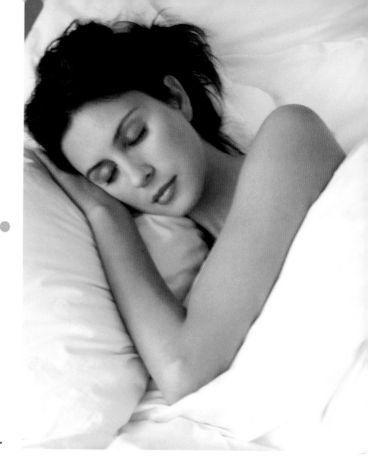

Good blood sugar control and weight loss come easier when you add restful sleep and relaxation to your eating and exercise program. Nurturing your mind and spirit keeps you motivated and reduces stress hormones that raise blood sugar and pack on belly fat. On the Choose plan you'll also learn to plan ahead for sick days and travel.

what to do

GOAL 1
Enjoy seven to eight hours of sleep a night

We're starting the Choose plan with sleep for three great reasons: First, sweet repose is now proven to help people with diabetes control their blood sugar. Second, research shows it is also a powerful strategy for shedding unwanted pounds and keeping them off. Being well-rested also will help you accomplish every other Choose goal with ease.

GOAL 2
Make time to unwind every day

Indulging in a little "me" time—and using it to melt away the day's anxieties and tensions— is much more than a frill. It's a necessity for healthy blood sugar, for maintaining or achieving a healthy weight, and for staying on track as you make healthy lifestyle changes. Learning the art of relaxation is worth the investment in time, as you'll discover.

GOAL 3
Keep your motivation stoked

Reversing diabetes begins in your mind—with a strategy for keeping your emotional commitment and energy levels high as you face the day-to-day challenges of managing your blood sugar and weight. Strong motivation has been proven to help people with diabetes not only keep blood sugar within a healthy range but also prevent diabetes complications.

what to record

1. HOW MUCH SLEEP YOU GOT LAST NIGHT

Every day for the next 12 weeks, record the number of hours you slept the night before in the Planner section. Aim for seven to eight hours, and notice how you're feeling if you get more or less. You'll begin to see how your sleep affects your blood sugar and your success with healthy eating and exercise.

2. WHETHER YOU KEPT TV TIME UNDER TWO HOURS A DAY

Limiting TV viewing ensures that you have plenty of time for sleep, exercise, and relaxation. Need extra incentive to turn off the tube? Harvard University researchers estimate that TV viewing burns even fewer calories than reading a magazine, sewing, or playing a board game!

3. WHETHER YOU MADE TIME FOR RELAXATION AND/OR SOCIALIZING

They're every bit as important to your health as eating well and exercising. A daily dose could be as simple as coffee with a friend.

4. YOUR ATTITUDE RATING

Was it excellent or pretty good today, or are you glad that you'll get a fresh start tomorrow? Rating your attitude every day is a great reminder that attitude counts—and an opportunity for an honest self-evaluation of your outlook. Paying attention to your attitude can help you cultivate the art of supporting your own best efforts—another powerful tool for great diabetes self-care.

5. SUCCESSES AND CONFESSIONS

At the end of each of the 12 weeks, it's time to spill. You'll find space in the Planner where you can crow about anything and everything that went well that week—and to write down the low points. Recording this information will help you understand how you're doing on the Eat, Move, Choose Plan, including which areas are going well for you and which need some improvement.

GOAL 4

Nurture resilience

Studies show that resilient people are better able to weather the ups and downs of life with diabetes. The best news: You can learn and practice the ability to draw on your inner strength and to bounce back from whatever life throws in your path. Developing a positive attitude, maintaining a sense of humor, and knowing when to reach out for help are crucial. You'll learn how to master all three.

GOAL 5

Plan ahead for sick days and travel

Being consistent from day to day, especially when it comes to diet and exercise, is key to managing diabetes. But when you're sick or on the road, your routine will change, and you'll face some special challenges that can affect your blood sugar and other aspects of your health. We'll show you how to manage both circumstances so that your diabetes doesn't suffer.

before you begin

Take the quiz on the next page.
This quiz will help you assess whether your sleep habits, mindset, and planning skills are helping you manage your diabetes—or getting in the way of your success. As always, answer as frankly as possible, and take your results seriously: They'll tell you in which areas of your life you'll want to make some changes in order to choose to reverse diabetes. If the results hint at burnout or emotional problems, these merit a visit to your doctor. So does a serious sleep problem such as insomnia or sleep apnea.

the quiz

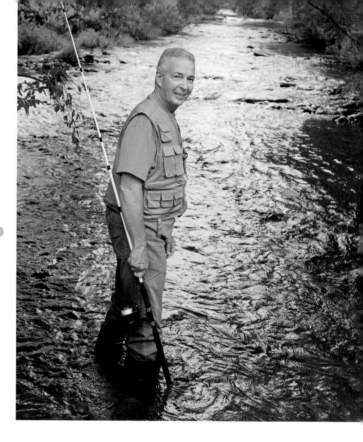

Are you making the everyday choices and putting plans in place so that blood sugar control fits easily into your day, no matter what? Or are stress, burnout, low motivation, depression, lack of sleep, or simply a lack of planning getting in your way? Take our quiz and find out.

1. **On a typical weeknight I:**
   a. Stay up late paying bills, surfing the Internet, or watching TV.
   b. Try my best to hit the hay in time for seven to eight hours of sleep.
   c. Dread the bed, knowing I'll lay awake for hours.

2. **In the morning I:**
   a. Usually wish I'd gone to bed earlier the night before.
   b. Feel pretty good.
   c. Am exhausted.

3. **During the night I:**
   a. Often wake up and can't get back to sleep.
   b. Sleep like a baby.
   c. Snore so loudly my spouse has to nudge or poke me.

4. **I would say my sleep quality is:**
   a. Not up to par because I'm doing the wrong things.
   b. Good or great.
   c. Poor despite my best efforts.

5. **My motivation for controlling my blood sugar is:**
   a. Starting to slip; keeping up with diabetes is becoming more difficult.
   b. Going strong.
   c. Nearly gone; I feel overwhelmed and tired of all this work.

6. **In the past two weeks I've felt:**
   a. Somewhat tense, irritated, or stressed out.
   b. Pretty good—I'm weathering difficult days and good days equally well.
   c. Down, depressed, or not interested in the things that I usually enjoy.

7. **When someone cuts me off in traffic or something else stressful happens, I:**
   a. Get mad and fume for a little while, then get over it.
   b. Feel a brief jolt of frustration, then forget about it.
   c. Become extremely angry and stay that way.

8. At the end of the day I:

a. Overeat, have several alcoholic drinks, or watch a lot of TV to drown out the stress.

b. Spend some time unwinding in my favorite way.

c. Replay the day's stresses over and over in my mind, or face new ones at home. There's no downtime.

9. When I get off course with managing my diabetes—by overeating, skipping exercise, or not testing my blood sugar enough—I tend to:

a. Feel guilty—but vow to do better.

b. Remind myself that ups and downs are normal, and I can make a fresh start tomorrow.

c. Feel defeated and make even more mistakes.

10. When I'm sick I:

a. Eat whatever's in the pantry, including junk food.

b. Consume regular doses of soup, crackers, tea, and other foods that I keep on hand to keep my blood sugar steady and prevent dehydration.

c. Don't pay any attention to what—or even whether—I eat or drink.

11. The last time I talked with my doctor about how often to check my blood sugar and take my medicine when I'm sick was:

a. Once, a long time ago.

b. Recently; we review my sick-day plan every year or so.

c. Never.

12. When I travel I:

a. Am never sure what to do with my medications and testing supplies.

b. Bring extra supplies and prescriptions and stay up to date with airline security regulations.

c. Throw all of my diabetes supplies into my suitcase and check it at the airport.

13. While traveling or away from home, I tell my companions this about my diabetes:

a. Nothing; they already know, and I assume someone would help me if I had a problem.

b. Everyone knows I have diabetes, and I talk to one person about where I keep my medications and how to help me if I have signs of low blood sugar.

c. Absolutely nothing; no one needs to know except me.

14. To protect my feet while on a trip I:

a. Pack a pair of comfy shoes.

b. Pack at least one pair of comfy shoes as well as some small bandages or moleskin to protect any "hot spots" that develop and check my feet often.

c. Do nothing and lament about my blisters when the trip is done.

your score

Give yourself 1 point for each "a" you circled, 2 points for each "b" answer, and 0 points for each "c."

24–28 points

You're choosing to reverse your diabetes.
You're taking pretty good care of yourself by getting enough sleep, keeping a positive attitude, controlling stress, and being smart about sick days and travel. But unless you scored a perfect 28, there's always room for improvement!

15–23 points

You're short-changing yourself a bit.
Giving higher priority to quality sleep and quality leisure time can help you get a better handle on your blood sugar and stave off stress and depression. You should also learn to take a little more care the next time you're sick or on the road.

0–14 points

You're sabotaging your efforts.
Lack of good rest and quality relaxation time are making it harder for you to control your weight and your blood sugar, not to mention maintain a positive outlook. Remember that taking care of your diabetes means taking care of yourself.

why the plan works

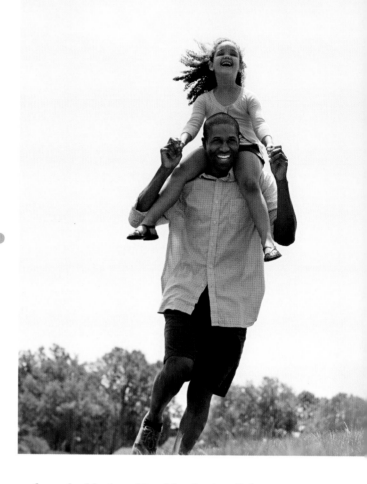

Refreshing sleep. Deep, daily serenity. Renewed motivation. Extra support if you're feeling burned out. Real help if you're depressed. The Choose plan will help you take care of your body and your mind in ways that make it easier for you to manage your diabetes and your overall health. Yes, taking care of your disease is a *choice* you make every day. We're here to help you make that choice again and again—and we'll stay with you over the next 12 weeks to make sure you're on track.

It Helps Lower Your Blood Sugar

The twin goals of the Eat, Move, Choose Plan are to lower your blood sugar and help you loose weight. The Eat and Move portions of the plan will take you a long way toward both goals. But if you're not taking care of your mind and giving yourself plenty of sleep to bolster your efforts, your chances of succeeding in reversing your diabetes shrink. Believe it or not, getting enough sleep and taming stress also work directly on your blood sugar to keep it in check.

Reversing diabetes with sleep. A chronic lack of sleep reduces your body's sensitivity to insulin and can double the odds of developing diabetes. In people who already have diabetes, it's associated with higher A1C scores, an indication of poor long-term blood sugar management, and a higher risk for diabetes complications. It doesn't take months or years of late nights to develop blood sugar problems due to lack of sleep. In a dramatic University of Chicago experiment, healthy young men who went without much sleep for just one week became 30 percent more insulin-resistant than they were at the start of the experiment. Researchers were stunned. It's enough to make you turn off Leno and Letterman and hit the hay!

On the Choose plan you'll learn how to set the stage for the deep, refreshing night's sleep your body needs. You'll also learn how to address two serious sleep problems that can interfere with your diabetes and your overall health: insomnia and obstructive sleep apnea (OSA). People with OSA are three times more likely to develop diabetes than those who don't have it. And once you have diabetes, apnea can make blood sugar control more difficult. Experts suspect that it raises levels of hormones that interfere with the action of insulin. Reversing apnea can do wonders for your blood sugar. When researchers tracked 25 people with diabetes and apnea who received treatment for this sleep disorder, they found that their blood sugar after breakfast was reduced from 191 mg/dl to 130 mg/dl.

Stress, the hidden blood sugar culprit. Cutting-edge diabetes management programs all include stress management, and it's no wonder why. When you're on edge, your body pumps out stress hormones, such as cortisol, to help you react to danger. Among other things, these hormones make your heartbeat and breathing speed up. They also send glucose stores into the blood to make energy immediately available to your muscles. The result: higher blood sugar. Stress hormones also make it more difficult for the pancreas to secrete the insulin that's needed to move glucose out of the blood. Some of these hormones may also contribute to insulin resistance—a triple whammy.

Taming tension is an effective way to bring down blood sugar. One groundbreaking study at Duke University in Durham, North Carolina, found that when people with diabetes used easy relaxation techniques like the ones you'll learn on the Choose plan, they dropped their A1C numbers significantly. In fact, about a third of the volunteers lowered their A1C levels by 1 percent or more after a year—an effect on a par with that of diabetes drugs.

It Helps You Lose Weight

Losing weight is usually a sure step toward reversing insulin resistance and lowering blood sugar. The Eat and Move portions of the Eat, Move, Choose Plan were designed largely to help you do just that. And the Choose plan supports your efforts so the pounds come off almost without trying.

Quality sleep keeps hunger in check. When you don't get enough sleep, the urge to eat bad-for-you foods can get out of control. Not only do late nights in front of the TV go hand in hand with mindless snacking, sleep deprivation can actually alter your body chemistry in ways that make you hungrier. In the same University of Chicago study we mentioned earlier, in which men went without much sleep for a week, the scientists discovered that levels of the appetite-stimulating hormone leptin rose as the study volunteers' sleep debt grew. The men began to crave high-carbohydrate foods such as candy, cookies, potato chips, and pasta.

And in an amazing study of 68,000 women conducted at Harvard Medical School, women who slept five hours a night were 32 percent more likely to gain 30 pounds or more as they aged than women who slept seven hours or more—even when the women who slept longer ate more than the other women!

But you can flip that switch the other way—saving yourself hundreds of extra calories per day—simply by snoozing. In one study, 32 university students kept diaries noting how much sleep they got and what foods they ate over a three-week period. The first week, students stuck to their normal eating and sleeping schedules. The second week, students were asked to sleep an extra two hours a day. The third week, students returned to their normal routine. When the students got an extra two hours of sleep per night, they ate nearly 300 calories a day *less* than they did the other weeks!

Stress control subdues appetite. Stress not only raises your blood sugar, it also stimulates your appetite. Yes, that's right: Stress makes you eat more—something anyone who's faced a work deadline fortified with doughnuts knows all too well. Cortisol's dirty little secret? It encourages cells in your abdomen to conserve fat. In other words, it packs on intra-abdominal fat, also known as visceral fat, the type that fuels insulin resistance.

Regularly practicing our relaxation methods will help lower your levels of stress hormones to reverse this trend. It should also help you stick to your eating and exercise goals. Think about it: When you're stressed, you're probably tempted to chow down on whatever fatty, high-calorie snacks are in reach. You're also less likely to stop and think about hitting the pavement for a nice, long walk when you're busy fretting over bills to pay, family problems, or that fight with your spouse. When you practice the art of relaxation, you'll step back and see the big picture, and your true priorities—including taking care of your body—will emerge.

Mastering stress has other beneficial side effects. Specifically, it helps ward off emotional problems that are linked with poor blood sugar control, particularly depression, burnout, and low motivation.

It Sidesteps Diabetes Burnout

Diabetes is a disease you deal with every day, and let's face it, that can be tough. But simply believing that you can stay on top of the condition—and even reverse it—is powerful medicine. When Denver Veterans Affairs Medical Center researchers assessed the mindsets of 88 people with diabetes, they found that those who reported a strong belief in their ability to take care of their diabetes were more likely to follow diet and exercise recommendations and, a year later, had lower blood sugar than people with low confidence.

Maintaining a positive, can-do attitude can also significantly cut your risk for diabetes complica-

tions. In a study of 165 people with type 2 diabetes, those who were motivated to take charge of their diabetes were 55 percent less likely to have a heart attack, 53 percent less likely to have a stroke, and 50 percent less likely to have severe kidney damage over 7 1/2 years. Their blood sugar levels were lower, and their blood pressure and cholesterol levels were healthier than people who were less motivated to care for themselves.

The Choose plan can help you keep the flames of motivation burning high or rekindle them if they've been dwindling lately. It can also help you avoid diabetes burnout—the feeling that the day-to-day responsibilities involved in handling this challenging medical condition are just too much. It's easy to push feelings of early burnout aside. But catching this kind of mental and emotional fatigue as soon as possible will help you refresh yourself—with emotional support, pampering, and a reassessment of your diabetes-management goals—so that you can keep your blood sugar under control. The quiz on page 134 should give you a sense of your burnout level, and you'll find plenty of ways to lower it in the following pages.

It Helps You Spot Depression and Get Help

You'll also find out how to spot depression early—and what to do to truly feel better. Diabetes and depression are deeply connected on many levels. Obviously if you're depressed you're much less likely to exercise and eat well. But the health dangers don't end there. Stanford University scientists think that depression itself alters body chemistry in profound ways that spell trouble for anyone at risk for diabetes. Rates of insulin resistance were 23 percent higher among depressed women than women who were not depressed, regardless of body weight, exercise habits, or age in one study.

The combination of depression and diabetes can be fatal: People with both are three times more likely to die from coronary artery disease than are people with diabetes who are not depressed. Experts have long debated which comes first. Now, there's new evidence that depression isn't just the *result* of coping with illness or of biochemical changes caused by diabetes: It may exist before you have diabetes and help trigger its development by raising levels of inflammation and stress hormones. These factors will also make blood sugar more difficult to control.

It Puts You in Control on Sick Days and When Traveling

A well-planned diabetes management routine will help you sail through your weeks and weekends with confidence, but what about times when life throws a curveball? Sick days and travel can change everything, by uprooting your meal plans, making exercise difficult or impossible, making it difficult to take medications on time and in the usual doses, and even by altering your body chemistry in ways that can raise your blood sugar.

The Choose plan can help you stay on track, so that these unusual days mean business as usual for your blood sugar. Planning ahead will help you avoid problems such as dehydration, undereating, or not being able to rest when you're sick. It will also help you sail through airport security with your diabetes medications (yes, even with insulin syringes and the lancets used to test blood sugar)—and avoid mishaps such as missed doses or a shortage of medication or testing supplies while you're away from home.

The result? Lower stress, better blood sugar, and a happier, healthier you.

Choosing to Quit

Of course we don't mean quit taking care of your diabetes; we mean quit smoking. If you're a smoker with diabetes, getting cigarettes out of your life should be your top priority. Diabetes is already putting your heart and blood vessels at risk; they don't need any more trouble from tobacco. Need even more incentive? Some 90 percent of people with diabetes who have to have a foot amputated are smokers. Your best quitting strategies:

Counseling programs and cognitive behavioral therapy. These train you to solve practical problems related to quitting (for instance, if you always light up when you pour your morning coffee, maybe you need to switch to tea or have your coffee in a nonsmoking environment); include social support, such as pairing you with a nonsmoking "buddy" you can call when you feel the need to smoke; and help you set up social support outside of therapy. Ask your doctor for a referral.

Nicotine replacement. These include gums, patches, lozenges, inhalers, and nasal spray. It doesn't matter if you get your nicotine fix with a prescription product or an over-the-counter product; both are equally effective.

Bupropion. This antidepressant doubles the success of the nicotine patch compared to using the patch alone. And it seems to reduce the weight gain so common after quitting.

Exercise. Exercising three times a week may work even better than a behavioral therapy program (of course, doing both is ideal). One study found that nearly 20 percent of the exercisers were still smoke free after a year compared to 11 percent of the therapy group.

GOAL 1

Enjoy seven to eight hours of sleep a night

WOULDN'T IT BE GREAT if you could go to bed tonight and wake up tomorrow morning with better blood sugar control and a slimmer waist? It's possible—if you make a good night's sleep a priority. But more and more of us are doing exactly the opposite: We're getting less and less shut-eye. Ten years ago at least 38 percent of us slept eight hours a night, which, depending on personal biology and life stage, is what most of us need. Five years ago that number dropped to 30 percent. Two years ago it was down to 26, and it's falling even further today.

The price for all of this sleeplessness goes way beyond feeling groggy instead of energetic in the morning. Sleep problems are deeply connected with insulin resistance, high blood sugar, and hormone changes that lead to weight gain. At the same time, the growing obesity epidemic is bringing on a new wave of sleep apnea—periods of breathlessness at night that also raise risk for being overweight and for developing diabetes and heart problems, too. A lack of sleep is also guaranteed to raise your stress levels during the day. It's tough staying calm and centered when a tired mind meets an emotional challenge—whether it's an angry boss, a rude driver on the road, or a broken dishwasher at home.

That's why we've made good sleep the first of the Choose plan's goals. Get this one right and the rest—from reducing stress to taking control of top blood sugar challenges—will be far easier.

STEP ONE
Set the Stage

Many of us don't get enough sleep simply because we choose to stay up late (there are always bills to pay and late-night TV for laughs). Or, if we do hit the hay on time, we toss and turn, replaying the day's worries, fighting the lingering effects of that late-afternoon cup of coffee, or trying to ignore the noise of a sleeping spouse or the discomfort of a sagging mattress. If that's you, a deep, refreshing night's sleep is just a few fixes away. These strategies will help you prepare your mind, body, and bedroom for a full dose of slumber.

Wake up at the same time every morning. This is one of the surest ways to train your body to fall asleep at the same time every night. Experts

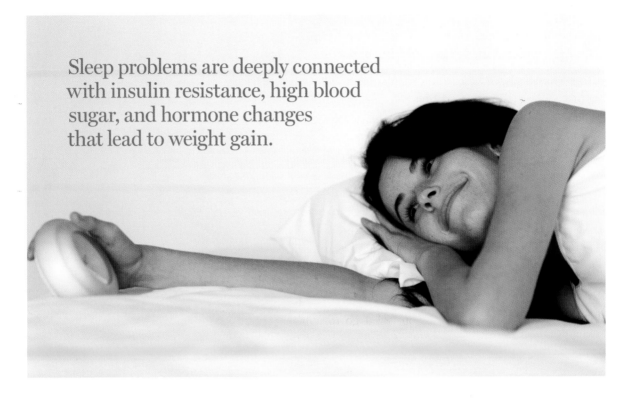

Sleep problems are deeply connected with insulin resistance, high blood sugar, and hormone changes that lead to weight gain.

say that keeping a regular sleep schedule is critical to keeping insomnia at bay.

Beware Sunday night insomnia. Staying up late on Friday and Saturday nights and sleeping in on Saturday and Sunday mornings is frequently the gift we give ourselves on weekends after a hard week at work. Yet that little gift—small as it is—is enough to screw up our biological clocks. Even if you get to bed early on Sunday night, you will not be ready to sleep, and you will not end up being the happy camper you were expecting come Monday morning.

Get some exercise every day. Physical activity improves sleep as effectively as powerful sleeping pills called benzodiazepines in some studies. On average it reduces the time it takes to get to sleep by 12 minutes, and it increases total sleep time by 42 minutes.

It doesn't take much: Studies at the University of Arizona show that walking six blocks at a normal pace during the day significantly improves sleep at night for women. Just make sure you finish your walk at least two hours before bed. Any later and the energizing effect of the activity can keep you up.

Sleep when the getting is good. Ever find that you get really sleepy at 10 p.m., that the sleepiness passes, and that by the time the late news comes on, you're wide awake? Some experts believe sleepiness comes in cycles. Push past a period of sleepiness and you likely won't be able to fall asleep very easily for a while. If you've noticed these kinds of rhythms in your own body, use them to your advantage. When sleepiness comes, get yourself to bed, pronto.

Allow at least three hours between dinner and bedtime. The brain does not sleep well on a full stomach. If you know that you have a busy day planned the following day, have your big meal at lunchtime and a lighter meal as early as possible in the evening. If you find you are still hungry before bedtime, avoid sugar; try a small handful of nuts.

Wind down an hour before you turn in. According to a National Sleep Foundation poll, during the hour before bed, around 60 percent of us do household chores, 37 percent take care of children, 36 percent do activities with other family members, 36 percent are on the Internet, and 21 percent do work related to their jobs. A better plan: Read a book, listen to music, take a warm bath, or do some light stretching. The goal is to build a routine that relaxes your body and tells your mind that sleep is up next.

Turn off the computer an hour before bed. Researchers at Stanford University have found that the light from your monitor right before bed is enough to reset your whole wake/sleep cycle—and postpone the onset of sleepiness by three hours.

Chill your bedroom. Lowering the temperature will signal to your body that it's time to sleep, experts say.

Shut the drapes. You sleep better in the dark. If your eyelids flutter open as you move from one stage of sleep to another, even streetlights or a full moon can wake you.

Ditch all night-lights. That goes for clocks, too. Turn your clock's face or digital readout away so you can't see it. We wake slightly throughout the night. Your brain can misinterpret even such dim lights and wonder if it should wake you up. Do all you can to keep things dark—researchers say it tells your brain to stay asleep. If you have to get up to visit the bathroom at night, keep the path from bed to toilet clear so you can navigate it with a minimum of light (use enough to stay safe, of course!). A night-light in the bathroom is a good idea.

Relax your body. If your mind is relaxed but your body is tense, do some low-intensity stretches and

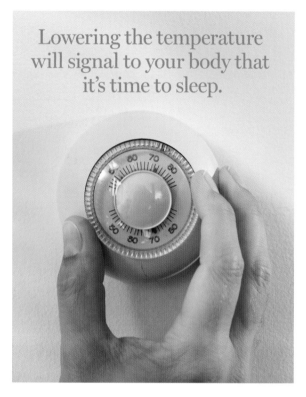

Lowering the temperature will signal to your body that it's time to sleep.

exercises to relax your muscles, especially those in your upper body, neck, and shoulders. The relaxation routine and progressive muscle relaxation exercise you'll find later in this chapter will both work.

Keep a worry book. Put a small journal and a pen on your bedside table. If you wake up in the wee, small hours and begin worrying, jot down your thoughts. Then close the book, put it on your nightstand, turn out the light, and go back to sleep.

Get up if you're not sleeping. Snoozing from 11:30 p.m. until 2:00 a.m., tossing and turning until 4, then sleeping until 6 gives you eight hours in bed but only 4 1/2 hours of sleep—and letting yourself toss and turn at night to the point of frustration creates anxiety about sleep that can make insomnia worse. If you wake at 2 a.m., get up and go read a book or magazine in the living room. Don't go back to bed until you feel sleepy enough to fall asleep.

It's tempting to stay in a warm, cozy bed even if you're not asleep, but remind yourself that it's important to get out of bed when you're awake. If you don't, a part of your mind will begin to associate the bed with being awake rather than being asleep, making falling asleep more difficult.

Banish Fido and Fluffy from the boudoir. Up to 25 percent of insomniacs may have their pets to blame for their lack of snooze time, say Mayo Clinic researchers who interviewed 300 patients at the clinic's Sleep Disorders Center. Pets wake us up by walking around at night, jumping on the bed, and demanding to be let outside for middle-of-the-night bathroom breaks. Consider investing in a white-noise machine to cover up their sounds, shut your door and insist they sleep elsewhere, or talk with your vet about introducing your animal to sleeping in a pet crate. Healthy pets can also be trained gradually to wait till morning for a bladder break; your vet can help you do this the right way.

Cut out caffeine. In a study of thousands of Australians, those who got 240 milligrams of caffeine a day—about the amount in two 8-ounce cups of coffee or 2 1/2 shots of espresso—had a 40 percent higher risk for insomnia than those who skipped it. Caffeine blocks the action of a sleep-inducing brain chemical called adenosine. It takes three to seven hours for your body to metabolize just half the caffeine in a cup of tea or coffee. If you can't live without it, relegate your caffeine to the morning.

STEP TWO
Tackle Insomnia

Staring at the ceiling all night? You're not alone. An estimated one in three adults has trouble falling asleep—or staying asleep—at least one night per week. When does "I can't get to sleep" qualify as insomnia? Experts say you've crossed the line

---

What Lies Beneath

When a consulting firm surveyed 400 adults for the Better Sleep Council, they found that 8 in 10 thought a bad mattress could cause sleep problems. Ironically, nearly half also confessed that their current mattress was "bad" or even "very bad."

You need a new mattress if:
▸ Yours is 10 years old or older.
▸ The topography of your mattress resembles a mountain range, with all its peaks, valleys, and slopes.
▸ You wake up feeling sore or stiff, despite not being physically active the day before.

How to buy a mattress you'll like:
▸ Try it in the store. Lie on it. Roll over. Get into your typical sleeping position and stay there for at least five minutes. Go by what's comfortable. *Consumer Reports* found that firmer mattresses don't resist permanent sagging any better than softer mattresses; that thicker mattresses sag more than thinner ones; and that the more padding there is, the greater the possibility the mattress will sag.
▸ Buy one that's larger than you think you will need, especially if you sleep with someone else. If you're used to a Queen and feel cramped when you sleep, invest in a King.
▸ Once you get it home, turn it over and upside down at least every three months.

---

and may need treatment if on three or more nights each week you need more than 30 minutes to fall asleep and/or you awaken in the middle of the night and have trouble getting back to sleep.

If that's you, be sure to start with all of the sleep tactics in Step One. Experts recommend them for people with insomnia, too, because they'll help your mind and body establish a healthier sleep schedule. If you still feel you're losing out on zzzzs, move on to these strategies.

Try sleeping pills for a few nights. Talk to your doctor and ask for a prescription. The new and widely advertised insomnia drugs—including zolpidem (Ambien), zaleplon (Sonata), and eszopiclone (Lunesta)—appear to be as effective as older, habit-forming sleeping pills, with fewer side effects, probably because the body metabolizes them faster. Taking them for a few nights can help quell your anxiety about being unable to fall asleep and get you out of the habit of dreading the bed. But don't rely on them as a long-term solution. A report from the National Institutes of Health warns that few prescription drugs for insomnia have been tested in long-term studies of a year or more—yet many people take them for years on end. And recently the FDA required warnings on 13 prescription sleep aids about risks that people may attempt to drive, cook, and eat while asleep.

Retrain your brain. The most successful treatment for insomnia is called cognitive behavioral therapy (CBT). In more than 20 studies involving 470 patients with insomnia from a variety of causes, CBT worked just as well as sleeping pills at increasing sleep and improving sleep quality—and it was better than sleeping pills at helping study participants fall asleep faster.

CBT involves meeting with a trained therapist to discover information about what keeps you from sleeping (the "cognitive" part) and learn how to alter your behavior (the "behavioral" part) so that you can improve your sleep. It generally takes just four or five 30-minute sessions to effect change.

Unfortunately, certified cognitive behavioral therapists are scarce. To find one, visit www.academyofct.org and click on "Find a Certified Cognitive Therapist." Fill in your zip code or city and state on the popup, and a list of therapists in your area will appear. If none do, or if you don't have time for even the small number of sessions CBT requires, you can visit www.cbtforinsomnia.com. For a fee ($24.95 at press time) you can take an online tutorial based on a Harvard University CBT insomnia program to retrain your brain for a better night's sleep.

Limit your time in bed. It sounds crazy, but one of the most effective strategies to combat insomnia is to restrict the number of hours you spend in bed.

The reason is that most people who have been struggling with insomnia will do seemingly practical things like go to bed a couple of hours early to try to sleep. It rarely works, researchers have found, so most of those people will spend, say, seven hours in bed and only sleep for five.

Don't go to bed until you truly feel like you can fall asleep. And remember what we said previously: Don't stay in bed when you're awake or the association you make (bed = awake) can program you for insomnia. Get up, go into another room, and do something boring and quiet for awhile. When you're really sleepy, go back to bed.

sugar buster quiz

Q: Sleeping pills or therapy?
A: Therapy

When researchers at Johns Hopkins University compared 21 studies using drugs or cognitive behavioral therapy for insomnia, the therapy emerged as the clear winner. It reduced the amount of time it took people to fall asleep 43 percent; drugs reduced it 30 percent. Therapy shortened the length of wake-ups at night 56 percent; drugs, 46 percent. Therapy improved overall sleep quality 28 percent; drugs, 20 percent. The therapy bonus: No side effects. And other studies show it keeps on working for months or years.

STEP THREE

Take Sleep Apnea Seriously

If you wake up in the morning feeling tired, irritable, sad, forgetful, and headachy, there's a good chance that you have sleep apnea, a sleep-related breathing disorder that affects millions of people—including many with diabetes.

When you have sleep apnea, your breathing actually stops or becomes very shallow as you sleep. Hundreds of times every night, your breathing may pause for 10 or more seconds, depriving your body of oxygen, increasing your heart rate, and preventing you from entering the important stages of deep sleep that restore mind and body. You may awaken slightly as you struggle to take a breath. By morning you may not recall any of your nighttime awakenings. But they have a profound affect on your blood sugar, your heart, and your brain.

Most sleep apnea is a type called obstructive sleep apnea, or OSA. It occurs when the soft tissue in the back of the throat relaxes and blocks the passage of air until your airway opens—often with a loud choking or gasping sound—and you begin to breathe again. Getting your sleep apnea diagnosed and treated will help you get a good night's sleep and feel refreshed. It can also help you control your blood sugar and reduce your odds for diabetes-related kidney damage, one recent study shows.

Here's how to find and fix sleep apnea.

Be alert for symptoms. You may have OSA if:

You snore loudly. About half of all people who snore loudly have OSA. It's a sign that your airway is partially blocked. Ask your sleep partner if you snore loudly at night, and whether he or she has noticed if you seem to stop breathing during sleep, then catch your breath again with a loud snort.

You have a large neck. The size of your neck can be a telltale sign because it's a reflection of being

Snoring Spouse? Sleep Alone!

Sure you love your spouse or partner, but studies find one of the greatest disruptors of sleep is that loved one dreaming away next to you. He might snore; she might kick or cry out or whatever. One study found that 86 percent of women surveyed said their husbands snored, and half had their sleep interrupted by it. Men have it a bit easier; 57 percent said their wives snored, while just 15 percent found their sleep bothered by it. The best solution? Have one of you sleep in the guest room. If you absolutely will not kick your partner out (or head to the guest room yourself), then consider these anti-snoring tips:

- ▶ Get him (or her) to stop smoking. Cigarette smoking contributes to snoring.
- ▶ Feed him (or her) a light meal for dinner and nix any alcohol, which can add to the snoring.
- ▶ Buy some earplugs and use them!
- ▶ Present your partner with a gift-wrapped box of Breathe Right strips, which work by pulling the nostrils open wider. A Swedish study found they significantly reduced snoring.
- ▶ Make an appointment for your sleeping partner at a sleep center. If nothing you do improves his or her snoring, your bedmate might be a candidate for a sleep test called polysomnography to see if sleep apnea is the cause.

overweight—and carrying extra pounds is a major risk factor for sleep apnea. Women with OSA often have a neck size of more than 16 inches; men, 17 inches.

You wake frequently for bathroom breaks. If you're not drinking loads of water before bed and you're not taking high-dose water pills, you shouldn't wake more than once or twice a night to use the bathroom. People with OSA often visit the bathroom three or more times each night.

145

You feel sleepy in the morning despite getting 8, 9, or 10 hours of sleep. Or you become dangerously drowsy during the day. People with OSA can become so sleepy that they fall asleep at the wheel.

See a sleep specialist. A sleep doctor will check your mouth, nose, and throat and make a recording of what happens with your breathing while you sleep. This may require an overnight stay at a sleep center.

Ask about continuous positive airway pressure (CPAP). This "gold standard" treatment uses a small, quiet air compressor to gently push air through a mask over the sleeper's nose. The extra pressure keeps airways open, so you breathe normally all night. When researchers analyzed 36 CPAP studies involving 1,718 people with sleep apnea, they found that those who used this system improved daytime sleepiness by nearly 50 percent, cut the number of sleep interruptions by eight per hour, and boosted the amount of oxygen in the blood significantly.

In one Chicago study, people with diabetes and apnea saw blood sugar levels drop three months after starting CPAP therapy. Other research shows it can also lower blood pressure and even improve the size, shape, and pumping action of the heart—good news because people with sleep apnea often have enlarged hearts. Talk to your doctor about this therapy and whether it might be right for you.

that's easy!

Trouble sleeping? Check your blood sugar more often this week to see if you're hitting the target goals you've set with your doctor. High and low blood sugar can affect sleep quality. And take one more step: Set your alarm for 3 a.m. for another check. If your levels are normal, that's great. If they're low, it might explain why you're waking up in the night. (If sugar levels are below 75 mg/dl, have a small snack. An ongoing pattern of low blood sugar at night should be discussed with your doctor.)

Lose weight. Following the rest of the Eat, Move, Choose Plan could help you reduce sleep apnea by helping you lose weight. When University of Wisconsin Medical School researchers tracked 690 Wisconsin residents for four years, they found those who lost 10 percent of their body weight saw apnea improve 26 percent. Almost any amount of weight loss helps. Extremely overweight people who underwent surgical weight loss procedures to drop 25 to 50 percent of their body weight saw a 70 to 98 percent drop in sleep apnea in one study. And among people who lost just 7 to 9 percent of their weight (about 14 to 18 pounds if you now weigh 200 pounds), sleep apnea scores fell by about 50 percent. Weight loss usually is not a replacement for CPAP or surgery, if you need them, but it can help make those treatments even more effective.

GOAL 2

Make time to unwind every day

YOU KNOW FIRSTHAND all about your body's responses to stress—the way you feel keyed-up or angry and how your head starts to throb, your armpits start to sweat, or your neck muscles tense up. You may be less familiar with your body's relaxation response—an innate, natural ability each of us has to enter into a physical state of thorough, sweet relaxation. It's that deep-down *ahhhh!* you may notice when you hold hands with your spouse, hug a child, hold a sleeping baby, watch the ocean waves, listen to soothing music, or engage in prayer or meditation. Believe it or not, you can teach yourself to elicit this relaxation response whenever you like, with a little practice. Here's how to get there.

STEP ONE
Learn a Relaxation Technique

No matter which of these tension-taming techniques you choose, commit to practicing it regularly—every day if possible. The more you do, the better and faster it will work, and the easier it will be for you to turn on your body's relaxation response when you need it. These are great ways to melt tension at the end of the day and can help you avoid spiraling into high anxiety when something stressful does happen in your life.

Try progressive relaxation. One study after another has demonstrated that progressive muscle relaxation blocks the chemical effects of stress, anxiety, and 24/7 living on your brain. To do it, lie down or sit in a comfortable chair that supports your head. Close your eyes and start by mentally scanning your body for places that feel tense. Now follow the serenity sequence below, tightly clenching each muscle area for 5 seconds. Take about 20 seconds to gradually release the tension, consciously relaxing your muscles as much as possible, then move on to the next area. When you've finished with the entire sequence, silently repeat a soothing thought, such as "I am totally relaxed."

Hands. Clench your fists, then relax.

Arms. Bend your dominant arm at the elbow and tense your biceps and lower arm as hard as you can without clenching your fist. Relax and repeat with the other arm.

Forehead. Raise your eyebrows and wrinkle your forehead as tightly as you can, then relax while

147

picturing your forehead becoming smooth. Next, deeply furrow your brow into a frown and relax.

Eyes. Squeeze your eyes shut as tightly as you can, then relax, keeping your eyelids closed.

Jaw. Tighten your jaw so your back teeth clench together (skip this if you have TMJ). Gradually relax, ending with your lips slightly parted.

Lips. Press your lips and front teeth together, then relax.

Neck. Press your head into the bed or the back of the chair, then relax. Move your chin to your chest. As you relax, let your head return to a comfortable position.

Shoulders. Shrug your shoulders up toward your ears as far as is comfortable. As you release, note the relaxation you feel in your neck.

Abdomen. Pull your navel in toward your backbone, then relax.

Buttocks. Squeeze your buttocks together, then relax.

Thighs. Push your heels against the floor or bed, then relax.

Shins. Raise your toes off the bed or floor, then relax.

Calves and feet. Point your toes hard, then relax.

Use imagery to erase tension. Perhaps you can't physically escape to a beautiful, peaceful place whenever stress rears its ugly head. But if you can *imagine* such a place—including all the sights, sounds, smells, and even the temperature— you can experience it. The scenario you choose is up to you. Here's one example.

Picture yourself on a mountaintop surrounded by lush tropical vegetation but open to the sky, so

Stress and Your Blood Sugar

Studies find that stress affects blood sugar differently from one person to the next. How do your sugar levels change when you're all charged up? To find out, each time you check your glucose level, rate how stressed you feel at that moment on a scale of 1 to 10, with 1 being a sunny day at the beach and 10 being just about he worst day of your life. Write the number down next to your reading. After two weeks, look at the numbers together (plotting them on a graph can help) to see how much your blood sugar swings in response to various levels of stress. If yours shoots up in response to stress, take the tips in this chapter seriously and make an extra effort to follow them.

you're bathed in sunlight. Note the deep blue color of the sky, feel the sun's rays soothing your body, smell the fragrance of the flowers all around, and hear the patter of drops falling off leaves after a recent rain. Look far below and see the shore of a tranquil beach on a placid lake. Take yourself to the shore of the lake and imagine walking along the soft sand. You're completely alone, but you find a boat tied to a dock. After untying the mooring rope, lie down on soft blankets inside the boat and watch the clouds as you drift on the calm water. The boat rocks gently, and waves gurgle under the hull as you drink in the warmth and feel the soft movement of a breeze. You feel a deep sense of relaxation as you drift between the water and the clouds.

Breathe in serenity, breathe out tension. A simple meditation that focuses on your breath can melt stress in as little as three to five minutes. Sit quietly with your feet flat on the floor and your back supported (don't slump). Close your eyes. Inhale slowly, feeling the air move through your mouth or nose and your abdomen filling up. Pause for a second or two, then exhale slowly. When your mind wanders (and it will!), gently direct your attention back to your breathing. This is a shortened version of mindfulness-based stress reduction, a meditation technique proven (when practiced for longer periods of time every day) to improve long-term blood sugar levels in one Duke University study.

STEP TWO
Use Movement to Relax

One of the most effective ways to defuse stress is to run away from it—or at least walk briskly. In one study that asked 38 men and 35 women to keep diaries of their activity, mood, and stress, volunteers reported that they felt less anxious on days when they were physically active than on days when they didn't exercise. Even when stressful events occurred, people in the study said they felt less troubled on their physically active days.

Turn your workouts into stress reducers. Virtually any kind of physical activity seems to relieve stress, although some researchers think that activities that involve repetitive movements—walking, running, cycling, or swimming, for instance—may offer the best defense. Many people consider swimming to be one of the most relaxing exercises, a soothing way to literally go with the flow. Repeating a physical movement over and over again somehow seems to ease mind and body.

Think about some ways to make your workout even more relaxing. If you're a walker, be aware of the way your arms swing from front to back and the rhythm of your gait. Repeat a soothing word or phrase each time you exhale. If you work out on

an exercise cycle or stair machine at a fitness club, ignore what's on the big TV screen in the room. Scientists have found that watching television makes people more jittery, not less. If you can't turn off the TV, look elsewhere and focus on your breathing, or plug yourself into some soothing music.

Discover yoga. Looking for a simple way to relax, refresh your energy, become more limber, and strengthen muscles at the same time? Yoga may be just the ticket. Exercise scientists have long known that yoga offers a great way to stretch, increase strength, and improve balance. Now psychologists are discovering it can also ease a troubled mind. At Oxford University, a researcher divided 71 men and women into three groups. One group practiced simple relaxation techniques like deep breathing. The second visualized themselves feeling less tense. The third did a half-hour yoga routine.

The relaxers and the visualizers felt sluggish afterward. The people in the yoga group reported feeling more energetic and emotionally content after their class.

How to get started? Several of the stretches you'll find in this section are based on yoga positions. If you find that you like doing these stretches, you may want to sign up for a yoga class at a local fitness center or yoga studio.

Establish a daily stretching routine. Stretching isn't just relaxing; it's also great for your whole body. Get in the habit of spending just 5 or 10 minutes stretching in the evenings, and you may find yourself sleeping better before you know it—and craving your stretches the next day. Try the stretches starting on the next page.

The *Reverse Diabetes* Stretching Routine

This series of 10 stretches takes just 5 to 10 minutes to complete and will make you feel as if a world-class massage therapist has just kneaded the tension out of every muscle in your body!

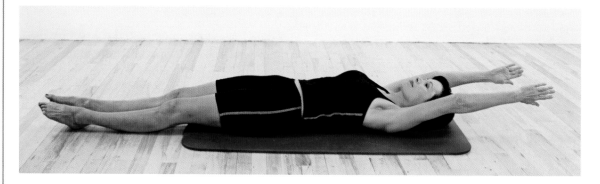

Lying Total Body Stretch

This stretch feels great and expands your whole body. It's particularly good for shoulders and abdominal muscles.

ONE Lie on your back with your legs extended and feet together or about hip-width apart.

TWO Extend your arms straight over your head and stretch your legs and toes, making your entire body as long as comfortably possible. Hold.

smart tip Take a deep breath before you begin the stretch, and exhale as you extend your hands and feet, then breathe normally as you hold, which enhances the stretch. Don't hold your breath; this prevents the abdominal muscles from relaxing.

Cross-Legged Seated Stretch

Sit up now for this soothing, classic back stretch, often used in yoga routines. It's great for lower back tension.

ONE Sit on the floor with your legs crossed and hands in front of you. Lean forward gently with your head down, rounding your back and "walking" your fingers forward until you feel a stretch in your lower and middle back. Hold.

TWO Walk your hands back to your legs and return to the starting position.

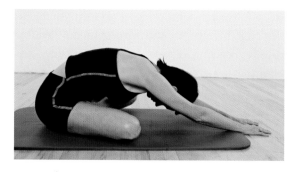

smart tip For a balanced stretch to both sides of the back, do this exercise twice, switching the leg that is crossed over the top.

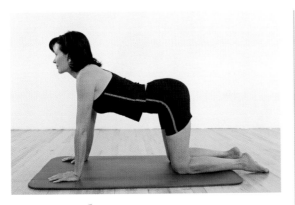

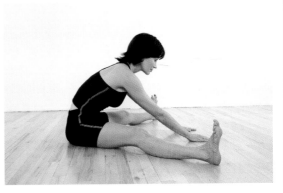

Cat Stretch

Pull yourself forward onto your hands and knees for another great stretch for your back.

ONE Get on your hands and knees. Tuck your chin toward your chest, and tighten your stomach muscles to arch your back. Hold.

TWO Relax, raising your head so you're looking straight ahead while letting your stomach drop toward the floor. Hold.

Seated V

This exercise lengthens the adductor muscles of the groin area in the inner thigh.

ONE Sit on the floor, back straight, legs extended, toes pointed toward the ceiling, and feet spread comfortably apart in a V.

TWO Keeping your back straight, gently "walk" your hands out in front of you until you feel a slight stretch in your inner thighs. Hold.

smart tip Use this position for a hamstring stretch by putting your left hand on the inside of your right thigh and the right hand on the outside, then moving both hands down your leg. Hold. Repeat on the left leg.

Lying Pelvis Rotation

Relax onto the ground for this gentle torso stretch. It uses gravity to stretch the abductor muscles on the outside of the hip.

ONE Lie on your right side, using your right arm as a pillow to support your head. Keeping your right leg straight, bend your left hip at a 90-degree angle so your knee is in front of you.

TWO Relax the muscles of your left leg so that your left knee slowly drops toward the ground. Stay relaxed and hold. Repeat with the other leg.

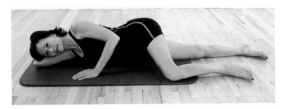

smart tip When you're more limber, try this variation: Lie on your back with your knees bent and your feet flat on floor. Keeping your shoulders on the ground, slowly lower both knees to the right to get a stretch in left hip and buttocks. Hold, return to the starting position. Repeat on the other side.

continued >>>

151

Calf Stretch

Popular with runners, this stretch is ideal for anyone who walks a lot, as you're doing on the Move plan.

ONE Stand with toes of both feet about 12 to 18 inches from a wall.

TWO Supporting yourself against the wall with one or both hands, take a big step back with your right foot, keeping your left foot in place.

THREE Bending your left knee, keep your right leg straight with your heel flat on the ground to produce a gentle tug at the back of your lower leg. Hold and return to the starting position. Repeat on the other side.

smart tip Move your hips forward to increase the stretch.

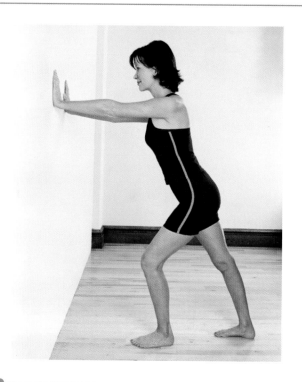

Forearm Flip

This stretch works muscles in your forearms that can hold tension after a day of typing or housework.

ONE Stand straight with your feet hip-width apart and knees slightly bent, arms hanging by your sides. Bend your elbows to 90 degrees with your palms facing upward as if you're holding a tray.

TWO Smoothly flip your hands over so the palms are facing the floor. Hold and return to the start position.

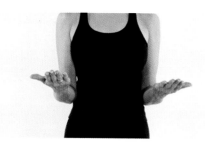

Knuckle Rub

Now it's on to your upper body to work out tension in your shoulder and neck muscles.

ONE Stand up straight with feet hip-width apart and knees slightly bent, hands down by your sides. Make a fist and, with knuckles facing forward, move your hands behind you and place them against your lower back.

TWO Gently move your knuckles up your back until you feel a stretch in the front part of your shoulder and your upper arms. Hold.

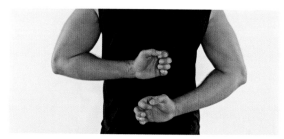

"Say Hello" Shoulder Stretch

Say hello to the world with this soothing shoulder stretch.

ONE Stand straight with your feet hip-width apart and knees slightly bent, arms hanging down and hands on the front part of the opposite thigh.

TWO Keeping your arms extended, lift your hands in a sideways and upward motion as high over your head as you can. Hold for one second and return to the starting position. Do 6 repetitions.

smart tip Breathe in as you slowly lift your arms, and exhale as you return; this helps you establish a rhythm and trains you to breathe more deeply.

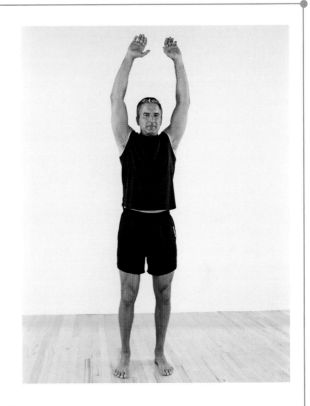

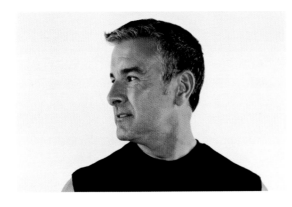

Neck Turn

If your neck is sensitive or in pain, do this exercise lying down to lessen the pressure.

ONE Sit or stand up straight with your eyes looking directly ahead.

TWO Slowly and smoothly move your head to the right side until you feel a slight stretch in the muscles on the opposite side of your neck. Relax and hold. Slowly return to the starting position and repeat on the other side.

Hold each stretch for 10 to 15 seconds. That's how long it usually takes for a muscle to relax and stay relaxed.

STEP THREE

Master an Instant Anxiety-Buster

There's big stress—moving, losing a job, getting divorced. Then there's nuisance stress—the daily stuff that can keep your anxiety level boiling all day if you let it. Fortunately, you don't have to let everyday living get your goat. By mastering a couple of instant tension-tamers you can head off stress before it gets a grip on your mind and body. All of these strategies work. Find two or three that seem to fit you best, then test-drive them for a few days to see if they melt the nuisance tensions in your life.

Force a smile. Studies show that the physical act of smiling—even if you don't really mean it—causes chemical changes in your body associated with happiness.

Count your blessings. Write down 5 or 10 things that make you happy or thankful—friends, a beloved pet, a roof over your head, a sunny day—and reflect on each of them for a minute.

Get a massage. Massages not only relieve muscle tension, they trigger the release of serotonin, a brain chemical associated with a feeling of well-being, and reduce levels of the stress hormone cortisol. Bonus: Lowering your stress hormones may even lower your blood sugar. If you can't get a massage from a professional, ask your partner to rub your shoulders, or rub your own feet.

Sniff a scent. Scents have an amazing impact on your mood. Sprinkle a few drops of an essential oil such as lavender, ylang-ylang, eucalyptus, sandalwood, or rose on a tissue or handkerchief and inhale the scent. If you don't have any essential oil, sniff a flower, light a scented candle, or brew a cup of peppermint tea and breathe in the steam.

Put on a great song. Whether it's soothing classical music, soulful blues, cool jazz, or rousing rock and roll, music can change your mood faster than you can say "feeling groovy" or "here comes the sun."

See molehills, not mountains. When something goes wrong, ask yourself whether it's really a big deal. Will you remember it years from now? What's the worst thing that can happen as a result? Is it likely to happen?

Think of your children or your pet. Sometimes diverting your thoughts momentarily to those who love you, who matter more, who bring you pleasure, helps you instantly put things in perspective during very stressful moments.

Play with a dog. Playing with a dog for just a few minutes raises levels of the brain chemicals serotonin and oxytocin—both mood elevators. You don't need to own a dog to experience these feel-good effects. Your neighbor's dog would probably love the attention. Or stop by your local pet store. Who knows? You may even end up taking a pooch or kitty home.

Post a stop sign in your brain. When you catch yourself in the midst of stressful thinking, shout "Stop!" to yourself and picture a stop sign. Replace the distressing thought with another thought that's more positive and rational. For example, if the stressful thought is, "I can't do this; I'm worthless," instead say to yourself, "There are many valuable things I can do."

Buy yourself flowers. If you'd buy them for someone else, why not for yourself? You're worth it! Put them on your desk or table to put a little joy in your heart.

GOAL 3

Keep your motivation stoked

DIABETES IS A CHRONIC CONDITION, something you have to live with for the rest of your life (though you *can* reverse both of the core problems behind it—insulin resistance and lack of insulin secretion—by following the Eat, Move, Choose Plan). It requires daily attention, which can seem burdensome. But a key fact to remember is this: The better you take care of yourself, the less likely you are to experience the complications that account for most of the suffering that goes with diabetes.

STEP ONE
Find Ways to Stay Inspired

These tips will help you maintain the emotional energy and commitment to stay in control of your diabetes.

Remind yourself that when it comes to blood sugar, better control equals a better life. One study, published in the *Journal of the American Medical Association,* compared quality of life in people with diabetes who had good blood sugar control with peers who didn't. Those with good control had milder symptoms, felt better, and were more likely to feel mentally sharp than the other group. As a result, they tended to be more productive and less restricted in every aspect of life. Don't you want to be one of those people?

Know what's at stake. An estimated three out of five people with diabetes have one or more complications associated with the disease, ranging from heart disease to vision loss to nerve pain to kidney damage. The key to avoiding complications is keeping your blood sugar levels in check—which the Eat, Move, Choose Plan will help you do. Stick with it and you'll see results—we promise!

that's easy!

Feeling burned out or downright depressed? Take a short walk. Numerous studies show that regular exercise improves depression. In one, getting 30 minutes of moderately intense activity three times a week for four months was as effective as antidepressant medication. (If you have depression and take medication, a walk is a great add-on therapy.) A single walk can boost your mood and give you motivation to do it again tomorrow.

Choose to fight. We didn't call it the Choose plan for nothing! Remember that diabetes is very manageable and that most aspects of diabetes management are under your direct control. Don't accept complications or worsening blood sugar as inevitabilities—even if friends or relatives with diabetes have suffered serious diabetes-related complications. It doesn't have to happen to you.

Visualize success. Thinking about your dreams and aspirations for the future can help stoke the fire that keeps your motivation strong. Sit down, close your eyes, and imagine what you want to be doing in the future. Do you want to be alive and healthy in 20 years to enjoy your grandchildren? In 10 years for a healthy, active retirement? In five years, so that you can start a family or enjoy the one you have?

Spend five minutes in the morning planning your day. Over your morning coffee or tea, use a paper and pen to write out your intentions and action plan for the day. When will you fit in a daily walk? Have you packed a healthy lunch? If not, what's the plan for buying one? If there's a hectic day ahead, how will you stay calm? Feeling in control is a great way to stay motivated.

Recognize your successes. In the Planner section we've even given you a place to write them down at the end of every week. When you have

that's easy! ←

When life with diabetes starts to get you down, talk about it with a friend, relative, or your spouse. Ask first if he or she would mind listening, and reassure your trusted companion that you're not asking for answers. Just an open ear can work wonders. In fact, studies show that a supportive spouse can help you keep your blood sugar under better control.

diabetes, signs that you're managing it well go beyond your blood sugar numbers. Include any of these in your mental "success log": lower blood sugar peaks, fewer episodes of hypoglycemia, improved cholesterol levels, lower blood pressure, greater energy, better-fitting clothes, better sleep, and improved moods.

STEP TWO
Battle Diabetes Burnout

Over time, a creeping sense of fatigue and frustration can set in when you have diabetes—what some experts call "diabetes burnout." When you're burned out, you may not feel outright depressed, just sick and tired of what can seem like a never-ending grind. Even though burnout won't directly cause physical changes in the body, feeling frustrated—often because you may sense that you're not making progress against your disease—can have an impact on your health. You may start to slack off your diet, exercise, drug regimen, or blood-sugar monitoring. Of course, by following the Eat, Move, Choose Plan you *will* see results, and your diabetes should seem much more manageable. But if you do start to feel a bit defeated at any point, use these tips to get yourself back on track.

Define yourself as a person first. You're a person with diabetes, not a diabetic. The difference is crucial, because it means diabetes is just part of your life—a life in which there's so much more going on that's wonderful and positive. View diabetes as you would being nearsighted. It's something you must account for, but it doesn't define who you are.

Talk with your doctor or certified diabetes educator. Your doctor may be able to make adjustments in your treatment—fewer shots using different combinations of insulin, for example—to ease your burden. And a certified diabetes educator will be able to suggest specific strategies for dealing with issues that are challenging you and help you understand why you're not seeing better results.

Evaluate your progress. Maybe you haven't made as much progress as you would like—or perhaps you're making terrific progress but just feel tired from all the effort. Be objective about what you have accomplished. How has your blood sugar control improved? How about your weight or your overall fitness? Have you managed to be disciplined about testing and taking medication? You may find that you've done better than you give yourself credit for. On the other hand, your frustration may be a good sign: It means you actually are motivated to do better.

Identify specific problem areas. You may have more success with some areas of the Eat, Move, Choose Plan, or with your overall diabetes care,

than with others. But don't let weakness or lack of progress in one area color the entire picture. Instead, try to isolate the aspects of your care with which you have the most trouble. Is it a challenge to control your appetite? Are you forgetting to take your medication or insulin? Is finding time for exercise a constant battle? Once you isolate the problem you can work on finding a solution. For instance, can't seem to get out for your walks? Many malls have walking clubs that encourage people to step out in their climate-controlled, security-patrolled, bathroom-equipped corridors. Call your local mall to see if it has a club.

Join a support group, in person or online. You're not in this battle alone. Talk to other people with diabetes for perspective, ideas, and encouragement. Ask your doctor or diabetes educator to recommend a local support group, or find an Internet chat group. The American Diabetes Association (www.diabetes.org) and the renowned Joslin Diabetes Center (www.joslin.org) both run online diabetes support groups.

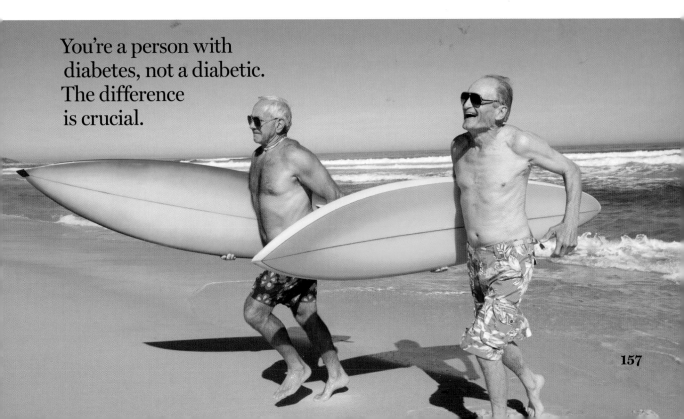

You're a person with diabetes, not a diabetic. The difference is crucial.

157

GOAL 4

Nurture resilience

IT'S ONE THING to feel happy on a carefree Saturday morning in the summer, when the sun is shining, the birds are singing, and you haven't a care in the world. It's quite another to remain joyful, content, and upbeat on a slushy winter day when your car's broken down, your blood sugar is too high, there's little time for exercise or choosing healthy foods, or you haven't quite reached the goals you've set for yourself.

That's when you need resilience, the ability to deal with life's curveballs and challenges. It's a trait anyone can cultivate—and one that helps people with diabetes to thrive. In one recent University of Texas at Austin study of people with type 2 diabetes, those who took weekly resilience-training classes for just one month saw improvements in their cholesterol levels, blood pressure, and fasting blood sugar levels—and they felt less stressed.

Researchers have identified four common traits of resilient people, traits that this chapter will help you develop:

- Seeing a challenge as an opportunity, not a threat.
- Having a strong value system to guide their decisions and actions.
- Being genuinely committed to the people in their lives and activities in which they're involved.

- Feeling a sense of control and believing they have the power to make things better.

Even if you're on the low end of the resiliency scale now, you can take steps today to build your inner resiliency. The following tips provide a good start.

STEP ONE
Cultivate a Positive Attitude

How do resilient people meet challenges? They draw on the strengths in their lives to build a positive, optimistic attitude. These include friendship, gratitude, self-confidence, and more. These tips can help you identify and "grow" these building blocks for yourself.

View diabetes as a blessing in disguise. Some people who've managed their diabetes well say they are healthier now than they were before their diagnoses; that the disease helped them "get their priorities straight." They have better habits and happier lives, and they're enjoying brighter moods, greater energy, and a stronger sense of personal control. You can, too, and it may take less effort than you think.

Focus on the reasons you'll succeed in managing your diabetes. You're a competent person who's succeeded in other ways in life. And you're on track for success with diabetes, too. The reasons? We know there are many. They may include the fact that you're eating better, exercising, reducing stress, working with your doctor on the best dosages of your medications, checking your blood sugar regularly, and getting plenty of sleep.

Say no to your inner critic. When negative thoughts threaten to drag you into darkness, fight back. If you hear your inner skeptic saying that you'll never lose weight or improve your blood sugar control, tell yourself NO! in a firm, commanding voice. Say it out loud if possible. Sometimes this is all it takes to stop nagging, negative thoughts from snowballing into a defeatist attitude.

Now insert a positive message. Once you've stopped your internal naysayer, it's time to replace gloomy thoughts with realistic, positive ones. Counter a thought like "I'll never change" with something objective, specific, and fair to yourself, such as, "I always eat a healthy breakfast now," or "I lost a pound last week." And look for other causes

for critical thinking, such as low blood sugar. Test yourself and have a snack if necessary.

Evoke feelings of love. Do something each day to bring a sustained, loving smile to your face. Download a couple of great photos of your kids when they were toddlers to your computer and call them up when you need a break. Provide hugs galore to your spouse. Listen to some classic Sinatra love songs. Don't want to leave this to chance? Try something called the loving-kindness meditation, which you can do anywhere. Simply:

- Take a break from what you're doing and focus on your heart.
- Recall an experience during which you felt happiness, love, and appreciation.
- Breathe deeply and feel your heart lighten as you re-experience those feelings.

List your strengths. This could be everything from your ability to interact with anyone at any time to your talent for baking. Don't do this on your

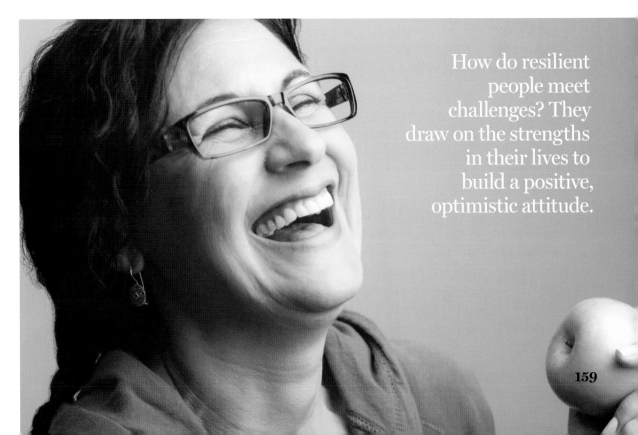

How do resilient people meet challenges? They draw on the strengths in their lives to build a positive, optimistic attitude.

159

own; ask people who know you well to contribute to the list. Becoming aware of your strengths is like putting money into the resilience bank. When it's time for a withdrawal, you'll know just how much you have to use.

Manage your expectations. Don't expect that every aspect of managing your health, or your life, will always go perfectly; it won't. For instance, if you expect everything to be smooth when you travel by airplane these days, you're setting yourself up for disappointment. Instead, anticipate delays and lost luggage; bring extra reading material or playing cards, and don't put anything you can't live without—especially your diabetes medications—in your checked luggage.

Pinch yourself every time you hear yourself using words like "never" and "always." As in, "I always seem to eat foods I shouldn't" or "I'm never going to get my blood sugar under control or lose weight." Such thinking leads to a black-and-white, all-or-nothing defeatist mentality that's sure to make you stumble in your efforts to Eat, Move, and Choose to reverse diabetes. If you mess up one day, forgive yourself. Remind yourself that everyone's human and that at least you're trying. Then vow to do better tomorrow!

Set daily goals. You need a sense of accomplishment every day to strengthen your own belief in yourself. These goals could be small—eating one extra vegetable serving, going to bed 15 minutes earlier—but don't worry, they'll add up. And remember that success often breeds more success.

Have fun! When is the last time you had fun? If a recent memory doesn't pop into your mind, it's time to ink some fun onto your calendar. It doesn't have to be elaborate, just something you look forward to. Once a week, set up a golf date, rent a funny movie, or take your kids or grandkids to the park. You'll feel less bogged down by daily life if you regularly reward yourself with good times.

Maintain Your Sense of Humor

A sense of humor is part of the resiliency toolbox. And when it comes to your blood sugar, laughter is good medicine, too. That's the conclusion drawn by scientists at the University of Tsukuba in Japan who kept tabs on the blood sugar levels of 19 men and women with high blood sugar after they attended two radically different events: a boring lecture and a hilarious comedy show. The study was published in the journal *Diabetes Care*.

Before both events, volunteers each ate a 500-calorie meal. Afterward, their blood sugar was tested. Sugar levels were significantly lower after the comedy. Why is mirth magic for your sugar levels? Laughter makes us move (ever try to sit perfectly still while you laugh? Impossible!)—and muscle cells absorb more blood sugar when they're active, the researchers speculate. Comic relief may also influence hormones that play a role in blood sugar absorption.

Of course, having a sense of humor also makes it far easier to sail through the ups and downs of daily life. It vaporizes fear, relaxes your mind and body, helps you keep things in perspective, and gives you an outlet for negative emotions. It might even help you lose weight!

Watch a comedy instead of a tearjerker. University of Mississippi researchers have found that study volunteers munched 30 percent more buttered popcorn while watching the classic romance *Love Story* compared to when they guffawed their way through the comedy *Sweet Home Alabama*. So put comedies at the top of your list when you're heading to the video store or choosing a movie on TV or online. These 10 top the American Film Institute's list of the 100 Funniest Films: *Some Like It Hot, Tootsie, Dr. Strangelove, Annie Hall, Duck Soup, Blazing Saddles, M*A*S*H, It Happened One Night, The Graduate,* and *Airplane!*

Call your funniest friend. Everybody has someone who makes them laugh. Keep your funniest pal's phone number on speed dial so you can chat regularly—both of you will get a boost.

Choose funny books. Act like a kid at the library or bookstore and head for the humor section instead of the serious literature. Stock up on a few by your favorite humor writers, such as Dave Barry or David Sedaris. Or try a few authors you've never read before. Not only will you get a few laughs, you'll also get an education in seeing the hilarious side of things that would normally frustrate or upset you.

Laugh at your foibles. Finding humor in your own life doesn't mean laughing at who you are. It means finding the funny side of what you're doing, what you're thinking, or what's happening *to* you. Did you get lost on your walk when exploring a new neighborhood? Silly you! But hey, it made you walk a few extra blocks—so you benefited in the end.

Anytime something annoying occurs, turn it on its head and find the humor. Sure, if you took the trouble to pack your lunch and then left it on the kitchen table, that's annoying. You could get mad—but it doesn't accomplish anything other than to put you in a sour mood. Instead, chuckle at your own feeble-mindedness for just a second, then pretend your lunch has a life of its own back home. Imagine the grapes dancing across the table and the sandwich meat fighting with the lettuce.

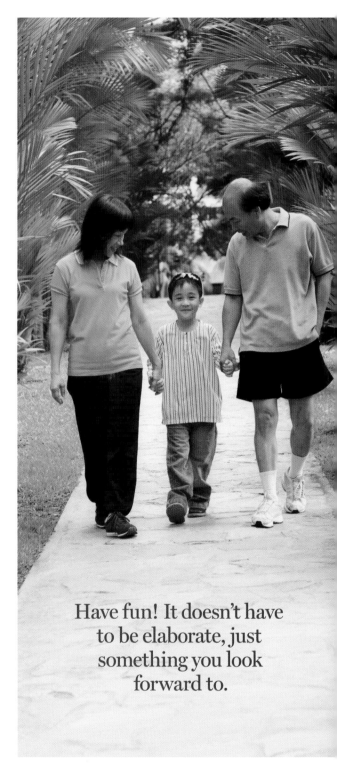

Have fun! It doesn't have to be elaborate, just something you look forward to.

When a person offends you or makes you angry, respond with humor rather than hostility. For instance, if someone is always late, say, "Well, I'm glad you're not running an airline." Life is too short to turn every personal affront into a battle. If you are constantly offended by someone in particular, yes, take it seriously and take appropriate action. But for occasional troubles, or if nothing you do can change the person or situation, take the humor response.

Cultivate the humor habit. Have a ha-ha bulletin board where you post funny sayings or signs. Every night at dinner, ask family members to share one funny moment of their day. Develop a silly routine to break a dark mood. It could be something as silly as speaking in a crazy accent, doing a little dance, or repeating a funny punch line from a movie or TV show that always cracks you up. And add an item to your daily to-do list: Find something humorous. Don't mark it off until you do it.

STEP THREE
Deal with Depression

More than a passing bad mood, depression interferes with your life, your relationships, your sense of yourself, and your health. Often, people with diabetes are also battling this mental health challenge—and researchers are still trying to figure out whether diabetes leads to depression or depression leads to diabetes. They do know this: Up to 30 percent of people with diabetes also have depression—a rate three times higher than for people who do not have diabetes. That's dangerous because depression doesn't just affect you emotionally by making life miserable and sapping your motivation to take care of yourself; people who feel chronically blue also tend to have higher blood pressure and are more prone to heart disease than others.

While building resiliency may help you lower your risk for depression, it's important to watch out for signs of depression, understand when it's time to seek help, and know what you can do on your own (*not* in place of seeing your doctor).

Recognize the symptoms. How do you know if you're just feeling blue or if you're truly depressed? After all, everybody has a day or two when they feel some sadness. Maybe you're a little under the weather; maybe something unpleasant happened. While these feelings tend to be temporary, depression, on the other hand, drags on for weeks or months. It affects your mood, thoughts, and even physical body, including the way you eat and sleep. If you have several of these symptoms for two weeks or more, make an appointment to see your doctor.

If you're depressed, repeat this sentence: *I deserve to feel better.* The trouble is, most people with depression aren't getting the help they need. Thanks to punishing and flat-out wrong beliefs that this mental health problem is a sign of weak-

Is It Depression?

Some classic symptoms of the condition are:

- ▶ Feelings of sadness, emptiness, or worthlessness
- ▶ Difficulty concentrating
- ▶ Short-term memory loss
- ▶ Pessimism
- ▶ Loss of enjoyment of activities you once found pleasurable
- ▶ Fatigue
- ▶ Irritability or agitation
- ▶ Changes in appetite
- ▶ Lack of sexual desire
- ▶ Difficulty sleeping

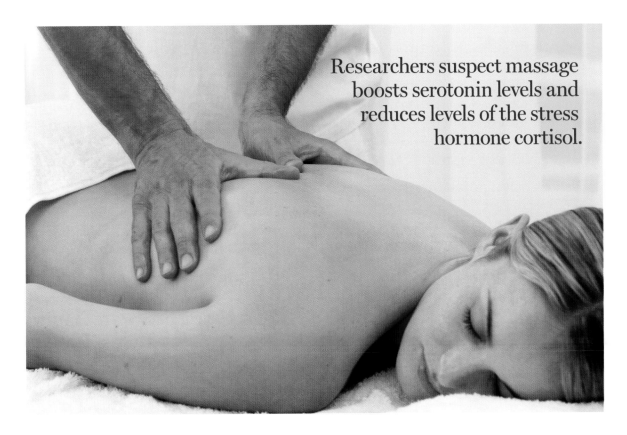

Researchers suspect massage boosts serotonin levels and reduces levels of the stress hormone cortisol.

ness (or something you can "tough out" on your own) and to doctors who don't always check or treat depression, millions of us slog along on our own. If that sounds like you or someone you know, stop now. Call your doctor, ask for an evaluation, and sign up for treatment. No one should go through life feeling sad and hopeless. There's just too much at stake.

Be patient with treatment. Nearly 70 percent of the 3,700 people in a recent landmark study of depression treatments eventually felt as good as new. Just 37 percent got there with the first treatment they tried (an antidepressant). What eventually worked? For some, a combination of two drugs. For others, therapy was the turning point. You won't know what works for you until you try—and try again.

Have high expectations. Expect to feel completely better. If you have lingering down times after giving a therapy a good try (usually 8 to 12 weeks), talk to your doctor again about what else she can do to help you.

Be persistent. Plenty of people stop taking antidepressants or going to therapy as soon as they begin to feel better. But many relapse. The reason: A single episode of depression can last for 9 to 12 months. Stopping early leaves you vulnerable. Stick with the treatment that's making your life better. If you think you're ready to go it alone, talk with your doctor about the best way to taper off a drug and how to decide whether you need to resume treatment.

Spend at least an hour each week with a close friend. In a British study, when 86 depressed women were paired with a volunteer friend, 65 percent of the women felt better. In fact, regular social contact worked as effectively as antidepressant medication and psychotherapy. Spending time regularly with a close friend may boost your self-confidence and encourage you to make other positive changes that will help lift depression, such as starting an exercise program.

Get a quick massage three times a week. Ask your spouse to do it or get one from the masseuses you sometimes see at the mall or at your nail salon. It doesn't have to cost a lot. In a study of depressed dialysis patients, participants who received a 12-minute massage three times a week were less depressed than those who didn't get the soothing rub. Another study of 84 depressed pregnant women found those who received two 20-minute massages a week from their partners reduced their incidence of depression 70 percent. Researchers suspect massage boosts serotonin levels (which jumped 17 percent in the women who received twice-weekly massages) and reduces levels of the stress hormone cortisol.

Exercise! A study of older adults found 10 weeks of regular exercise was 20 percent more effective at reducing depressive symptoms than medication. However, because depression may make you want to do anything but exercise, many physicians recommend combining the two treatments.

Take a 10-minute walk three times a day during the winter. Many people feel depressed during the winter months, when they travel to and from work in darkness and don't get enough natural sunlight. Physical exercise encourages the release of hormones and neurochemicals that boost mood. Walking outside during the day will give you a few short doses of sunlight, also shown to boost mood, particularly in the winter.

Invest in a light box for winter depression. Bright light therapy has been shown to relieve depression, especially seasonal affective disorder, a type of depression some people experience during the winter months when sunlight is in short supply. The therapy involves sitting in front of a specially designed light box shortly after waking each morning for 20 minutes to an hour. You can purchase a light box for home use. They range in price from $200 to $400.

Eat seafood at least twice a week. A Dutch study found that people who consume diets rich in omega-3 fatty acids, a type of fat found in cold-water fish such as salmon and mackerel, were less likely to suffer from depression than people whose diets were low in this important fat. Another study, this one conducted in England, found that pregnant women who didn't eat fish had twice the rate of depression as women who ate 10 ounces of fish a day. In fact, one reason researchers think the rate of depression has skyrocketed in this country is that we get so few omega-3 fatty acids in our diets. If you don't like fish, take enough fish oil capsules to get 1,000 milligrams of the omega-3s called DHA and EPA (they're on the label) once or twice a day. Talk with your doctor first.

GOAL 5

Plan ahead for sick days and travel

EVEN THE BEST diabetes management can be temporarily thrown off course by two special circumstances: illness and travel. Both can alter your eating habits and make it more difficult to take medications at the right times, and both pose special threats that can either raise your blood sugar or subject you to hypoglycemia. Planning ahead will help you take good care of yourself should either one arise. Here's what you need to know and to do.

STEP ONE
Have a Sick-Day Strategy

Being sick is no fun for anyone, but it takes a special toll if you have diabetes because it can throw off your blood sugar and put you at risk for short-term complications. The best way to deal with sick days is to plan for them before you're laid up. Speak with your primary-care physician, endocrinologist, and dietitian to work out the details of a strategy you can put into action the next time a cold, the flu, or something else strikes.

Illness is a form of stress that—like emotional stress—rouses the body's defenses. One effect is that the liver steps up glucose production to provide more energy. At the same time, stress hormones are released that make cells more insulin resistant. The net result is that blood sugar can rise dramatically when you're ill. To keep your blood sugar in check and help yourself feel better faster, follow these steps.

Step up your monitoring. It's more important than ever to keep careful track of your blood sugar levels, so you'll probably need to test yourself more often than you usually do—at least every three to four hours. If your blood sugar goes higher than 240 mg/dl, do a urine ketone test as well. If ketone results are positive, or if your blood sugar consistently hovers above 240, call your doctor.

Talk to your doctor. Call the doctor's office if you're unable to eat, have diarrhea, have been vomiting for more than six hours, have a fever that's not improving, or have flushed skin for more than two days. Know the signs of ketoacidosis (which include stomach pain, vomiting, chest

165

pain, difficulty breathing, feelings of weakness, sleepiness, fruity-smelling breath, blurry vision) and of dehydration (extreme thirst, dry mouth, cracked lips, sunken eyes, mental confusion, dry skin). Call your doctor right away if you experience symptoms of either of these conditions.

Stock up on sick-day foods in advance. Even if you don't have an appetite, it's important to eat regularly to keep your blood sugar steady. Start with foods that are already part of your healthy diet, such as oatmeal, chicken soup, applesauce, or toast. Keep a supply of broth-based soups, along with saltine-type crackers.

Get plenty of fluids. This familiar advice is doubly critical when you have diabetes because water is drawn into excess glucose and excreted in the urine, which can cause dehydration. Aim to drink a cup of fluid (which includes soup broth) every half hour or so. If lack of appetite is making it difficult for you to consume enough food to meet your energy needs, sip sugared drinks like non-diet soda, fruit juices, or sports beverages instead of plain water to make sure you're getting at least some calories into your body.

Stay the drug course. Unless your doctor instructs you otherwise, it's important to keep taking your medications or giving yourself insulin even if you're not up to eating. In fact, your doctor may want you to take more insulin when you're feeling under the weather, with the exact amounts depending on your blood sugar readings and how sick you are. Even if you have type 2 diabetes and don't normally take insulin, your doctor may want you to keep a vial of short-acting insulin on hand in case he thinks it's necessary when illness strikes.

Watch the OTC remedies. Some common over-the-counter medicines, such as decongestants with pseudoephedrine, can raise blood sugar. Check with your doctor before taking any drug, herbal remedy, or dietary supplement when you're ill.

Rest in bed. It isn't safe to exercise when you're sick, diabetes experts say. Instead, do your immune system and blood sugar a favor by dimming the lights and hopping into bed. It's a good idea to arrange in advance to have your spouse or a close friend or neighbor take over household responsibilities when you're sick, so that you can rest and recover. See if the kids can spend the evening with a neighbor (offer to reciprocate as soon as you can) and if your spouse can make dinner and do laundry.

that's easy! ←

Catching a plane involves a whole lot of hurry up and wait. While you're waiting to board your plane, use that spare half-hour to tool around the terminal rather than heading to the news-stand for an overpriced candy bar. If you combine the calories you'll burn moving your feet and the calories you save *not* chomping the chocolate, you'll end up a grand total of 420 calories behind where you would have been.

STEP TWO
Travel Safely with Diabetes

Planning a family vacation or business trip? There's no reason diabetes should hold you back from traveling, as long as you take some reasonable precautions to make sure that while you're getting away from it all, your blood sugar isn't. Your mantra is "Plan ahead." Let your doctor know your itinerary. Depending on how long you'll be gone, she may want to give you a thorough examination before you depart. And to ensure smooth sailing, heed the following advice.

Anticipate airport security. With the increased security at airports, expect your supplies to get a thorough once-over. The U.S. Transportation Security Administration (TSA), as of press time, allows you to board a plane with insulin, syringes, and insulin-delivery systems. It's okay to carry lancets on board as well, as long as they're capped and you also carry a glucose meter with a manufacturer's name printed on it. The American Diabetes Association recommends that you notify the screener at security checkpoints that you have diabetes and are carrying your supplies with you.

At press time, the TSA didn't require prescription labels or a doctor's letter, but it's a good idea to have prescription labels for your supplies and to be sure that nonprescription items essential for your diabetes care are also clearly labeled in original containers. It will make security screening faster. Be sure to call ahead for current policies before you leave or check the TSA Web site, www.tsa.gov.

Keep glucose goods close at hand. If you are traveling by plane, pack your medications, insulin, syringes, test strips, lancets, ketone strips, and other supplies in your carry-on bag so there's no chance of losing them. Consider bringing extra supplies in your checked luggage. Some experts recommend packing twice as much as you think you'll need—it's easier to carry extra than to get more on the road. Also ask your doctor if he wants to prescribe a glucagon kit, which contains an emergency dose of a hormone that someone with you can inject to make your liver pump out glucose if you have a hypoglycemic emergency that leaves you unable to swallow or makes you lose consciousness. Again, make sure all medications bear the original pharmacy prescription labels.

There's no reason diabetes should hold you back from traveling, as long as you take some reasonable precautions.

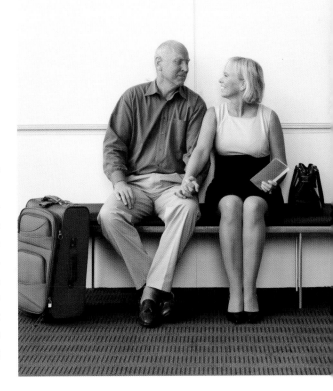

Bring extra prescriptions and a medication list, too. In case you do need to restock while you're away, have your doctor give you prescriptions for refills. It's also a good idea to have him provide a printout of all your medications in case you need to see a doctor while on the road.

Wear a medical-alert bracelet. If you don't already have one, get a medical ID bracelet or necklace that alerts people that you have diabetes and provides a number to call in an emergency.

Pack a snack. Wherever you go, take a tote-able snack like an apple, an energy bar, a banana, raisins, or cheese and crackers in case your blood sugar starts to dip when you don't have immediate access to other food. If you sample your snacks en route, replenish your supplies as soon as you can.

Maintain regular mealtimes. When traveling, try to stick to your regular mealtime schedule to keep your blood sugar stable. If that's not possible, carry glucose tablets along with you and be alert to symptoms of low blood sugar, such as nervousness, sweating, and crankiness. If you feel a hypoglycemic episode coming on, pull over and take several glucose tablets. Wait at least 10 to 15 minutes for the feeling to pass before continuing on.

Get in the zone. Traveling across different time zones can throw your normal insulin and meal schedule completely out of kilter, but you can compensate for the disruption if you're careful. When adding hours to your day by traveling west, you may need to take more insulin. When losing hours by traveling east, you may need less. Check with your doctor for specific recommendations. As for timing your injections and meals, keep your watch set to your home time as you travel to your destination, then switch your watch—and your schedule—to the local time the morning after you arrive.

Exercising on the Road

It's tough to stay physically active when traveling—but not impossible. Try to keep your body in gear by planning ahead and snatching opportunities as they arise:

▶ If your hotel doesn't have an exercise room or pool, bring along a jump rope or elastic resistance band so you can exercise in your room. Definitely pack your walking shoes, and ask at the front desk about where you can take a safe and scenic stroll.

▶ Pack comfortable "nice" clothes. If you're not attending a formal event, try to pack outfits that do double duty as walking gear and meeting or travel clothing. That way, you'll be able to seize small amounts of walking time with ease. Do the same for your feet, by bringing shoes you can wear to meetings and events and also walk in.

Organize for overseas. If you're traveling outside the country, be aware that insulin you find abroad may be sold in weaker strengths than the insulin available in the United States, which has standardized its insulin in a dose known as U-100. Each insulin strength (such as U-40 and U-80) requires specially matched syringes. Filling a different type of syringe with your U.S. insulin will make your dose inaccurate. Best bet: Stick to your own supplies. If you must buy insulin that's a different strength, also buy syringes to match.

Bring sunscreen. Certain diabetes drugs and blood pressure drugs make the skin more sensitive to the sun, so it's especially important that you protect yourself. A bad sunburn can even raise your blood sugar and may take longer to heal than it would for someone else. Choose a sunscreen that has an SPF of at least 15 and look for a "broad-spectrum" brand that protects against both UVA and UVB light. These often contain ingredients such as Mexoryl, Helioplex, zinc oxide, or avobenzone (aka Parsol 1789).

Pack two pairs of comfortable shoes. This way you can air out one pair while you tool around town in the other. Also bring a pair of brown or black closed-toe flats for dinners and other more formal occasions. All the shoes you bring should be broken in before your trip, so leave your new ones at home. If you're heading to the beach, bring aqua shoes. These stretchy-soled booties will protect your feet from hot sand, rough sidewalks around the pool, and sharp pebbles underfoot.

Put together a small foot-care kit. When you're traveling, you want to see and do everything you can in a short time. But zipping from vista to landmark not only can wear out your feet, it can make you susceptible to "hot spots" and blisters. Although they seem innocent enough, blisters can

sugar buster quiz

Q: Rub-on or spray-on sunscreen?

A: Spray-on.
Using a spray-on product will allow you to cover hard-to-reach spots like your legs, feet, and back.

lead to infections that can turn serious for someone with diabetes. To keep your feet feeling fine, fill a sandwich bag with several sheets of moleskin, several large and small adhesive bandages, and round-tipped scissors. As soon as you feel a hot spot developing, cut off a piece of moleskin that's large enough to cover the spot and stick it on. If you discover a full-fledged blister, cover it with a bandage.

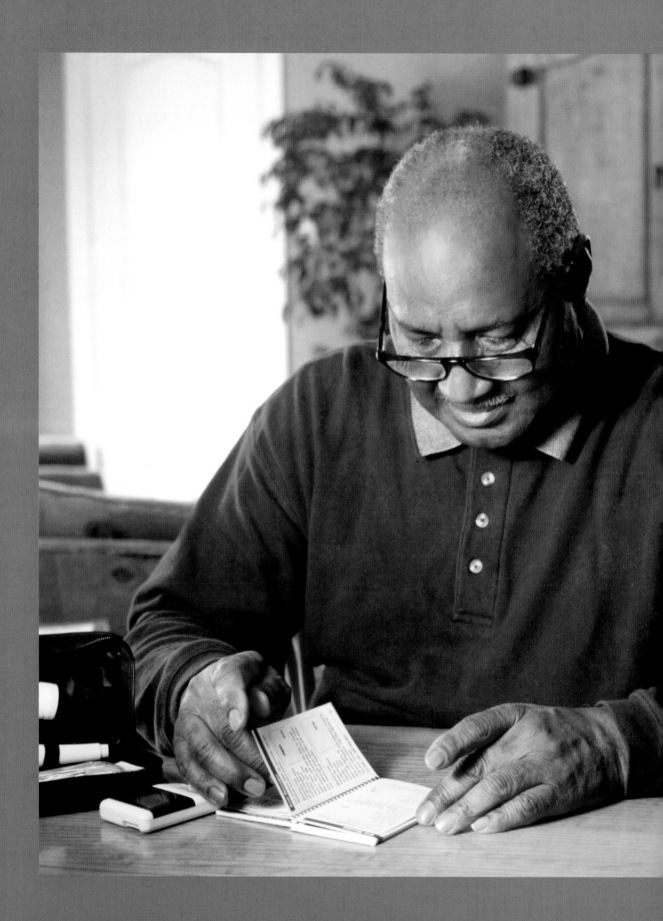

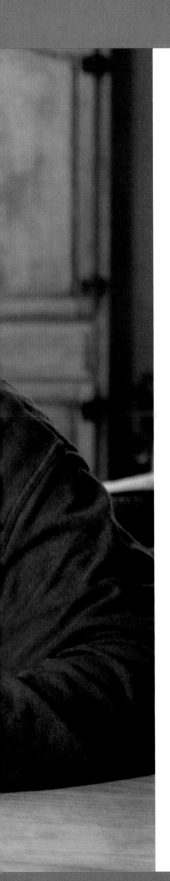

4

reverse diabetes
PLANNER

- Weekly Meal Planning
- Daily Progress Checks
- Successes and Confessions

- Better Health

week ❶ meal planner

The key to healthy eating is planning ahead. Plotting your dinners is most important. The trick is to find 8 or 10 healthy recipes you love (you may even want to keep a list on your refrigerator), then rotate them in.

If you don't mind leftovers, make extra and serve leftovers, either for lunch or dinner, at least once or twice a week. If you're planning to take leftovers for lunch, store them in single-serving containers so your lunch is ready to go when you are.

For other lunches, buy sliced turkey, whole-wheat bread or rolls, and a bag of pre-washed lettuce at the beginning of the week, and stock the pantry with cans of tuna fish and lentil or black bean soup.

monday	tuesday	wednesday
breakfast		
lunch		
dinner		

thursday	friday	saturday	sunday

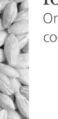

food fact
One cup of pearl barley (which doesn't require any soaking before cooking) has 10 grams of fiber, nearly half your daily target.

1 monday

My numbers:

weight _____

blood sugar (time/level) _____ / _____
_____ / _____ • _____ / _____

Servings I ate today:

vegetables 0 1 2 3 4 **5 6 7**
fruit 0 1 2 **3**
whole grains 0 1 2 3 **4 5 6**
calcium-rich foods 0 1 **2 3**

Times I ate out of boredom, stress, or habit:

0 1 2 3 4 5

How I took charge:

eat
☐ ate a healthy breakfast
☐ had protein at every meal
☐ avoided refined carbohydrates
  and sugary drinks
☐ swapped saturated fats for good fats

move
☐ walked _____ minutes / _____ steps
☐ performed Sugar Buster exercises
☐ got other exercise _____

choose
☐ got enough sleep (_____ hours)
☐ kept TV time under 2 hours
☐ found time for relaxation and/or socializing

My attitude today:

☐ excellent
☐ pretty good
☐ not my best day; I'll do better tomorrow

1 tuesday

My numbers:

weight _____

blood sugar (time/level) _____ / _____
_____ / _____ • _____ / _____

Servings I ate today:

vegetables 0 1 2 3 4 **5 6 7**
fruit 0 1 2 **3**
whole grains 0 1 2 3 **4 5 6**
calcium-rich foods 0 1 **2 3**

Times I ate out of boredom, stress, or habit:

0 1 2 3 4 5

How I took charge:

eat
☐ ate a healthy breakfast
☐ had protein at every meal
☐ avoided refined carbohydrates
  and sugary drinks
☐ swapped saturated fats for good fats

move
☐ walked _____ minutes / _____ steps
☐ performed Sugar Buster exercises
☐ got other exercise _____

choose
☐ got enough sleep (_____ hours)
☐ kept TV time under 2 hours
☐ found time for relaxation and/or socializing

My attitude today:

☐ excellent
☐ pretty good
☐ not my best day; I'll do better tomorrow

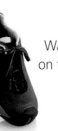

smart tip When you go for your walk, seek soft surfaces. Walking or jogging on hard surfaces such as concrete can be hard on the joints and the feet. Whenever possible, walk on grass, a dirt road, or a running track at the local high school or YMCA.

① wednesday

My numbers:

weight _____

blood sugar (time/level) _____ / _____
_____ / _____ • _____ / _____

Servings I ate today:

vegetables 0 1 2 3 4 **5 6 7**
fruit 0 1 2 **3**
whole grains 0 1 2 3 **4 5 6**
calcium-rich foods 0 1 **2 3**

**Times I ate out of boredom,
stress, or habit:**

0 1 2 3 4 5

How I took charge:

eat
☐ ate a healthy breakfast
☐ had protein at every meal
☐ avoided refined carbohydrates
  and sugary drinks
☐ swapped saturated fats for good fats

move
☐ walked _____ minutes / _____steps
☐ performed Sugar Buster exercises
☐ got other exercise _____

choose
☐ got enough sleep (_____ hours)
☐ kept TV time under 2 hours
☐ found time for relaxation and/or socializing

My attitude today:

☐ excellent
☐ pretty good
☐ not my best day; I'll do better tomorrow

① thursday

My numbers:

weight _____

blood sugar (time/level) _____ / _____
_____ / _____ • _____ / _____

Servings I ate today:

vegetables 0 1 2 3 4 **5 6 7**
fruit 0 1 2 **3**
whole grains 0 1 2 3 **4 5 6**
calcium-rich foods 0 1 **2 3**

**Times I ate out of boredom,
stress, or habit:**

0 1 2 3 4 5

How I took charge:

eat
☐ ate a healthy breakfast
☐ had protein at every meal
☐ avoided refined carbohydrates
  and sugary drinks
☐ swapped saturated fats for good fats

move
☐ walked _____ minutes / _____steps
☐ performed Sugar Buster exercises
☐ got other exercise _____

choose
☐ got enough sleep (_____ hours)
☐ kept TV time under 2 hours
☐ found time for relaxation and/or socializing

My attitude today:

☐ excellent
☐ pretty good
☐ not my best day; I'll do better tomorrow

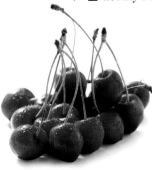

smart tip For quick, nutrient-rich, low-calorie snacking throughout the week, wash, cut, and bag hardy fruits and vegetables such as cucumbers, carrots, celery, bell peppers, melon balls, grapes, and berries. The easier they are to grab, the more likely you'll be to eat them.

175

1 friday

My numbers:

weight _____

blood sugar (time/level) _____ / _____
_____ / _____ • _____ / _____

Servings I ate today:

vegetables 0 1 2 3 4 **5 6 7**
fruit 0 1 2 **3**
whole grains 0 1 2 3 **4 5 6**
calcium-rich foods 0 1 **2 3**

Times I ate out of boredom, stress, or habit:

0 1 2 3 4 5

How I took charge:

eat
☐ ate a healthy breakfast
☐ had protein at every meal
☐ avoided refined carbohydrates and sugary drinks
☐ swapped saturated fats for good fats

move
☐ walked _____ minutes / _____steps
☐ performed Sugar Buster exercises
☐ got other exercise _____

choose
☐ got enough sleep (_____ hours)
☐ kept TV time under 2 hours
☐ found time for relaxation and/or socializing

My attitude today:

☐ excellent
☐ pretty good
☐ not my best day; I'll do better tomorrow

1 saturday

My numbers:

weight _____

blood sugar (time/level) _____ / _____
_____ / _____ • _____ / _____

Servings I ate today:

vegetables 0 1 2 3 4 **5 6 7**
fruit 0 1 2 **3**
whole grains 0 1 2 3 **4 5 6**
calcium-rich foods 0 1 **2 3**

Times I ate out of boredom, stress, or habit:

0 1 2 3 4 5

How I took charge:

eat
☐ ate a healthy breakfast
☐ had protein at every meal
☐ avoided refined carbohydrates and sugary drinks
☐ swapped saturated fats for good fats

move
☐ walked _____ minutes / _____steps
☐ performed Sugar Buster exercises
☐ got other exercise _____

choose
☐ got enough sleep (_____ hours)
☐ kept TV time under 2 hours
☐ found time for relaxation and/or socializing

My attitude today:

☐ excellent
☐ pretty good
☐ not my best day; I'll do better tomorrow

smart tip Believe that you can succeed. Build faith by setting very small goals at first—taking two short walks in a week, for example, or skipping dessert two nights in a row. As you succeed at achieving small goals, build on your successes.

① sunday

My numbers:

weight _____

blood sugar (time/level) _____ / _____

_____ / _____ • _____ / _____

Servings I ate today:

vegetables 0 1 2 3 4 **5 6 7**

fruit 0 1 2 **3**

whole grains 0 1 2 3 **4 5 6**

calcium-rich foods 0 1 **2 3**

Times I ate out of boredom, stress, or habit:

0 1 2 3 4 5

How I took charge:

eat
☐ ate a healthy breakfast
☐ had protein at every meal
☐ avoided refined carbohydrates and sugary drinks
☐ swapped saturated fats for good fats

move
☐ walked _____ minutes / _____ steps
☐ performed Sugar Buster exercises
☐ got other exercise _____

choose
☐ got enough sleep (_____ hours)
☐ kept TV time under 2 hours
☐ found time for relaxation and/or socializing

My attitude today:

☐ excellent
☐ pretty good
☐ not my best day; I'll do better tomorrow

> "We never repent of having eaten too little."
> —Thomas Jefferson

① the week in review

Successes and confessions

_____

_____

_____

_____

_____

_____

My numbers:

weight loss: _____ pounds
waist measurement: _____ inches

Next week's goals

eat
Dinner should be 450-550 calories. This may be quite a bit less than you're eating now. To help you bring your calories in line, start dinners this week with either a green salad or a bowl of clear soup to help fill you up.

move
You should have started the walking plan by now. Next week, walk for 15 minutes at least 5 days a week. Put your walks on your calendar, and be sure to keep all your "appointments."

choose
Enlist a support team. Ask your spouse to join you in your walks next week. Tell all your friends and family that you've started to improve your diet, and solicit their encouragement.

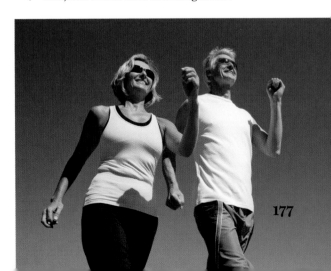

week ② meal planner

It's easier to eat home-cooked meals if they're already cooked before you get home! The key is to make big meals on a weekend day with an eye toward the week ahead. Making a stew, chili, or soup? Freeze one- or two-person servings as soon as you're done. You'll not only have a microwavable meal, you'll also have a portion-controlled one.

Sunday's broiled shrimp can be Tuesday's egg-white shrimp frittata. Roast chicken can reappear in any number of dishes. Remove the skin and sauté the meat with tomatoes and onions for a quick mid-week meal. If you have lean sirloin for dinner on Saturday, use the sliced refrigerated leftovers for a quick main-dish salad or stir-fry later in the week.

monday	tuesday	wednesday
breakfast		
lunch		
dinner		

thursday	friday	saturday	sunday

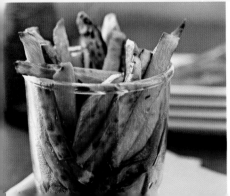

food fact
Sweet potatoes are higher in fiber and nutrients than white potatoes and have less impact on blood sugar.

② monday

My numbers:

weight _____

blood sugar (time/level) _____ / _____
_____ / _____ • _____ / _____

Servings I ate today:

vegetables 0 1 2 3 4 **5 6 7**
fruit 0 1 2 **3**
whole grains 0 1 2 3 **4 5 6**
calcium-rich foods 0 1 **2 3**

Times I ate out of boredom, stress, or habit:

0 1 2 3 4 5

How I took charge:

eat
☐ ate a healthy breakfast
☐ had protein at every meal
☐ avoided refined carbohydrates and sugary drinks
☐ swapped saturated fats for good fats

move
☐ walked _____ minutes / _____steps
☐ performed Sugar Buster exercises
☐ got other exercise _____

choose
☐ got enough sleep (_____hours)
☐ kept TV time under 2 hours
☐ found time for relaxation and/or socializing

My attitude today:

☐ excellent
☐ pretty good
☐ not my best day; I'll do better tomorrow

② tuesday

My numbers:

weight _____

blood sugar (time/level) _____ / _____
_____ / _____ • _____ / _____

Servings I ate today:

vegetables 0 1 2 3 4 **5 6 7**
fruit 0 1 2 **3**
whole grains 0 1 2 3 **4 5 6**
calcium-rich foods 0 1 **2 3**

Times I ate out of boredom, stress, or habit:

0 1 2 3 4 5

How I took charge:

eat
☐ ate a healthy breakfast
☐ had protein at every meal
☐ avoided refined carbohydrates and sugary drinks
☐ swapped saturated fats for good fats

move
☐ walked _____ minutes / _____steps
☐ performed Sugar Buster exercises
☐ got other exercise _____

choose
☐ got enough sleep (_____hours)
☐ kept TV time under 2 hours
☐ found time for relaxation and/or socializing

My attitude today:

☐ excellent
☐ pretty good
☐ not my best day; I'll do better tomorrow

smart tip Share the news. Tell family and friends that you are starting an exercise/weight-loss program and that you would like their support. Who knows—they may join you in your efforts to eat better. Perhaps they'd even like to be your exercise buddy.

② wednesday

My numbers:

weight _____

blood sugar (time/level) _____ / _____

_____ / _____ • _____ / _____

Servings I ate today:

vegetables 0 1 2 3 4 **5 6 7**
fruit 0 1 2 **3**
whole grains 0 1 2 3 **4 5 6**
calcium-rich foods 0 1 **2 3**

Times I ate out of boredom, stress, or habit:

0 1 2 3 4 5

How I took charge:

eat
☐ ate a healthy breakfast
☐ had protein at every meal
☐ avoided refined carbohydrates and sugary drinks
☐ swapped saturated fats for good fats

move
☐ walked _____ minutes / _____steps
☐ performed Sugar Buster exercises
☐ got other exercise _____

choose
☐ got enough sleep (_____ hours)
☐ kept TV time under 2 hours
☐ found time for relaxation and/or socializing

My attitude today:

☐ excellent
☐ pretty good
☐ not my best day; I'll do better tomorrow

② thursday

My numbers:

weight _____

blood sugar (time/level) _____ / _____

_____ / _____ • _____ / _____

Servings I ate today:

vegetables 0 1 2 3 4 **5 6 7**
fruit 0 1 2 **3**
whole grains 0 1 2 3 **4 5 6**
calcium-rich foods 0 1 **2 3**

Times I ate out of boredom, stress, or habit:

0 1 2 3 4 5

How I took charge:

eat
☐ ate a healthy breakfast
☐ had protein at every meal
☐ avoided refined carbohydrates and sugary drinks
☐ swapped saturated fats for good fats

move
☐ walked _____ minutes / _____steps
☐ performed Sugar Buster exercises
☐ got other exercise _____

choose
☐ got enough sleep (_____ hours)
☐ kept TV time under 2 hours
☐ found time for relaxation and/or socializing

My attitude today:

☐ excellent
☐ pretty good
☐ not my best day; I'll do better tomorrow

smart tip For recipes that call for the smoky taste of bacon (soups, chowders, egg dishes, and bean dishes), choose lean turkey bacon instead of pork bacon. It delivers plenty of flavor while saving significantly on calories and fat. Experiment to find a brand you like.

2 friday

My numbers:

weight _____

blood sugar (time/level) _____ / _____
_____ / _____ • _____ / _____

Servings I ate today:

vegetables 0 1 2 3 4 **5 6 7**
fruit 0 1 2 **3**
whole grains 0 1 2 3 **4 5 6**
calcium-rich foods 0 1 **2 3**

Times I ate out of boredom, stress, or habit:

0 1 2 3 4 5

How I took charge:

eat
☐ ate a healthy breakfast
☐ had protein at every meal
☐ avoided refined carbohydrates
   and sugary drinks
☐ swapped saturated fats for good fats

move
☐ walked _____ minutes / _____ steps
☐ performed Sugar Buster exercises
☐ got other exercise _____

choose
☐ got enough sleep (_____ hours)
☐ kept TV time under 2 hours
☐ found time for relaxation and/or socializing

My attitude today:

☐ excellent
☐ pretty good
☐ not my best day; I'll do better tomorrow

2 saturday

My numbers:

weight _____

blood sugar (time/level) _____ / _____
_____ / _____ • _____ / _____

Servings I ate today:

vegetables 0 1 2 3 4 **5 6 7**
fruit 0 1 2 **3**
whole grains 0 1 2 3 **4 5 6**
calcium-rich foods 0 1 **2 3**

Times I ate out of boredom, stress, or habit:

0 1 2 3 4 5

How I took charge:

eat
☐ ate a healthy breakfast
☐ had protein at every meal
☐ avoided refined carbohydrates
   and sugary drinks
☐ swapped saturated fats for good fats

move
☐ walked _____ minutes / _____ steps
☐ performed Sugar Buster exercises
☐ got other exercise _____

choose
☐ got enough sleep (_____ hours)
☐ kept TV time under 2 hours
☐ found time for relaxation and/or socializing

My attitude today:

☐ excellent
☐ pretty good
☐ not my best day; I'll do better tomorrow

smart tip Avoid all-or-nothing thinking. If you aim to exercise for 25 minutes but find you only have 10 minutes, don't feel that because you don't have time for your entire walk or workout you should do nothing. If all you have is 10 minutes, then exercise for 10 minutes.

② sunday

My numbers:

weight _____

blood sugar (time/level) _____ / _____

_____ / _____ • _____ / _____

Servings I ate today:

vegetables 0 1 2 3 4 **5 6 7**
fruit 0 1 2 **3**
whole grains 0 1 2 3 **4 5 6**
calcium-rich foods 0 1 **2 3**

Times I ate out of boredom, stress, or habit:

0 1 2 3 4 5

How I took charge:

eat
☐ ate a healthy breakfast
☐ had protein at every meal
☐ avoided refined carbohydrates
   and sugary drinks
☐ swapped saturated fats for good fats

move
☐ walked _____ minutes / _____ steps
☐ performed Sugar Buster exercises
☐ got other exercise _____

choose
☐ got enough sleep (_____ hours)
☐ kept TV time under 2 hours
☐ found time for relaxation and/or socializing

My attitude today:

☐ excellent
☐ pretty good
☐ not my best day; I'll do better tomorrow

> "To eat is a necessity, but to eat intelligently is an art."
> — François de La Rochefoucauld

② the week in review

Successes and confessions

_____
_____
_____
_____
_____
_____

My numbers:

weight loss: _____ pounds
waist measurement: _____ inches

Next week's goals

eat
Eat breakfast every day next week, and make it a good one. Stock up on cereals that contain 5 grams of fiber per serving, and top them with fresh fruit.

move
Increase your walking time. Your goal next week: 20 minutes of walking on five days. Any pace is fine for now.

choose
Getting a good night's sleep is critical to helping you stay the course. If you're not getting a full 8 hours (or however many hours you need to feel truly rested), move up your bedtime by an hour.

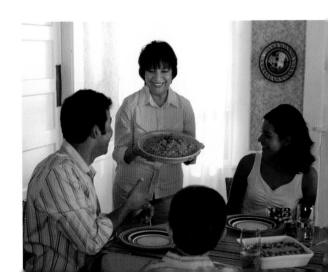

week ③ meal planner

Plan at least one vegetarian meal this week. Try Couscous-Stuffed Peppers (see recipe, page 293). Need more recipe ideas? *The Moosewood Restaurant* cookbook series is popular, and for good reason. Other good options: *Cooking Vegetarian: Healthy, Delicious, and Easy Vegetarian Cuisine*, and *Becoming Vegetarian: The Complete Guide to Adopting a Healthy Vegetarian Diet.*

To get more vegetables into your meals, take advantage of prepared veggies such as bagged salads, prewashed spinach, and chopped bell peppers and onions, etc. Also, stock the freezer with bags of frozen vegetables and use them in stir-fries.

monday	tuesday	wednesday
breakfast		
lunch		
dinner		

thursday	friday	saturday	sunday

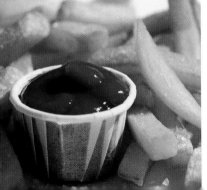

food fact
One tablespoon of ketchup contains about half a teaspoon of sugar. Buying sugar-free condiments can make a dent in your overall sugar consumption.

(3) monday

My numbers:

weight _____

blood sugar (time/level) _____ / _____
_____ / _____ • _____ / _____

Servings I ate today:

vegetables 0 1 2 3 4 **5 6 7**
fruit 0 1 2 **3**
whole grains 0 1 2 3 **4 5 6**
calcium-rich foods 0 1 **2 3**

Times I ate out of boredom, stress, or habit:

0 1 2 3 4 5

How I took charge:

eat
☐ ate a healthy breakfast
☐ had protein at every meal
☐ avoided refined carbohydrates
   and sugary drinks
☐ swapped saturated fats for good fats

move
☐ walked _____ minutes / _____ steps
☐ performed Sugar Buster exercises
☐ got other exercise _____

choose
☐ got enough sleep (_____ hours)
☐ kept TV time under 2 hours
☐ found time for relaxation and/or socializing

My attitude today:
☐ excellent
☐ pretty good
☐ not my best day; I'll do better tomorrow

(3) tuesday

My numbers:

weight _____

blood sugar (time/level) _____ / _____
_____ / _____ • _____ / _____

Servings I ate today:

vegetables 0 1 2 3 4 **5 6 7**
fruit 0 1 2 **3**
whole grains 0 1 2 3 **4 5 6**
calcium-rich foods 0 1 **2 3**

Times I ate out of boredom, stress, or habit:

0 1 2 3 4 5

How I took charge:

eat
☐ ate a healthy breakfast
☐ had protein at every meal
☐ avoided refined carbohydrates
   and sugary drinks
☐ swapped saturated fats for good fats

move
☐ walked _____ minutes / _____ steps
☐ performed Sugar Buster exercises
☐ got other exercise _____

choose
☐ got enough sleep (_____ hours)
☐ kept TV time under 2 hours
☐ found time for relaxation and/or socializing

My attitude today:
☐ excellent
☐ pretty good
☐ not my best day; I'll do better tomorrow

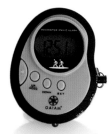

smart tip Buy a pedometer. These little gadgets keep track of all of your steps during the day—not only when you're walking for exercise. Pedometers are available at sporting goods stores. Aim for an ultimate goal of 10,000 steps a day.

③ wednesday

My numbers:

weight _____

blood sugar (time/level) _____ / _____

_____ / _____ • _____ / _____

Servings I ate today:

vegetables 0 1 2 3 4 **5 6 7**
fruit 0 1 2 **3**
whole grains 0 1 2 3 **4 5 6**
calcium-rich foods 0 1 **2 3**

Times I ate out of boredom, stress, or habit:

0 1 2 3 4 5

How I took charge:

eat
☐ ate a healthy breakfast
☐ had protein at every meal
☐ avoided refined carbohydrates
   and sugary drinks
☐ swapped saturated fats for good fats

move
☐ walked _____ minutes / _____ steps
☐ performed Sugar Buster exercises
☐ got other exercise _____

choose
☐ got enough sleep (_____ hours)
☐ kept TV time under 2 hours
☐ found time for relaxation and/or socializing

My attitude today:

☐ excellent
☐ pretty good
☐ not my best day; I'll do better tomorrow

③ thursday

My numbers:

weight _____

blood sugar (time/level) _____ / _____

_____ / _____ • _____ / _____

Servings I ate today:

vegetables 0 1 2 3 4 **5 6 7**
fruit 0 1 2 **3**
whole grains 0 1 2 3 **4 5 6**
calcium-rich foods 0 1 **2 3**

Times I ate out of boredom, stress, or habit:

0 1 2 3 4 5

How I took charge:

eat
☐ ate a healthy breakfast
☐ had protein at every meal
☐ avoided refined carbohydrates
   and sugary drinks
☐ swapped saturated fats for good fats

move
☐ walked _____ minutes / _____ steps
☐ performed Sugar Buster exercises
☐ got other exercise _____

choose
☐ got enough sleep (_____ hours)
☐ kept TV time under 2 hours
☐ found time for relaxation and/or socializing

My attitude today:

☐ excellent
☐ pretty good
☐ not my best day; I'll do better tomorrow

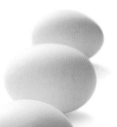

smart tip In recipes that call for whole eggs, save calories, saturated fat, and cholesterol by substituting egg whites instead. Replace each egg in the recipe with two egg whites. Or use a cholesterol-free liquid egg product instead.

③ friday

My numbers:

weight _____

blood sugar (time/level) _____ / _____

_____ / _____ • _____ / _____

Servings I ate today:

vegetables 0 1 2 3 4 **5 6 7**
fruit 0 1 2 **3**
whole grains 0 1 2 3 **4 5 6**
calcium-rich foods 0 1 **2 3**

Times I ate out of boredom, stress, or habit:

0 1 2 3 4 5

How I took charge:

eat
☐ ate a healthy breakfast
☐ had protein at every meal
☐ avoided refined carbohydrates
   and sugary drinks
☐ swapped saturated fats for good fats

move
☐ walked _____ minutes / _____ steps
☐ performed Sugar Buster exercises
☐ got other exercise _____

choose
☐ got enough sleep (_____ hours)
☐ kept TV time under 2 hours
☐ found time for relaxation and/or socializing

My attitude today:

☐ excellent
☐ pretty good
☐ not my best day; I'll do better tomorrow

③ saturday

My numbers:

weight _____

blood sugar (time/level) _____ / _____

_____ / _____ • _____ / _____

Servings I ate today:

vegetables 0 1 2 3 4 **5 6 7**
fruit 0 1 2 **3**
whole grains 0 1 2 3 **4 5 6**
calcium-rich foods 0 1 **2 3**

Times I ate out of boredom, stress, or habit:

0 1 2 3 4 5

How I took charge:

eat
☐ ate a healthy breakfast
☐ had protein at every meal
☐ avoided refined carbohydrates
   and sugary drinks
☐ swapped saturated fats for good fats

move
☐ walked _____ minutes / _____ steps
☐ performed Sugar Buster exercises
☐ got other exercise _____

choose
☐ got enough sleep (_____ hours)
☐ kept TV time under 2 hours
☐ found time for relaxation and/or socializing

My attitude today:

☐ excellent
☐ pretty good
☐ not my best day; I'll do better tomorrow

smart tip Do you tend to eat when you're bored? If so, make a list of other things you can do in those instances, and post it on your refrigerator. Your list may include calling a friend, taking your dog for a walk, knitting, organizing your photos, or spending time on an old or new hobby.

③ sunday

My numbers:

weight _____

blood sugar (time/level) _____ / _____

_____ / _____ • _____ / _____

Servings I ate today:

vegetables 0 1 2 3 4 **5 6 7**

fruit 0 1 2 **3**

whole grains 0 1 2 3 **4 5 6**

calcium-rich foods 0 1 **2 3**

Times I ate out of boredom, stress, or habit:

0 1 2 3 4 5

How I took charge:

eat

☐ ate a healthy breakfast
☐ had protein at every meal
☐ avoided refined carbohydrates and sugary drinks
☐ swapped saturated fats for good fats

move

☐ walked _____ minutes / _____ steps
☐ performed Sugar Buster exercises
☐ got other exercise _____

choose

☐ got enough sleep (_____ hours)
☐ kept TV time under 2 hours
☐ found time for relaxation and/or socializing

My attitude today:

☐ excellent
☐ pretty good
☐ not my best day; I'll do better tomorrow

> "There is no failure except in no longer trying."
> —Elbert Hubbard

③ the week in review

Successes and confessions

_____

_____

_____

_____

_____

_____

My numbers:

weight loss: _____ pounds
waist measurement: _____ inches

Next week's goals

eat

Focus on eating more vegetables. Start lunch and dinner with a salad, and add color (in the form of veggies) to every meal you make.

move

Walk 25 minutes at least 5 days a week, and start the Sugar Buster Routine: Do each sequence at least once during the week. If some of the exercises are too difficult for you right now, do fewer repetitions. You'll get stronger as you go.

choose

Practice deep breathing for 5 minutes every day next week. Breathe deeply through your nose, expanding your belly and filling your lungs from the bottom up. Exhale slowly.

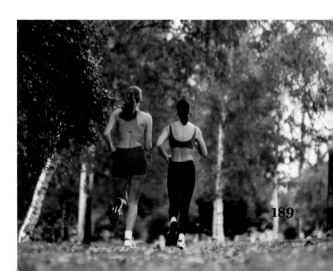

week ④ meal planner

Cook up a whole grain to go with dinner. Try pearl barley (which doesn't require any soaking before cooking) as a side dish. Or mix in some steamed carrots and broccoli, toss with olive oil and a bit of Parmesan or feta cheese, maybe throw in a can of tuna or a couple of ounces of cut-up chicken, and you've got the whole dinner.

For a delicious high-fiber meal, make Barley Risotto with Asparagus and Mushrooms (see recipe, page 293). Other interesting grains to experiment with include amaranth and wheat berries.

	monday	tuesday	wednesday
breakfast			
lunch			
dinner			

thursday	friday	saturday	sunday

food fact
One-half cup of vanilla frozen yogurt has just 100 calories compared with 160 calories or more for one-half cup of premium ice cream.

(4) monday

My numbers:

weight _____

blood sugar (time/level) _____ / _____

_____ / _____ • _____ / _____

Servings I ate today:

vegetables 0 1 2 3 4 **5 6 7**
fruit 0 1 2 **3**
whole grains 0 1 2 3 **4 5 6**
calcium-rich foods 0 1 **2 3**

Times I ate out of boredom, stress, or habit:

0 1 2 3 4 5

How I took charge:

eat
☐ ate a healthy breakfast
☐ had protein at every meal
☐ avoided refined carbohydrates
    and sugary drinks
☐ swapped saturated fats for good fats

move
☐ walked _____ minutes / _____ steps
☐ performed Sugar Buster exercises
☐ got other exercise _____

choose
☐ got enough sleep (_____ hours)
☐ kept TV time under 2 hours
☐ found time for relaxation and/or socializing

My attitude today:

☐ excellent
☐ pretty good
☐ not my best day; I'll do better tomorrow

(4) tuesday

My numbers:

weight _____

blood sugar (time/level) _____ / _____

_____ / _____ • _____ / _____

Servings I ate today:

vegetables 0 1 2 3 4 **5 6 7**
fruit 0 1 2 **3**
whole grains 0 1 2 3 **4 5 6**
calcium-rich foods 0 1 **2 3**

Times I ate out of boredom, stress, or habit:

0 1 2 3 4 5

How I took charge:

eat
☐ ate a healthy breakfast
☐ had protein at every meal
☐ avoided refined carbohydrates
    and sugary drinks
☐ swapped saturated fats for good fats

move
☐ walked _____ minutes / _____ steps
☐ performed Sugar Buster exercises
☐ got other exercise _____

choose
☐ got enough sleep (_____ hours)
☐ kept TV time under 2 hours
☐ found time for relaxation and/or socializing

My attitude today:

☐ excellent
☐ pretty good
☐ not my best day; I'll do better tomorrow

smart tip Exercise while you watch TV. Whenever a commercial comes on, get up and walk up and down the stairs, do jumping jacks, or march in place until the program comes back on. Remember: Even small bursts of physical activity add up to weight loss and increased insulin sensitivity.

④ wednesday

My numbers:

weight _____

blood sugar (time/level) _____ / _____
_____ / _____ • _____ / _____

Servings I ate today:

vegetables 0 1 2 3 4 **5 6 7**
fruit 0 1 2 **3**
whole grains 0 1 2 3 **4 5 6**
calcium-rich foods 0 1 **2 3**

Times I ate out of boredom, stress, or habit:

0 1 2 3 4 5

How I took charge:

eat
☐ ate a healthy breakfast
☐ had protein at every meal
☐ avoided refined carbohydrates
   and sugary drinks
☐ swapped saturated fats for good fats

move
☐ walked _____ minutes / _____ steps
☐ performed Sugar Buster exercises
☐ got other exercise _____

choose
☐ got enough sleep (_____ hours)
☐ kept TV time under 2 hours
☐ found time for relaxation and/or socializing

My attitude today:

☐ excellent
☐ pretty good
☐ not my best day; I'll do better tomorrow

④ thursday

My numbers:

weight _____

blood sugar (time/level) _____ / _____
_____ / _____ • _____ / _____

Servings I ate today:

vegetables 0 1 2 3 4 **5 6 7**
fruit 0 1 2 **3**
whole grains 0 1 2 3 **4 5 6**
calcium-rich foods 0 1 **2 3**

Times I ate out of boredom, stress, or habit:

0 1 2 3 4 5

How I took charge:

eat
☐ ate a healthy breakfast
☐ had protein at every meal
☐ avoided refined carbohydrates
   and sugary drinks
☐ swapped saturated fats for good fats

move
☐ walked _____ minutes / _____ steps
☐ performed Sugar Buster exercises
☐ got other exercise _____

choose
☐ got enough sleep (_____ hours)
☐ kept TV time under 2 hours
☐ found time for relaxation and/or socializing

My attitude today:

☐ excellent
☐ pretty good
☐ not my best day; I'll do better tomorrow

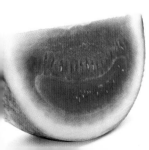

smart tip Eat "wet" foods. Studies show that foods that contain liquid—grapes, soups, stews, and smoothies, for example—make you feel fuller than a dry food with the same number of calories. A 100-calorie bowl of soup will leave you feeling fuller than a 100-calorie bag of pretzels.

193

4 friday

My numbers:

weight _____

blood sugar (time/level) _____ / _____
_____ / _____ • _____ / _____

Servings I ate today:

vegetables 0 1 2 3 4 **5 6 7**
fruit 0 1 2 **3**
whole grains 0 1 2 3 **4 5 6**
calcium-rich foods 0 1 **2 3**

**Times I ate out of boredom,
stress, or habit:**

0 1 2 3 4 5

How I took charge:

eat
☐ ate a healthy breakfast
☐ had protein at every meal
☐ avoided refined carbohydrates
and sugary drinks
☐ swapped saturated fats for good fats

move
☐ walked _____ minutes / _____ steps
☐ performed Sugar Buster exercises
☐ got other exercise _____

choose
☐ got enough sleep (_____ hours)
☐ kept TV time under 2 hours
☐ found time for relaxation and/or socializing

My attitude today:
☐ excellent
☐ pretty good
☐ not my best day; I'll do better tomorrow

4 saturday

My numbers:

weight _____

blood sugar (time/level) _____ / _____
_____ / _____ • _____ / _____

Servings I ate today:

vegetables 0 1 2 3 4 **5 6 7**
fruit 0 1 2 **3**
whole grains 0 1 2 3 **4 5 6**
calcium-rich foods 0 1 **2 3**

**Times I ate out of boredom,
stress, or habit:**

0 1 2 3 4 5

How I took charge:

eat
☐ ate a healthy breakfast
☐ had protein at every meal
☐ avoided refined carbohydrates
and sugary drinks
☐ swapped saturated fats for good fats

move
☐ walked _____ minutes / _____ steps
☐ performed Sugar Buster exercises
☐ got other exercise _____

choose
☐ got enough sleep (_____ hours)
☐ kept TV time under 2 hours
☐ found time for relaxation and/or socializing

My attitude today:
☐ excellent
☐ pretty good
☐ not my best day; I'll do better tomorrow

smart tip Exercise with a friend. Your walk, jog, or swim will be much
more enjoyable—and probably longer—if you go with a companion.
Also, a friend can be a great motivator: You're much less likely to skip a
workout if you know your buddy is waiting for you.

④ sunday

My numbers:

weight _____

blood sugar (time/level) _____ / _____
_____ / _____ • _____ / _____

Servings I ate today:

vegetables 0 1 2 3 4 **5 6 7**
fruit 0 1 2 **3**
whole grains 0 1 2 3 **4 5 6**
calcium-rich foods 0 1 **2 3**

Times I ate out of boredom, stress, or habit:

0 1 2 3 4 5

How I took charge:

eat
☐ ate a healthy breakfast
☐ had protein at every meal
☐ avoided refined carbohydrates and sugary drinks
☐ swapped saturated fats for good fats

move
☐ walked _____ minutes / _____ steps
☐ performed Sugar Buster exercises
☐ got other exercise _____

choose
☐ got enough sleep (_____ hours)
☐ kept TV time under 2 hours
☐ found time for relaxation and/or socializing

My attitude today:

☐ excellent
☐ pretty good
☐ not my best day; I'll do better tomorrow

"The first wealth is health."
—Ralph Waldo Emerson

④ the week in review

Successes and confessions

_____
_____
_____
_____
_____
_____

My numbers:

weight loss: _____pounds
waist measurement: _____inches

Next week's goals

eat
It's time to start switching to whole grains. Buy bread with the word whole in the first ingredient. Also buy a bag of brown rice, a bag of barley, and a box of whole-wheat pasta to try.

move
Walk for 25 minutes at least 5 days next week, and do each sequence of the Sugar Buster Routine at least once during the week. Outside of your walks, look for other opportunities to move. Unless you're sick, don't let yourself go a day without some physical activity.

choose
Keep a can-do attitude. Think of all the ways in which your health is improving, and congratulate yourself for all the progress you've made.

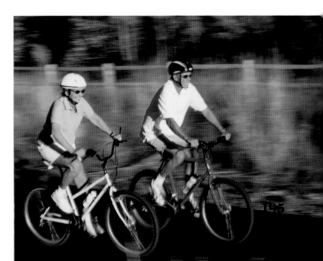

week ⑤ meal planner

Higher in protein and lower in saturated fat than either beef or pork, chicken breast is one of the best foods to use as the center of your meal. Plan at least one chicken-breast meal this week. Cook extra chicken and use it the next day to top a salad or include in a sandwich.

When cooking chicken, make sure to remove the skin, where most of the fat is. If you're roasting a chicken, either cook the vegetables separately so they don't soak up all the fat from the chicken, or wait until you've skimmed the fat from the meat juices before adding the vegetables.

For sandwiches, choose roasted turkey, which is even lower in calories than chicken.

	monday	tuesday	wednesday
breakfast			
lunch			
dinner			

thursday	friday	saturday	sunday

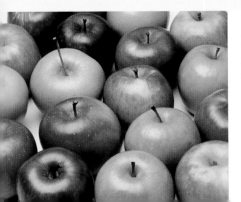

food fact
Apples are low in calories and rich in fiber, especially the soluble fiber that lowers blood sugar. And the skin is rich in heart-protective compounds called flavonoids.

5 monday

My numbers:

weight _____

blood sugar (time/level) _____ / _____

_____ / _____ • _____ / _____

Servings I ate today:

vegetables 0 1 2 3 4 **5 6 7**
fruit 0 1 2 **3**
whole grains 0 1 2 3 **4 5 6**
calcium-rich foods 0 1 **2 3**

Times I ate out of boredom, stress, or habit:

0 1 2 3 4 5

How I took charge:

eat
☐ ate a healthy breakfast
☐ had protein at every meal
☐ avoided refined carbohydrates
   and sugary drinks
☐ swapped saturated fats for good fats

move
☐ walked _____ minutes / _____ steps
☐ performed Sugar Buster exercises
☐ got other exercise _____

choose
☐ got enough sleep (_____ hours)
☐ kept TV time under 2 hours
☐ found time for relaxation and/or socializing

My attitude today:

☐ excellent
☐ pretty good
☐ not my best day; I'll do better tomorrow

5 tuesday

My numbers:

weight _____

blood sugar (time/level) _____ / _____

_____ / _____ • _____ / _____

Servings I ate today:

vegetables 0 1 2 3 4 **5 6 7**
fruit 0 1 2 **3**
whole grains 0 1 2 3 **4 5 6**
calcium-rich foods 0 1 **2 3**

Times I ate out of boredom, stress, or habit:

0 1 2 3 4 5

How I took charge:

eat
☐ ate a healthy breakfast
☐ had protein at every meal
☐ avoided refined carbohydrates
   and sugary drinks
☐ swapped saturated fats for good fats

move
☐ walked _____ minutes / _____ steps
☐ performed Sugar Buster exercises
☐ got other exercise _____

choose
☐ got enough sleep (_____ hours)
☐ kept TV time under 2 hours
☐ found time for relaxation and/or socializing

My attitude today:

☐ excellent
☐ pretty good
☐ not my best day; I'll do better tomorrow

smart tip Stay hydrated. Drink a glass of water before and after exercise. Keep a water bottle at hand during your workout and drink water whether or not you feel thirsty. Dehydration can leave you feeling lethargic and too tired to exercise.

5 wednesday

My numbers:

weight _____

blood sugar (time/level) _____ / _____

_____ / _____ • _____ / _____

Servings I ate today:

vegetables 0 1 2 3 4 **5 6 7**

fruit 0 1 2 **3**

whole grains 0 1 2 3 **4 5 6**

calcium-rich foods 0 1 **2 3**

Times I ate out of boredom, stress, or habit:

0 1 2 3 4 5

How I took charge:

eat
- ☐ ate a healthy breakfast
- ☐ had protein at every meal
- ☐ avoided refined carbohydrates and sugary drinks
- ☐ swapped saturated fats for good fats

move
- ☐ walked _____ minutes / _____ steps
- ☐ performed Sugar Buster exercises
- ☐ got other exercise _____

choose
- ☐ got enough sleep (_____ hours)
- ☐ kept TV time under 2 hours
- ☐ found time for relaxation and/or socializing

My attitude today:
- ☐ excellent
- ☐ pretty good
- ☐ not my best day; I'll do better tomorrow

5 thursday

My numbers:

weight _____

blood sugar (time/level) _____ / _____

_____ / _____ • _____ / _____

Servings I ate today:

vegetables 0 1 2 3 4 **5 6 7**

fruit 0 1 2 **3**

whole grains 0 1 2 3 **4 5 6**

calcium-rich foods 0 1 **2 3**

Times I ate out of boredom, stress, or habit:

0 1 2 3 4 5

How I took charge:

eat
- ☐ ate a healthy breakfast
- ☐ had protein at every meal
- ☐ avoided refined carbohydrates and sugary drinks
- ☐ swapped saturated fats for good fats

move
- ☐ walked _____ minutes / _____ steps
- ☐ performed Sugar Buster exercises
- ☐ got other exercise _____

choose
- ☐ got enough sleep (_____ hours)
- ☐ kept TV time under 2 hours
- ☐ found time for relaxation and/or socializing

My attitude today:
- ☐ excellent
- ☐ pretty good
- ☐ not my best day; I'll do better tomorrow

smart tip When it comes to snacks such as pretzels, peanuts, or popcorn, consider buying individual snack-size packages, even if the big bag is a better value. Studies find that when you buy larger sizes, you eat more. It's just human nature. Limit yourself to one snack-size bag a day.

5 friday

My numbers:

weight _____

blood sugar (time/level) _____ / _____
_____ / _____ • _____ / _____

Servings I ate today:

vegetables 0 1 2 3 4 **5 6 7**
fruit 0 1 2 **3**
whole grains 0 1 2 3 **4 5 6**
calcium-rich foods 0 1 **2 3**

Times I ate out of boredom, stress, or habit:

0 1 2 3 4 5

How I took charge:

eat
☐ ate a healthy breakfast
☐ had protein at every meal
☐ avoided refined carbohydrates
  and sugary drinks
☐ swapped saturated fats for good fats

move
☐ walked _____ minutes / _____ steps
☐ performed Sugar Buster exercises
☐ got other exercise _____

choose
☐ got enough sleep (_____ hours)
☐ kept TV time under 2 hours
☐ found time for relaxation and/or socializing

My attitude today:

☐ excellent
☐ pretty good
☐ not my best day; I'll do better tomorrow

5 saturday

My numbers:

weight _____

blood sugar (time/level) _____ / _____
_____ / _____ • _____ / _____

Servings I ate today:

vegetables 0 1 2 3 4 **5 6 7**
fruit 0 1 2 **3**
whole grains 0 1 2 3 **4 5 6**
calcium-rich foods 0 1 **2 3**

Times I ate out of boredom, stress, or habit:

0 1 2 3 4 5

How I took charge:

eat
☐ ate a healthy breakfast
☐ had protein at every meal
☐ avoided refined carbohydrates
  and sugary drinks
☐ swapped saturated fats for good fats

move
☐ walked _____ minutes / _____ steps
☐ performed Sugar Buster exercises
☐ got other exercise _____

choose
☐ got enough sleep (_____ hours)
☐ kept TV time under 2 hours
☐ found time for relaxation and/or socializing

My attitude today:

☐ excellent
☐ pretty good
☐ not my best day; I'll do better tomorrow

smart tip Hunger isn't the only reason we reach for food. Boredom, anger, sadness, and stress sometimes inspire an eating spree even when we're not really hungry. The next time you find yourself reaching for a chocolate bar, think about why you want it.

⑤ sunday

My numbers:

weight _____

blood sugar (time/level) _____ / _____

_____ / _____ • _____ / _____

Servings I ate today:

vegetables 0 1 2 3 4 **5 6 7**
fruit 0 1 2 **3**
whole grains 0 1 2 3 **4 5 6**
calcium-rich foods 0 1 **2 3**

Times I ate out of boredom, stress, or habit:

0 1 2 3 4 5

How I took charge:

eat
☐ ate a healthy breakfast
☐ had protein at every meal
☐ avoided refined carbohydrates and sugary drinks
☐ swapped saturated fats for good fats

move
☐ walked _____ minutes / _____ steps
☐ performed Sugar Buster exercises
☐ got other exercise _____

choose
☐ got enough sleep (_____ hours)
☐ kept TV time under 2 hours
☐ found time for relaxation and/or socializing

My attitude today:

☐ excellent
☐ pretty good
☐ not my best day; I'll do better tomorrow

> "Happiness is nothing more than good health and a bad memory."
> —Albert Schweitzer

⑤ the week in review

Successes and confessions

_____
_____
_____
_____
_____
_____

My numbers:

weight loss: _____ pounds
waist measurement: _____ inches

Next week's goals

eat
Take aim at fat. The answer isn't low-fat cookies. It's buying low-fat or nonfat milk and yogurt and choosing the leanest cuts of meat. Find three chicken breast recipes you like. Avoid ground beef!

move
Walk for 30 minutes at least 5 days next week. Do all the Sugar Buster Routine exercises twice.

choose
Develop a relaxation ritual. Sit outside in your garden for 10 minutes a day. Add lavender oil to a diffuser and inhale the scent before you go to bed. Remember, lowering your stress hormones can lower your blood sugar.

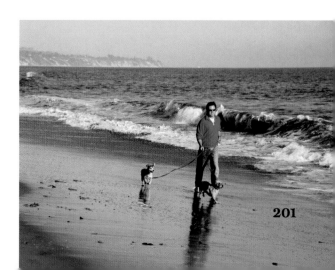

week ⑥ meal planner

When cooking beef, choose round (eye of round, top round, ground round) or loin (tenderloin, sirloin). Flank steak (good for stir-frying) and filet mignon are also lean cuts. When serving beef, make sure to include plenty of vegetables. Sauté beef with peppers and onions, or cook steak pieces in a wok with lots of peppers or broccoli.

If you buy ground beef, don't think that using the fatty kind and pouring off the grease makes it fine. Much of the fat is bound in with the meat. Good quality, 90-percent-or-more ground sirloin is the best choice.

When making beef stew, make it in advance if you can, then chill it and remove the congealed fat before reheating.

monday	tuesday	wednesday
breakfast		
lunch		
dinner		

thursday	friday	saturday	sunday

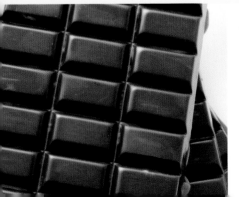

food fact
Dark chocolate contains significantly more antioxidants than milk chocolate—and less fat. Milk chocolate contains milk fat that is highly saturated.

⑥ monday

My numbers:

weight _____

blood sugar (time/level) _____ / _____

_____ / _____ • _____ / _____

Servings I ate today:

vegetables 0 1 2 3 4 **5 6 7**
fruit 0 1 2 **3**
whole grains 0 1 2 3 **4 5 6**
calcium-rich foods 0 1 **2 3**

Times I ate out of boredom, stress, or habit:

0 1 2 3 4 5

How I took charge:

eat
☐ ate a healthy breakfast
☐ had protein at every meal
☐ avoided refined carbohydrates
  and sugary drinks
☐ swapped saturated fats for good fats

move
☐ walked _____ minutes / _____ steps
☐ performed Sugar Buster exercises
☐ got other exercise _____

choose
☐ got enough sleep (_____ hours)
☐ kept TV time under 2 hours
☐ found time for relaxation and/or socializing

My attitude today:

☐ excellent
☐ pretty good
☐ not my best day; I'll do better tomorrow

⑥ tuesday

My numbers:

weight _____

blood sugar (time/level) _____ / _____

_____ / _____ • _____ / _____

Servings I ate today:

vegetables 0 1 2 3 4 **5 6 7**
fruit 0 1 2 **3**
whole grains 0 1 2 3 **4 5 6**
calcium-rich foods 0 1 **2 3**

Times I ate out of boredom, stress, or habit:

0 1 2 3 4 5

How I took charge:

eat
☐ ate a healthy breakfast
☐ had protein at every meal
☐ avoided refined carbohydrates
  and sugary drinks
☐ swapped saturated fats for good fats

move
☐ walked _____ minutes / _____ steps
☐ performed Sugar Buster exercises
☐ got other exercise _____

choose
☐ got enough sleep (_____ hours)
☐ kept TV time under 2 hours
☐ found time for relaxation and/or socializing

My attitude today:

☐ excellent
☐ pretty good
☐ not my best day; I'll do better tomorrow

smart tip Watch your posture when you walk. Hold your body fully upright, with your shoulders pulled slightly back and down. Keep your arms bent at a 90-degree angle. Don't thrust your head forward. Instead, keep your ears aligned with your shoulders. Your hands should be lightly clenched.

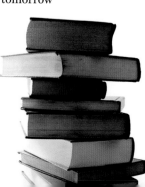

6 wednesday

My numbers:

weight _____

blood sugar (time/level) _____ / _____

_____ / _____ • _____ / _____

Servings I ate today:

vegetables 0 1 2 3 4 **5 6 7**
fruit 0 1 2 **3**
whole grains 0 1 2 3 **4 5 6**
calcium-rich foods 0 1 **2 3**

Times I ate out of boredom, stress, or habit:

0 1 2 3 4 5

How I took charge:

eat
☐ ate a healthy breakfast
☐ had protein at every meal
☐ avoided refined carbohydrates and sugary drinks
☐ swapped saturated fats for good fats

move
☐ walked _____ minutes / _____ steps
☐ performed Sugar Buster exercises
☐ got other exercise _____

choose
☐ got enough sleep (_____ hours)
☐ kept TV time under 2 hours
☐ found time for relaxation and/or socializing

My attitude today:

☐ excellent
☐ pretty good
☐ not my best day; I'll do better tomorrow

6 thursday

My numbers:

weight _____

blood sugar (time/level) _____ / _____

_____ / _____ • _____ / _____

Servings I ate today:

vegetables 0 1 2 3 4 **5 6 7**
fruit 0 1 2 **3**
whole grains 0 1 2 3 **4 5 6**
calcium-rich foods 0 1 **2 3**

Times I ate out of boredom, stress, or habit:

0 1 2 3 4 5

How I took charge:

eat
☐ ate a healthy breakfast
☐ had protein at every meal
☐ avoided refined carbohydrates and sugary drinks
☐ swapped saturated fats for good fats

move
☐ walked _____ minutes / _____ steps
☐ performed Sugar Buster exercises
☐ got other exercise _____

choose
☐ got enough sleep (_____ hours)
☐ kept TV time under 2 hours
☐ found time for relaxation and/or socializing

My attitude today:

☐ excellent
☐ pretty good
☐ not my best day; I'll do better tomorrow

smart tip Discover fresh herbs. Add flavor to vegetables, salads, meat, poultry, and fish with fresh herbs such as basil, rosemary, parsley, oregano, and cilantro. Most grocery stores carry fresh herbs— or grow your own on a sunny windowsill.

(6) friday

My numbers:

weight _____

blood sugar (time/level) _____ / _____

_____ / _____ • _____ / _____

Servings I ate today:

vegetables 0 1 2 3 4 **5 6 7**

fruit 0 1 2 **3**

whole grains 0 1 2 3 **4 5 6**

calcium-rich foods 0 1 **2 3**

Times I ate out of boredom, stress, or habit:

0 1 2 3 4 5

How I took charge:

eat

☐ ate a healthy breakfast

☐ had protein at every meal

☐ avoided refined carbohydrates and sugary drinks

☐ swapped saturated fats for good fats

move

☐ walked _____ minutes / _____ steps

☐ performed Sugar Buster exercises

☐ got other exercise _____

choose

☐ got enough sleep (_____ hours)

☐ kept TV time under 2 hours

☐ found time for relaxation and/or socializing

My attitude today:

☐ excellent

☐ pretty good

☐ not my best day; I'll do better tomorrow

(6) saturday

My numbers:

weight _____

blood sugar (time/level) _____ / _____

_____ / _____ • _____ / _____

Servings I ate today:

vegetables 0 1 2 3 4 **5 6 7**

fruit 0 1 2 **3**

whole grains 0 1 2 3 **4 5 6**

calcium-rich foods 0 1 **2 3**

Times I ate out of boredom, stress, or habit:

0 1 2 3 4 5

How I took charge:

eat

☐ ate a healthy breakfast

☐ had protein at every meal

☐ avoided refined carbohydrates and sugary drinks

☐ swapped saturated fats for good fats

move

☐ walked _____ minutes / _____ steps

☐ performed Sugar Buster exercises

☐ got other exercise _____

choose

☐ got enough sleep (_____ hours)

☐ kept TV time under 2 hours

☐ found time for relaxation and/or socializing

My attitude today:

☐ excellent

☐ pretty good

☐ not my best day; I'll do better tomorrow

smart tip If you make a mistake—you gobble up a huge serving of cherry pie, for example, or you skip your daily walk and go out for ice cream instead—forgive yourself, try to learn from your mistake, and move on.

⑥ sunday

My numbers:

weight _____

blood sugar (time/level) _____ / _____

_____ / _____ • _____ / _____

Servings I ate today:

vegetables 0 1 2 3 4 **5 6 7**

fruit 0 1 2 **3**

whole grains 0 1 2 3 **4 5 6**

calcium-rich foods 0 1 **2 3**

Times I ate out of boredom, stress, or habit:

0 1 2 3 4 5

How I took charge:

eat
☐ ate a healthy breakfast
☐ had protein at every meal
☐ avoided refined carbohydrates and sugary drinks
☐ swapped saturated fats for good fats

move
☐ walked _____ minutes / _____ steps
☐ performed Sugar Buster exercises
☐ got other exercise _____

choose
☐ got enough sleep (_____ hours)
☐ kept TV time under 2 hours
☐ found time for relaxation and/or socializing

My attitude today:

☐ excellent
☐ pretty good
☐ not my best day; I'll do better tomorrow

> "Health is the thing that makes you feel that now is the best time of the year."
>
> —Franklin P. Adams

⑥ the week in review

Successes and confessions

_____
_____
_____
_____
_____
_____

My numbers:

weight loss: _____ pounds
waist measurement: _____ inches

Next week's goals

eat
Zero in on portion sizes, especially when you're eating meat. Remember, a dinner serving of meat is just the size of a deck of cards. Fill the rest of your plate with veggies and a starch or a serving of whole grains.

move
Walk for 30 minutes at least 5 days next week. Do all the Sugar Buster Routine exercises twice. Plan one extra activity that involves being active. Sign up for a tennis lesson, schedule a short hike with the family, or test out the pool at the local YMCA.

choose
Try practicing meditation for 10 minutes a day. When thoughts enter your mind, don't actively push them away, just focus on your breathing and let them drift away on their own.

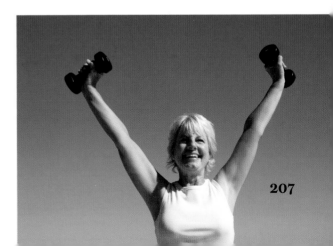

207

week ⑦ meal planner

Use prepared or packaged foods to give yourself a head start on dinner. Buy marinated chicken breasts. Top frozen pizza crust with plenty of vegetables and low-fat cheese for a fast meal.

Open a bag of frozen vegetables and stir-fry with some quick-peel shrimp for a low-cal dinner, or sauté in a little olive oil and add to pasta along with a little bit of Parmesan cheese for an easy pasta primavera. (Add leftover sliced chicken breast for a heartier meal.)

Cook frozen veggie burgers and top with sliced tomato, onion, mustard, lettuce, salsa, or low-fat feta cheese.

monday	tuesday	wednesday
breakfast		
lunch		
dinner		

thursday	friday	saturday	sunday

food fact

One slice of Swiss cheese contains abut 100 calories. Leave
it off your sandwich every day for a year and you'll lose 10 pounds.

(7) monday

My numbers:

weight _____

blood sugar (time/level) _____ / _____

_____ / _____ • _____ / _____

Servings I ate today:

vegetables 0 1 2 3 4 **5 6 7**
fruit 0 1 2 **3**
whole grains 0 1 2 3 **4 5 6**
calcium-rich foods 0 1 **2 3**

Times I ate out of boredom, stress, or habit:

0 1 2 3 4 5

How I took charge:

eat
☐ ate a healthy breakfast
☐ had protein at every meal
☐ avoided refined carbohydrates
  and sugary drinks
☐ swapped saturated fats for good fats

move
☐ walked _____ minutes / _____ steps
☐ performed Sugar Buster exercises
☐ got other exercise _____

choose
☐ got enough sleep (_____ hours)
☐ kept TV time under 2 hours
☐ found time for relaxation and/or socializing

My attitude today:
☐ excellent
☐ pretty good
☐ not my best day; I'll do better tomorrow

(7) tuesday

My numbers:

weight _____

blood sugar (time/level) _____ / _____

_____ / _____ • _____ / _____

Servings I ate today:

vegetables 0 1 2 3 4 **5 6 7**
fruit 0 1 2 **3**
whole grains 0 1 2 3 **4 5 6**
calcium-rich foods 0 1 **2 3**

Times I ate out of boredom, stress, or habit:

0 1 2 3 4 5

How I took charge:

eat
☐ ate a healthy breakfast
☐ had protein at every meal
☐ avoided refined carbohydrates
  and sugary drinks
☐ swapped saturated fats for good fats

move
☐ walked _____ minutes / _____ steps
☐ performed Sugar Buster exercises
☐ got other exercise _____

choose
☐ got enough sleep (_____ hours)
☐ kept TV time under 2 hours
☐ found time for relaxation and/or socializing

My attitude today:
☐ excellent
☐ pretty good
☐ not my best day; I'll do better tomorrow

smart tip Have a goal. Exercise is more fun when you're working toward something specific. Sign up for a charity walk, a 5K run, or a golf tournament. Or keep track of how much time you spend exercising and treat yourself to a massage or new songs for your MP3 player when you reach, say, 500 minutes of exercise.

7 wednesday

My numbers:

weight _____

blood sugar (time/level) _____ / _____

_____ / _____ • _____ / _____

Servings I ate today:

vegetables 0 1 2 3 4 **5 6 7**
fruit 0 1 2 **3**
whole grains 0 1 2 3 **4 5 6**
calcium-rich foods 0 1 **2 3**

Times I ate out of boredom, stress, or habit:

0 1 2 3 4 5

How I took charge:

eat
☐ ate a healthy breakfast
☐ had protein at every meal
☐ avoided refined carbohydrates
  and sugary drinks
☐ swapped saturated fats for good fats

move
☐ walked _____ minutes / _____ steps
☐ performed Sugar Buster exercises
☐ got other exercise _____

choose
☐ got enough sleep (_____ hours)
☐ kept TV time under 2 hours
☐ found time for relaxation and/or socializing

My attitude today:

☐ excellent
☐ pretty good
☐ not my best day; I'll do better tomorrow

7 thursday

My numbers:

weight _____

blood sugar (time/level) _____ / _____

_____ / _____ • _____ / _____

Servings I ate today:

vegetables 0 1 2 3 4 **5 6 7**
fruit 0 1 2 **3**
whole grains 0 1 2 3 **4 5 6**
calcium-rich foods 0 1 **2 3**

Times I ate out of boredom, stress, or habit:

0 1 2 3 4 5

How I took charge:

eat
☐ ate a healthy breakfast
☐ had protein at every meal
☐ avoided refined carbohydrates
  and sugary drinks
☐ swapped saturated fats for good fats

move
☐ walked _____ minutes / _____ steps
☐ performed Sugar Buster exercises
☐ got other exercise _____

choose
☐ got enough sleep (_____ hours)
☐ kept TV time under 2 hours
☐ found time for relaxation and/or socializing

My attitude today:

☐ excellent
☐ pretty good
☐ not my best day; I'll do better tomorrow

smart tip Leave peels on. Unpeeled fruits and vegetables contain more filling fiber than those with their skin and membranes removed. Wash or scrub unpeeled produce carefully with warm water. If you're concerned about pesticide residue, buy organic produce when you can afford it.

7 friday

My numbers:

weight _____

blood sugar (time/level) _____ / _____
_____ / _____ • _____ / _____

Servings I ate today:

vegetables 0 1 2 3 4 **5 6 7**
fruit 0 1 2 **3**
whole grains 0 1 2 3 **4 5 6**
calcium-rich foods 0 1 **2 3**

Times I ate out of boredom, stress, or habit:

0 1 2 3 4 5

How I took charge:

eat
☐ ate a healthy breakfast
☐ had protein at every meal
☐ avoided refined carbohydrates
   and sugary drinks
☐ swapped saturated fats for good fats

move
☐ walked _____ minutes / _____ steps
☐ performed Sugar Buster exercises
☐ got other exercise _____

choose
☐ got enough sleep (_____ hours)
☐ kept TV time under 2 hours
☐ found time for relaxation and/or socializing

My attitude today:
☐ excellent
☐ pretty good
☐ not my best day; I'll do better tomorrow

7 saturday

My numbers:

weight _____

blood sugar (time/level) _____ / _____
_____ / _____ • _____ / _____

Servings I ate today:

vegetables 0 1 2 3 4 **5 6 7**
fruit 0 1 2 **3**
whole grains 0 1 2 3 **4 5 6**
calcium-rich foods 0 1 **2 3**

Times I ate out of boredom, stress, or habit:

0 1 2 3 4 5

How I took charge:

eat
☐ ate a healthy breakfast
☐ had protein at every meal
☐ avoided refined carbohydrates
   and sugary drinks
☐ swapped saturated fats for good fats

move
☐ walked _____ minutes / _____ steps
☐ performed Sugar Buster exercises
☐ got other exercise _____

choose
☐ got enough sleep (_____ hours)
☐ kept TV time under 2 hours
☐ found time for relaxation and/or socializing

My attitude today:
☐ excellent
☐ pretty good
☐ not my best day; I'll do better tomorrow

smart tip Be your own benchmark. Pay no attention to the next person's bulging biceps, trim waistline, or marathon medals. The exercise you're doing has nothing to do with anybody but you. Stay focused on your own goals, and don't compare yourself with others.

7 sunday

My numbers:

weight _____

blood sugar (time/level) _____ / _____

_____ / _____ • _____ / _____

Servings I ate today:

vegetables 0 1 2 3 4 **5 6 7**

fruit 0 1 2 **3**

whole grains 0 1 2 3 **4 5 6**

calcium-rich foods 0 1 **2 3**

Times I ate out of boredom, stress, or habit:

0 1 2 3 4 5

How I took charge:

eat

☐ ate a healthy breakfast

☐ had protein at every meal

☐ avoided refined carbohydrates and sugary drinks

☐ swapped saturated fats for good fats

move

☐ walked _____ minutes / _____ steps

☐ performed Sugar Buster exercises

☐ got other exercise _____

choose

☐ got enough sleep (_____ hours)

☐ kept TV time under 2 hours

☐ found time for relaxation and/or socializing

My attitude today:

☐ excellent

☐ pretty good

☐ not my best day; I'll do better tomorrow

> "He who has health, has hope. And he who has hope, has everything."
> —Arabian proverb

7 the week in review

Successes and confessions

_____

_____

_____

_____

_____

_____

My numbers:

weight loss: _____ pounds

waist measurement: _____ inches

Next week's goals

eat

Switch to olive oil and canola oil, which contain "good" fats that can help stabilize blood sugar levels. Use them in place of butter. Choose extra-virgin olive oil for best taste.

move

Walk for 35 minutes at least 5 days next week. Do all the Sugar Buster Routine exercises twice. If you're getting bored with walking, find a new park to walk through, or explore a new neighborhood (preferably a hilly one!).

move

Taking good care of yourself means taking time for yourself. Plan to spend at least three hours next week doing something you enjoy.

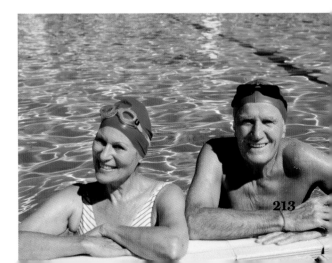

week ⑧ meal planner

How to get more vegetables into your meals? There are countless ways. First, get in the habit of starting just about every dinner with a green salad.

Sneak chopped vegetables into other foods. Add chopped or pureed carrots to meat loaf. Put chopped or pureed spinach in lasagna or pasta sauce. Add finely chopped mushrooms to beef up burgers.

You can also use vegetables in sauces. Open a jar of herb-seasoned roasted red peppers, puree, and add to tomato sauce or drizzle over fish. Puree butternut or acorn squash with carrots, grated ginger, and a bit of brown sugar for a yummy topping for chicken or turkey.

	monday	tuesday	wednesday
breakfast			
lunch			
dinner			

thursday	friday	saturday	sunday

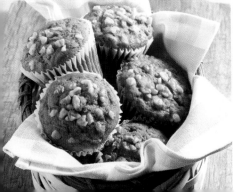

food fact
Some artificial sweeteners break down under high heat, so use brands such as Equal Spoonful or Splenda Granular for baking.

(8) monday

My numbers:

weight _____

blood sugar (time/level) _____ / _____
_____ / _____ • _____ / _____

Servings I ate today:

vegetables 0 1 2 3 4 **5 6 7**
fruit 0 1 2 **3**
whole grains 0 1 2 3 **4 5 6**
calcium-rich foods 0 1 **2 3**

Times I ate out of boredom, stress, or habit:

0 1 2 3 4 5

How I took charge:

eat
☐ ate a healthy breakfast
☐ had protein at every meal
☐ avoided refined carbohydrates and sugary drinks
☐ swapped saturated fats for good fats

move
☐ walked _____ minutes / _____ steps
☐ performed Sugar Buster exercises
☐ got other exercise _____

choose
☐ got enough sleep (_____ hours)
☐ kept TV time under 2 hours
☐ found time for relaxation and/or socializing

My attitude today:

☐ excellent
☐ pretty good
☐ not my best day; I'll do better tomorrow

(8) tuesday

My numbers:

weight _____

blood sugar (time/level) _____ / _____
_____ / _____ • _____ / _____

Servings I ate today:

vegetables 0 1 2 3 4 **5 6 7**
fruit 0 1 2 **3**
whole grains 0 1 2 3 **4 5 6**
calcium-rich foods 0 1 **2 3**

Times I ate out of boredom, stress, or habit:

0 1 2 3 4 5

How I took charge:

eat
☐ ate a healthy breakfast
☐ had protein at every meal
☐ avoided refined carbohydrates and sugary drinks
☐ swapped saturated fats for good fats

move
☐ walked _____ minutes / _____ steps
☐ performed Sugar Buster exercises
☐ got other exercise _____

choose
☐ got enough sleep (_____ hours)
☐ kept TV time under 2 hours
☐ found time for relaxation and/or socializing

My attitude today:

☐ excellent
☐ pretty good
☐ not my best day; I'll do better tomorrow

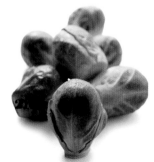

smart tip Don't love vegetables? Serve "baby" versions of vegetables such as carrots, spinach and other greens, and brussels sprouts. They tend to have more appealing texture and slightly sweeter flavor. Also, cooking vegetables a little less than usual will change the texture and perhaps even the taste.

(8) wednesday

My numbers:

weight _____

blood sugar (time/level) _____ / _____

_____ / _____ • _____ / _____

Servings I ate today:

vegetables 0 1 2 3 4 **5 6 7**
fruit 0 1 2 **3**
whole grains 0 1 2 3 **4 5 6**
calcium-rich foods 0 1 **2 3**

Times I ate out of boredom, stress, or habit:

0 1 2 3 4 5

How I took charge:

eat
☐ ate a healthy breakfast
☐ had protein at every meal
☐ avoided refined carbohydrates
  and sugary drinks
☐ swapped saturated fats for good fats

move
☐ walked _____ minutes / _____ steps
☐ performed Sugar Buster exercises
☐ got other exercise _____

choose
☐ got enough sleep (_____ hours)
☐ kept TV time under 2 hours
☐ found time for relaxation and/or socializing

My attitude today:

☐ excellent
☐ pretty good
☐ not my best day; I'll do better tomorrow

(8) thursday

My numbers:

weight _____

blood sugar (time/level) _____ / _____

_____ / _____ • _____ / _____

Servings I ate today:

vegetables 0 1 2 3 4 **5 6 7**
fruit 0 1 2 **3**
whole grains 0 1 2 3 **4 5 6**
calcium-rich foods 0 1 **2 3**

Times I ate out of boredom, stress, or habit:

0 1 2 3 4 5

How I took charge:

eat
☐ ate a healthy breakfast
☐ had protein at every meal
☐ avoided refined carbohydrates
  and sugary drinks
☐ swapped saturated fats for good fats

move
☐ walked _____ minutes / _____ steps
☐ performed Sugar Buster exercises
☐ got other exercise _____

choose
☐ got enough sleep (_____ hours)
☐ kept TV time under 2 hours
☐ found time for relaxation and/or socializing

My attitude today:

☐ excellent
☐ pretty good
☐ not my best day; I'll do better tomorrow

smart tip Be safe when you exercise outdoors. When you walk or jog, face oncoming traffic. Whenever possible, walk on a sidewalk rather than the road. Carry a cell phone to call for help if you need it. Carry identification. Wear a reflective vest if you walk on a road at night.

(8) friday

My numbers:

weight _____

blood sugar (time/level) _____ / _____

_____ / _____ • _____ / _____

Servings I ate today:

vegetables 0 1 2 3 4 **5 6 7**
fruit 0 1 2 **3**
whole grains 0 1 2 3 **4 5 6**
calcium-rich foods 0 1 **2 3**

Times I ate out of boredom, stress, or habit:

0 1 2 3 4 5

How I took charge:

eat
☐ ate a healthy breakfast
☐ had protein at every meal
☐ avoided refined carbohydrates
  and sugary drinks
☐ swapped saturated fats for good fats

move
☐ walked _____ minutes / _____ steps
☐ performed Sugar Buster exercises
☐ got other exercise _____

choose
☐ got enough sleep (_____ hours)
☐ kept TV time under 2 hours
☐ found time for relaxation and/or socializing

My attitude today:

☐ excellent
☐ pretty good
☐ not my best day; I'll do better tomorrow

(8) saturday

My numbers:

weight _____

blood sugar (time/level) _____ / _____

_____ / _____ • _____ / _____

Servings I ate today:

vegetables 0 1 2 3 4 **5 6 7**
fruit 0 1 2 **3**
whole grains 0 1 2 3 **4 5 6**
calcium-rich foods 0 1 **2 3**

Times I ate out of boredom, stress, or habit:

0 1 2 3 4 5

How I took charge:

eat
☐ ate a healthy breakfast
☐ had protein at every meal
☐ avoided refined carbohydrates
  and sugary drinks
☐ swapped saturated fats for good fats

move
☐ walked _____ minutes / _____ steps
☐ performed Sugar Buster exercises
☐ got other exercise _____

choose
☐ got enough sleep (_____ hours)
☐ kept TV time under 2 hours
☐ found time for relaxation and/or socializing

My attitude today:

☐ excellent
☐ pretty good
☐ not my best day; I'll do better tomorrow

smart tip If you like to buy in bulk to save money, be sure to divide the food into single-serving bags or containers as soon as you get home. For example, divide a large jar of peanuts into 1-ounce servings and store in plastic snack bags. Limit yourself to one bag at each snack.

8 sunday

My numbers:

weight _____

blood sugar (time/level) _____ / _____

_____ / _____ • _____ / _____

Servings I ate today:

vegetables 0 1 2 3 4 **5 6 7**

fruit 0 1 2 **3**

whole grains 0 1 2 3 **4 5 6**

calcium-rich foods 0 1 **2 3**

Times I ate out of boredom, stress, or habit:

0 1 2 3 4 5

How I took charge:

eat
- ☐ ate a healthy breakfast
- ☐ had protein at every meal
- ☐ avoided refined carbohydrates and sugary drinks
- ☐ swapped saturated fats for good fats

move
- ☐ walked _____ minutes / _____ steps
- ☐ performed Sugar Buster exercises
- ☐ got other exercise _____

choose
- ☐ got enough sleep (_____ hours)
- ☐ kept TV time under 2 hours
- ☐ found time for relaxation and/or socializing

My attitude today:
- ☐ excellent
- ☐ pretty good
- ☐ not my best day; I'll do better tomorrow

> "Take care of your body. It's the only place you have to live."
> —Jim Rohn

8 the week in review

Successes and confessions

_____

_____

_____

_____

_____

_____

My numbers:

weight loss: _____ pounds

waist measurement: _____ inches

Next week's goals

eat

Stock up on smart snacks. Remember, healthy snacking requires some preparation. Have on hand nuts, fresh fruit, cut-up raw vegetables, and low-fat yogurt.

move

Walk for 35 minutes at least 5 days next week. Do all the Sugar Buster Routine exercises twice. And make use of your time in front of the TV. Walk on your treadmill or, if you don't have one, do arm circles or march in place during the commercials.

choose

Practice waiting until you're truly hungry to eat. If there's just one food you want (especially if it's something sweet or greasy), it's a craving, not hunger. Go for a walk instead.

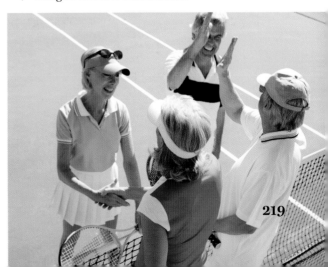

week ❾ meal planner

Many of us just aren't used to eating fish. But it's fast and easy to cook, in addition to being good for you, so we think you'll get "hooked" once you try it. Aim to eat fish twice a week. Broil it under the broiler, lightly sauté it in a pan, poach it by simmering it in a bit of broth or wine, or steam it. Try Asian Steamed Fish Fillets with Vegetable Sticks (see recipe, page 289).

Shrimp, which once had a bad reputation, is actually very low in saturated fat and relatively low in calories. So are scallops. Try Sea Scallop and Cherry Tomato Sauté (see recipe, page 288).

monday	tuesday	wednesday
breakfast		
lunch		
dinner		

thursday	friday	saturday	sunday

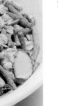

food fact
A food's glycemic load (GL) indicates the impact it has on blood sugar. Often, the more fiber and protein a cereal contains, the lower its GL.

(9) monday

My numbers:

weight _____

blood sugar (time/level) _____ / _____
_____ / _____ • _____ / _____

Servings I ate today:

vegetables 0 1 2 3 4 **5 6 7**
fruit 0 1 2 **3**
whole grains 0 1 2 3 **4 5 6**
calcium-rich foods 0 1 **2 3**

Times I ate out of boredom, stress, or habit:

0 1 2 3 4 5

How I took charge:

eat
☐ ate a healthy breakfast
☐ had protein at every meal
☐ avoided refined carbohydrates
   and sugary drinks
☐ swapped saturated fats for good fats

move
☐ walked _____ minutes / _____ steps
☐ performed Sugar Buster exercises
☐ got other exercise _____

choose
☐ got enough sleep (_____ hours)
☐ kept TV time under 2 hours
☐ found time for relaxation and/or socializing

My attitude today:

☐ excellent
☐ pretty good
☐ not my best day; I'll do better tomorrow

(9) tuesday

My numbers:

weight _____

blood sugar (time/level) _____ / _____
_____ / _____ • _____ / _____

Servings I ate today:

vegetables 0 1 2 3 4 **5 6 7**
fruit 0 1 2 **3**
whole grains 0 1 2 3 **4 5 6**
calcium-rich foods 0 1 **2 3**

Times I ate out of boredom, stress, or habit:

0 1 2 3 4 5

How I took charge:

eat
☐ ate a healthy breakfast
☐ had protein at every meal
☐ avoided refined carbohydrates
   and sugary drinks
☐ swapped saturated fats for good fats

move
☐ walked _____ minutes / _____ steps
☐ performed Sugar Buster exercises
☐ got other exercise _____

choose
☐ got enough sleep (_____ hours)
☐ kept TV time under 2 hours
☐ found time for relaxation and/or socializing

My attitude today:

☐ excellent
☐ pretty good
☐ not my best day; I'll do better tomorrow

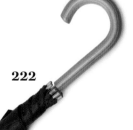

smart tip If you can't stand the weather, head for the mall. Many malls open early for walkers. Inside a mall, the temperature is always right, it never rains or snows, and you never have to worry about slipping on ice. What's more, many malls offer discounts and special offers to walkers.

⑨ wednesday

My numbers:

weight _____

blood sugar (time/level) _____ / _____
_____ / _____ • _____ / _____

Servings I ate today:

vegetables 0 1 2 3 4 **5 6 7**
fruit 0 1 2 **3**
whole grains 0 1 2 3 **4 5 6**
calcium-rich foods 0 1 **2 3**

Times I ate out of boredom, stress, or habit:

0 1 2 3 4 5

How I took charge:

eat
☐ ate a healthy breakfast
☐ had protein at every meal
☐ avoided refined carbohydrates and sugary drinks
☐ swapped saturated fats for good fats

move
☐ walked _____ minutes / _____ steps
☐ performed Sugar Buster exercises
☐ got other exercise _____

choose
☐ got enough sleep (_____ hours)
☐ kept TV time under 2 hours
☐ found time for relaxation and/or socializing

My attitude today:

☐ excellent
☐ pretty good
☐ not my best day; I'll do better tomorrow

⑨ thursday

My numbers:

weight _____

blood sugar (time/level) _____ / _____
_____ / _____ • _____ / _____

Servings I ate today:

vegetables 0 1 2 3 4 **5 6 7**
fruit 0 1 2 **3**
whole grains 0 1 2 3 **4 5 6**
calcium-rich foods 0 1 **2 3**

Times I ate out of boredom, stress, or habit:

0 1 2 3 4 5

How I took charge:

eat
☐ ate a healthy breakfast
☐ had protein at every meal
☐ avoided refined carbohydrates and sugary drinks
☐ swapped saturated fats for good fats

move
☐ walked _____ minutes / _____ steps
☐ performed Sugar Buster exercises
☐ got other exercise _____

choose
☐ got enough sleep (_____ hours)
☐ kept TV time under 2 hours
☐ found time for relaxation and/or socializing

My attitude today:

☐ excellent
☐ pretty good
☐ not my best day; I'll do better tomorrow

smart tip Keep sugarless gum everywhere—in your car, purse, briefcase, desk drawer. When you are tempted to eat an unplanned, bad-for-you snack, grab a piece of gum instead. Chewing gum provides a distraction and may buy you time to wait out your junk-food craving.

⑨ friday

My numbers:

weight _____

blood sugar (time/level) _____ / _____
_____ / _____ • _____ / _____

Servings I ate today:

vegetables 0 1 2 3 4 **5 6 7**
fruit 0 1 2 **3**
whole grains 0 1 2 3 **4 5 6**
calcium-rich foods 0 1 **2 3**

Times I ate out of boredom, stress, or habit:

0 1 2 3 4 5

How I took charge:

eat
☐ ate a healthy breakfast
☐ had protein at every meal
☐ avoided refined carbohydrates and sugary drinks
☐ swapped saturated fats for good fats

move
☐ walked _____ minutes / _____ steps
☐ performed Sugar Buster exercises
☐ got other exercise _____

choose
☐ got enough sleep (_____ hours)
☐ kept TV time under 2 hours
☐ found time for relaxation and/or socializing

My attitude today:
☐ excellent
☐ pretty good
☐ not my best day; I'll do better tomorrow

⑨ saturday

My numbers:

weight _____

blood sugar (time/level) _____ / _____
_____ / _____ • _____ / _____

Servings I ate today:

vegetables 0 1 2 3 4 **5 6 7**
fruit 0 1 2 **3**
whole grains 0 1 2 3 **4 5 6**
calcium-rich foods 0 1 **2 3**

Times I ate out of boredom, stress, or habit:

0 1 2 3 4 5

How I took charge:

eat
☐ ate a healthy breakfast
☐ had protein at every meal
☐ avoided refined carbohydrates and sugary drinks
☐ swapped saturated fats for good fats

move
☐ walked _____ minutes / _____ steps
☐ performed Sugar Buster exercises
☐ got other exercise _____

choose
☐ got enough sleep (_____ hours)
☐ kept TV time under 2 hours
☐ found time for relaxation and/or socializing

My attitude today:
☐ excellent
☐ pretty good
☐ not my best day; I'll do better tomorrow

smart tip Commit to getting plenty of sleep. Studies show that people are more likely to exercise and stick to their eating plan when they are well rested. Aim for seven to eight hours a night, or more if that's what you need to feel fully refreshed. If you need more sleep, move up your bedtime rather than sleeping later in the morning.

⑨ sunday

My numbers:

weight _____

blood sugar (time/level) _____ / _____

_____ / _____ • _____ / _____

Servings I ate today:

vegetables 0 1 2 3 4 **5 6 7**

fruit 0 1 2 **3**

whole grains 0 1 2 3 **4 5 6**

calcium-rich foods 0 1 **2 3**

Times I ate out of boredom, stress, or habit:

0 1 2 3 4 5

How I took charge:

eat

☐ ate a healthy breakfast

☐ had protein at every meal

☐ avoided refined carbohydrates and sugary drinks

☐ swapped saturated fats for good fats

move

☐ walked _____ minutes / _____ steps

☐ performed Sugar Buster exercises

☐ got other exercise _____

choose

☐ got enough sleep (_____ hours)

☐ kept TV time under 2 hours

☐ found time for relaxation and/or socializing

My attitude today:

☐ excellent

☐ pretty good

☐ not my best day; I'll do better tomorrow

> ## "If you don't like what's happening in your life, change your mind."
>
> —The Dalai Lama

⑨ the week in review

Successes and confessions

_____

_____

_____

_____

_____

_____

My numbers:

weight loss: _____ pounds

waist measurement: _____ inches

Next week's goals

eat

Eat fish or shellfish twice next week. Fresh fish is best eaten the day you buy it, but it will keep for up to a day or two if kept very cold.

move

Walk for 40 minutes at least 5 days next week. Do all the Sugar Buster Routine exercises twice. If you're getting bored of walking, substitute a new activity—like biking, ballroom dancing, cross-country skiing—on one or two days.

choose

Banish negative thoughts. When you have a negative thought, write it down, then write down a more positive version of the same thought and choose to believe it.

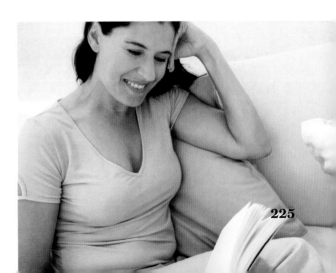

225

week ❿ meal planner

They may not be glamorous, but canned beans are convenient, cheap, and versatile. They are also highly nutritious—and a powerful way to lower your cholesterol. Plan one bean-based dinner this week.

Easy ways to use beans:

▓ Spread nonfat re-fried beans on a whole wheat burrito and sprinkle with chopped chicken and shredded cheese.

▓ Use a half-cup of black beans and salsa as a filling for your omelet.

▓ Make a bean salad with canned black beans, fresh or frozen corn kernels, chopped cilantro, chopped onion, and chopped tomato. Drizzle with olive oil and a dash of vinegar, salt, and pepper.

▓ Stock up on cans of black bean and lentil soup for lunch.

monday	tuesday	wednesday
breakfast		
lunch		
dinner		

thursday	friday	saturday	sunday

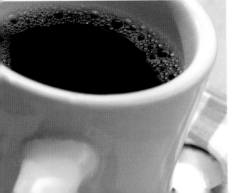

food fact
Studies have shown that coffee can lower blood sugar. It's not the caffeine that does it but other compounds, most likely chlorogenic acids. Decaf is best, since caffeine hampers insulin's effectiveness.

⑩ monday

My numbers:

weight _____

blood sugar (time/level) _____ / _____
_____ / _____ • _____ / _____

Servings I ate today:

vegetables 0 1 2 3 4 **5 6 7**
fruit 0 1 2 **3**
whole grains 0 1 2 3 **4 5 6**
calcium-rich foods 0 1 **2 3**

Times I ate out of boredom, stress, or habit:

0 1 2 3 4 5

How I took charge:

eat
☐ ate a healthy breakfast
☐ had protein at every meal
☐ avoided refined carbohydrates
　 and sugary drinks
☐ swapped saturated fats for good fats

move
☐ walked _____ minutes / _____ steps
☐ performed Sugar Buster exercises
☐ got other exercise _____

choose
☐ got enough sleep (_____ hours)
☐ kept TV time under 2 hours
☐ found time for relaxation and/or socializing

My attitude today:
☐ excellent
☐ pretty good
☐ not my best day; I'll do better tomorrow

⑩ tuesday

My numbers:

weight _____

blood sugar (time/level) _____ / _____
_____ / _____ • _____ / _____

Servings I ate today:

vegetables 0 1 2 3 4 **5 6 7**
fruit 0 1 2 **3**
whole grains 0 1 2 3 **4 5 6**
calcium-rich foods 0 1 **2 3**

Times I ate out of boredom, stress, or habit:

0 1 2 3 4 5

How I took charge:

eat
☐ ate a healthy breakfast
☐ had protein at every meal
☐ avoided refined carbohydrates
　 and sugary drinks
☐ swapped saturated fats for good fats

move
☐ walked _____ minutes / _____ steps
☐ performed Sugar Buster exercises
☐ got other exercise _____

choose
☐ got enough sleep (_____ hours)
☐ kept TV time under 2 hours
☐ found time for relaxation and/or socializing

My attitude today:
☐ excellent
☐ pretty good
☐ not my best day; I'll do better tomorrow

smart tip Follow the 100/100 rule. Eat 100 fewer calories a day (the amount in half a candy bar) and burn 100 more calories a day (by walking 15–20 minutes) and you'll lose almost half a pound a week, or 20 pounds a year. It's not fast, but it's easy and it's definitely significant.

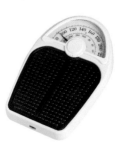

⑩ wednesday

My numbers:

weight _____

blood sugar (time/level) _____ / _____

_____ / _____ • _____ / _____

Servings I ate today:

vegetables 0 1 2 3 4 **5 6 7**
fruit 0 1 2 **3**
whole grains 0 1 2 3 **4 5 6**
calcium-rich foods 0 1 **2 3**

Times I ate out of boredom, stress, or habit:

0 1 2 3 4 5

How I took charge:

eat
☐ ate a healthy breakfast
☐ had protein at every meal
☐ avoided refined carbohydrates
  and sugary drinks
☐ swapped saturated fats for good fats

move
☐ walked _____ minutes / _____ steps
☐ performed Sugar Buster exercises
☐ got other exercise _____

choose
☐ got enough sleep (_____ hours)
☐ kept TV time under 2 hours
☐ found time for relaxation and/or socializing

My attitude today:

☐ excellent
☐ pretty good
☐ not my best day; I'll do better tomorrow

⑩ thursday

My numbers:

weight _____

blood sugar (time/level) _____ / _____

_____ / _____ • _____ / _____

Servings I ate today:

vegetables 0 1 2 3 4 **5 6 7**
fruit 0 1 2 **3**
whole grains 0 1 2 3 **4 5 6**
calcium-rich foods 0 1 **2 3**

Times I ate out of boredom, stress, or habit:

0 1 2 3 4 5

How I took charge:

eat
☐ ate a healthy breakfast
☐ had protein at every meal
☐ avoided refined carbohydrates
  and sugary drinks
☐ swapped saturated fats for good fats

move
☐ walked _____ minutes / _____ steps
☐ performed Sugar Buster exercises
☐ got other exercise _____

choose
☐ got enough sleep (_____ hours)
☐ kept TV time under 2 hours
☐ found time for relaxation and/or socializing

My attitude today:

☐ excellent
☐ pretty good
☐ not my best day; I'll do better tomorrow

smart tip Start dinner with soup or a big salad. Studies show that people who begin a meal with a clear soup (avoid cream-based soups) or green salad consume fewer calories overall at the meal. Soups and salads fill you up without a lot of calories.

229

10 friday

My numbers:

weight _____

blood sugar (time/level) _____ / _____

_____ / _____ • _____ / _____

Servings I ate today:

vegetables 0 1 2 3 4 **5 6 7**

fruit 0 1 2 **3**

whole grains 0 1 2 3 **4 5 6**

calcium-rich foods 0 1 **2 3**

Times I ate out of boredom, stress, or habit:

0 1 2 3 4 5

How I took charge:

eat
- ☐ ate a healthy breakfast
- ☐ had protein at every meal
- ☐ avoided refined carbohydrates and sugary drinks
- ☐ swapped saturated fats for good fats

move
- ☐ walked _____ minutes / _____ steps
- ☐ performed Sugar Buster exercises
- ☐ got other exercise _____

choose
- ☐ got enough sleep (_____ hours)
- ☐ kept TV time under 2 hours
- ☐ found time for relaxation and/or socializing

My attitude today:
- ☐ excellent
- ☐ pretty good
- ☐ not my best day; I'll do better tomorrow

10 saturday

My numbers:

weight _____

blood sugar (time/level) _____ / _____

_____ / _____ • _____ / _____

Servings I ate today:

vegetables 0 1 2 3 4 **5 6 7**

fruit 0 1 2 **3**

whole grains 0 1 2 3 **4 5 6**

calcium-rich foods 0 1 **2 3**

Times I ate out of boredom, stress, or habit:

0 1 2 3 4 5

How I took charge:

eat
- ☐ ate a healthy breakfast
- ☐ had protein at every meal
- ☐ avoided refined carbohydrates and sugary drinks
- ☐ swapped saturated fats for good fats

move
- ☐ walked _____ minutes / _____ steps
- ☐ performed Sugar Buster exercises
- ☐ got other exercise _____

choose
- ☐ got enough sleep (_____ hours)
- ☐ kept TV time under 2 hours
- ☐ found time for relaxation and/or socializing

My attitude today:
- ☐ excellent
- ☐ pretty good
- ☐ not my best day; I'll do better tomorrow

smart tip Set clear, immediate goals that are specific and oriented to what you can actually do, not where you want to end up. For example, it's better to set a goal of "I'll walk five minutes longer next time" than "I want to be able to run five miles by the holidays."

10 sunday

My numbers:

weight _____

blood sugar (time/level) _____ / _____
_____ / _____ • _____ / _____

Servings I ate today:

vegetables 0 1 2 3 4 **5 6 7**
fruit 0 1 2 **3**
whole grains 0 1 2 3 **4 5 6**
calcium-rich foods 0 1 **2 3**

Times I ate out of boredom, stress, or habit:

0 1 2 3 4 5

How I took charge:

eat
☐ ate a healthy breakfast
☐ had protein at every meal
☐ avoided refined carbohydrates and sugary drinks
☐ swapped saturated fats for good fats

move
☐ walked _____ minutes / _____ steps
☐ performed Sugar Buster exercises
☐ got other exercise _____

choose
☐ got enough sleep (_____ hours)
☐ kept TV time under 2 hours
☐ found time for relaxation and/or socializing

My attitude today:

☐ excellent
☐ pretty good
☐ not my best day; I'll do better tomorrow

> "The chains of habit are generally too small to be felt until they are too strong to be broken."
> —Samuel Johnson

10 the week in review

Successes and confessions

_____
_____
_____
_____
_____
_____

My numbers:

weight loss: _____ pounds
waist measurement: _____ inches

Next week's goals

eat
Eat beans at least three times next week. Add chickpeas or kidney beans to salads. Add white beans to pasta. Make turkey or vegetarian chili. Make a tasty black bean salad.

move
Walk for 40 minutes at least 5 days next week. Do all the Sugar Buster Routine exercises twice.

choose
Schedule any doctor's appointments you're due for. Remember, if you have diabetes, you should have an eye exam every year and see the dentist every six months.

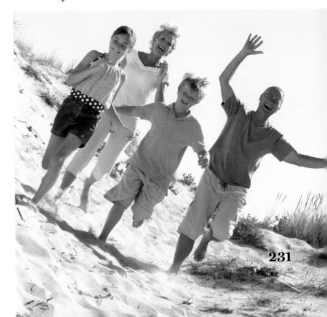

week ⑪ meal planner

Breakfast is the easiest meal to plan. If you want to lose weight and steady your blood sugar, just make sure it's high in fiber and contains protein. A high-fiber cereal (at least 5 grams per serving) with skim milk will do the trick. To boost fiber and cut sugar and calories, have a sliced orange instead of juice.

Other ideas:

- 3/4 cup oatmeal cooked in 1 1/2 cups skim milk. It'll be two servings—refrigerate one for tomorrow, then microwave.

- A half-cup low-fat cottage cheese with a cup of fresh fruit and 2 tablespoons sliced almonds.

- One hard-boiled egg with whole wheat toast.

- A 3-inch whole-wheat bagel topped with 2 tablespoons peanut butter plus one banana.

	monday	tuesday	wednesday
breakfast			
lunch			
dinner			

thursday	friday	saturday	sunday

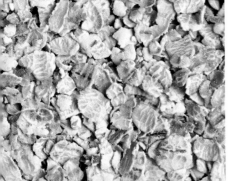

food fact
Thanks to oatmeal's soluble fiber, eating 1 1/2 cups a day can lower "bad" cholesterol by 12 to 24 percent.

⑪ monday

My numbers:

weight _____

blood sugar (time/level) _____ / _____
_____ / _____ • _____ / _____

Servings I ate today:

vegetables 0 1 2 3 4 **5 6 7**
fruit 0 1 2 **3**
whole grains 0 1 2 3 **4 5 6**
calcium-rich foods 0 1 **2 3**

Times I ate out of boredom, stress, or habit:

0 1 2 3 4 5

How I took charge:

eat
☐ ate a healthy breakfast
☐ had protein at every meal
☐ avoided refined carbohydrates
  and sugary drinks
☐ swapped saturated fats for good fats

move
☐ walked _____ minutes / _____ steps
☐ performed Sugar Buster exercises
☐ got other exercise _____

choose
☐ got enough sleep (_____ hours)
☐ kept TV time under 2 hours
☐ found time for relaxation and/or socializing

My attitude today:
☐ excellent
☐ pretty good
☐ not my best day; I'll do better tomorrow

⑪ tuesday

My numbers:

weight _____

blood sugar (time/level) _____ / _____
_____ / _____ • _____ / _____

Servings I ate today:

vegetables 0 1 2 3 4 **5 6 7**
fruit 0 1 2 **3**
whole grains 0 1 2 3 **4 5 6**
calcium-rich foods 0 1 **2 3**

Times I ate out of boredom, stress, or habit:

0 1 2 3 4 5

How I took charge:

eat
☐ ate a healthy breakfast
☐ had protein at every meal
☐ avoided refined carbohydrates
  and sugary drinks
☐ swapped saturated fats for good fats

move
☐ walked _____ minutes / _____ steps
☐ performed Sugar Buster exercises
☐ got other exercise _____

choose
☐ got enough sleep (_____ hours)
☐ kept TV time under 2 hours
☐ found time for relaxation and/or socializing

My attitude today:
☐ excellent
☐ pretty good
☐ not my best day; I'll do better tomorrow

smart tip Exercise can cause blood sugar levels to rise or fall, so it's important to monitor your blood sugar before and after exercising. If your blood sugar is less than 100 mg/dl, have a snack, such as a piece of fruit, before you exercise. Don't exercise if your blood sugar level is less than 100 mg/dl.

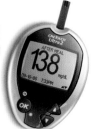

⑪ wednesday

My numbers:

weight _____

blood sugar (time/level) _____ / _____
_____ / _____ • _____ / _____

Servings I ate today:

vegetables 0 1 2 3 4 **5 6 7**
fruit 0 1 2 **3**
whole grains 0 1 2 3 **4 5 6**
calcium-rich foods 0 1 **2 3**

Times I ate out of boredom, stress, or habit:

0 1 2 3 4 5

How I took charge:

eat
☐ ate a healthy breakfast
☐ had protein at every meal
☐ avoided refined carbohydrates
   and sugary drinks
☐ swapped saturated fats for good fats

move
☐ walked _____minutes / _____steps
☐ performed Sugar Buster exercises
☐ got other exercise _____

choose
☐ got enough sleep (_____ hours)
☐ kept TV time under 2 hours
☐ found time for relaxation and/or socializing

My attitude today:

☐ excellent
☐ pretty good
☐ not my best day; I'll do better tomorrow

⑪ thursday

My numbers:

weight _____

blood sugar (time/level) _____ / _____
_____ / _____ • _____ / _____

Servings I ate today:

vegetables 0 1 2 3 4 **5 6 7**
fruit 0 1 2 **3**
whole grains 0 1 2 3 **4 5 6**
calcium-rich foods 0 1 **2 3**

Times I ate out of boredom, stress, or habit:

0 1 2 3 4 5

How I took charge:

eat
☐ ate a healthy breakfast
☐ had protein at every meal
☐ avoided refined carbohydrates
   and sugary drinks
☐ swapped saturated fats for good fats

move
☐ walked _____minutes / _____steps
☐ performed Sugar Buster exercises
☐ got other exercise _____

choose
☐ got enough sleep (_____ hours)
☐ kept TV time under 2 hours
☐ found time for relaxation and/or socializing

My attitude today:

☐ excellent
☐ pretty good
☐ not my best day; I'll do better tomorrow

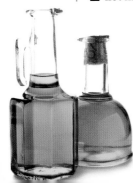

smart tip Make flavorful, extra-virgin olive oil a part of your diet. A recent study showed that people who used small amounts of olive oil in salad dressings and vegetable dishes lost more weight and ate more vegetables than those who used nonfat dressings.

⑪ friday

My numbers:

weight _____

blood sugar (time/level) _____ / _____
_____ / _____ • _____ / _____

Servings I ate today:

vegetables 0 1 2 3 4 **5 6 7**
fruit 0 1 2 **3**
whole grains 0 1 2 3 **4 5 6**
calcium-rich foods 0 1 **2 3**

Times I ate out of boredom, stress, or habit:

0 1 2 3 4 5

How I took charge:

eat
☐ ate a healthy breakfast
☐ had protein at every meal
☐ avoided refined carbohydrates
and sugary drinks
☐ swapped saturated fats for good fats

move
☐ walked _____ minutes / _____ steps
☐ performed Sugar Buster exercises
☐ got other exercise _____

choose
☐ got enough sleep (_____ hours)
☐ kept TV time under 2 hours
☐ found time for relaxation and/or socializing

My attitude today:

☐ excellent
☐ pretty good
☐ not my best day; I'll do better tomorrow

⑪ saturday

My numbers:

weight _____

blood sugar (time/level) _____ / _____
_____ / _____ • _____ / _____

Servings I ate today:

vegetables 0 1 2 3 4 **5 6 7**
fruit 0 1 2 **3**
whole grains 0 1 2 3 **4 5 6**
calcium-rich foods 0 1 **2 3**

Times I ate out of boredom, stress, or habit:

0 1 2 3 4 5

How I took charge:

eat
☐ ate a healthy breakfast
☐ had protein at every meal
☐ avoided refined carbohydrates
and sugary drinks
☐ swapped saturated fats for good fats

move
☐ walked _____ minutes / _____ steps
☐ performed Sugar Buster exercises
☐ got other exercise _____

choose
☐ got enough sleep (_____ hours)
☐ kept TV time under 2 hours
☐ found time for relaxation and/or socializing

My attitude today:

☐ excellent
☐ pretty good
☐ not my best day; I'll do better tomorrow

smart tip Don't get discouraged. Even if the numbers on the scale haven't budged much, as long as you're adding more exercise to your life, you're losing fat and replacing it with muscle, which will make it easier to keep the pounds off once you do start losing weight.

11 sunday

My numbers:

weight _____

blood sugar (time/level) _____ / _____

_____ / _____ • _____ / _____

Servings I ate today:

vegetables 0 1 2 3 4 **5 6 7**

fruit 0 1 2 **3**

whole grains 0 1 2 3 **4 5 6**

calcium-rich foods 0 1 **2 3**

Times I ate out of boredom, stress, or habit:

0 1 2 3 4 5

How I took charge:

eat
- ☐ ate a healthy breakfast
- ☐ had protein at every meal
- ☐ avoided refined carbohydrates and sugary drinks
- ☐ swapped saturated fats for good fats

move
- ☐ walked _____ minutes / _____ steps
- ☐ performed Sugar Buster exercises
- ☐ got other exercise _____

choose
- ☐ got enough sleep (_____ hours)
- ☐ kept TV time under 2 hours
- ☐ found time for relaxation and/or socializing

My attitude today:
- ☐ excellent
- ☐ pretty good
- ☐ not my best day; I'll do better tomorrow

> "The key to everything is patience. You get the chicken by hatching the egg, not by smashing it."
> —Arnold H. Glasow

11 the week in review

Successes and confessions

_____

_____

_____

_____

_____

_____

My numbers:

weight loss: _____ pounds

waist measurement: _____ inches

Next week's goals

eat

Identify three vegetable side dishes you like. Use them to start filling more of your plate with vegetables—a sure way to cut calories, as long as you don't drench your veggies in butter or cheese.

move

Next week, you should push your walks to 45 minutes—your ultimate walking goal. If you do, and you continue to walk consistently, you'll slash your risk of diabetes complications.

choose

Ask your doctor if it's okay for you to take fish oil to protect your heart. Ask over the phone if you don't have an appointment. If your doctor says yes, go out and buy the capsules, and start taking them.

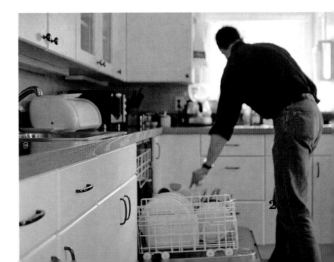

week ⑫ meal planner

A stir-fry is a quick way to make a balanced, flavorful meal. Use lots of crisp veggies with bite-size pieces of lean beef, pork, poultry, shrimp, or low-fat tofu. A wok makes it easier; for electric stoves, use a flat-bottomed wok. A nonstick stir-fry pan also works well.

To save time, buy frozen mixed vegetables such as broccoli, red peppers, onions, mushrooms, and snow peas. You can toss them directly into the hot pan. Or buy precut veggies at a salad bar. Use just a little peanut oil for extra flavor. Just two or three ounces of meat per person is fine. Cook it first, remove, and add back when the veggies are nearly done.

monday	tuesday	wednesday
breakfast		
lunch		
dinner		

thursday	friday	saturday	sunday

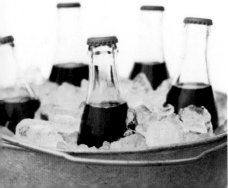

food fact
A 12-ounce can of regular soda has the equivalent of 10 teaspoons of sugar.

⑫ monday

● **My numbers:**

weight _____

blood sugar (time/level) _____ / _____

_____ / _____ • _____ / _____

● **Servings I ate today:**

vegetables 0 1 2 3 4 **5 6 7**
fruit 0 1 2 **3**
whole grains 0 1 2 3 **4 5 6**
calcium-rich foods 0 1 **2 3**

● **Times I ate out of boredom, stress, or habit:**

0 1 2 3 4 5

● **How I took charge:**

eat
☐ ate a healthy breakfast
☐ had protein at every meal
☐ avoided refined carbohydrates and sugary drinks
☐ swapped saturated fats for good fats

move
☐ walked _____ minutes / _____ steps
☐ performed Sugar Buster exercises
☐ got other exercise _____

choose
☐ got enough sleep (_____ hours)
☐ kept TV time under 2 hours
☐ found time for relaxation and/or socializing

● **My attitude today:**

☐ excellent
☐ pretty good
☐ not my best day; I'll do better tomorrow

⑫ tuesday

● **My numbers:**

weight _____

blood sugar (time/level) _____ / _____

_____ / _____ • _____ / _____

● **Servings I ate today:**

vegetables 0 1 2 3 4 **5 6 7**
fruit 0 1 2 **3**
whole grains 0 1 2 3 **4 5 6**
calcium-rich foods 0 1 **2 3**

● **Times I ate out of boredom, stress, or habit:**

0 1 2 3 4 5

● **How I took charge:**

eat
☐ ate a healthy breakfast
☐ had protein at every meal
☐ avoided refined carbohydrates and sugary drinks
☐ swapped saturated fats for good fats

move
☐ walked _____ minutes / _____ steps
☐ performed Sugar Buster exercises
☐ got other exercise _____

choose
☐ got enough sleep (_____ hours)
☐ kept TV time under 2 hours
☐ found time for relaxation and/or socializing

● **My attitude today:**

☐ excellent
☐ pretty good
☐ not my best day; I'll do better tomorrow

smart tip Cut down on alcohol. Beer, wine, and spirits are high in calories, and when you drink alcohol, you may be more likely to overeat. If you want to enjoy a drink, choose a low-calorie beer or make a spritzer—a half glass of wine mixed with club soda.

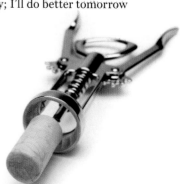

12 wednesday

My numbers:

weight _____

blood sugar (time/level) _____ / _____

_____ / _____ • _____ / _____

Servings I ate today:

vegetables 0 1 2 3 4 **5 6 7**
fruit 0 1 2 **3**
whole grains 0 1 2 3 **4 5 6**
calcium-rich foods 0 1 **2 3**

Times I ate out of boredom, stress, or habit:

0 1 2 3 4 5

How I took charge:

eat
☐ ate a healthy breakfast
☐ had protein at every meal
☐ avoided refined carbohydrates
   and sugary drinks
☐ swapped saturated fats for good fats

move
☐ walked _____minutes / _____steps
☐ performed Sugar Buster exercises
☐ got other exercise _____

choose
☐ got enough sleep (_____hours)
☐ kept TV time under 2 hours
☐ found time for relaxation and/or socializing

My attitude today:

☐ excellent
☐ pretty good
☐ not my best day; I'll do better tomorrow

12 thursday

My numbers:

weight _____

blood sugar (time/level) _____ / _____

_____ / _____ • _____ / _____

Servings I ate today:

vegetables 0 1 2 3 4 **5 6 7**
fruit 0 1 2 **3**
whole grains 0 1 2 3 **4 5 6**
calcium-rich foods 0 1 **2 3**

Times I ate out of boredom, stress, or habit:

0 1 2 3 4 5

How I took charge:

eat
☐ ate a healthy breakfast
☐ had protein at every meal
☐ avoided refined carbohydrates
   and sugary drinks
☐ swapped saturated fats for good fats

move
☐ walked _____minutes / _____steps
☐ performed Sugar Buster exercises
☐ got other exercise _____

choose
☐ got enough sleep (_____hours)
☐ kept TV time under 2 hours
☐ found time for relaxation and/or socializing

My attitude today:

☐ excellent
☐ pretty good
☐ not my best day; I'll do better tomorrow

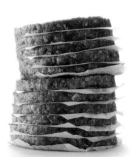

smart tip Cut calories by choosing the lowest-fat ground beef. A 3-ounce patty made with 95 percent lean ground beef contains 145 calories and 6 grams fat; the same size burger made with 73 percent lean ground beef weighs in at 248 calories and 18 grams fat.

241

(12) friday

My numbers:

weight _____

blood sugar (time/level) _____ / _____

_____ / _____ • _____ / _____

Servings I ate today:

vegetables 0 1 2 3 4 **5 6 7**
fruit 0 1 2 **3**
whole grains 0 1 2 3 **4 5 6**
calcium-rich foods 0 1 **2 3**

Times I ate out of boredom, stress, or habit:

0 1 2 3 4 5

How I took charge:

eat
☐ ate a healthy breakfast
☐ had protein at every meal
☐ avoided refined carbohydrates
   and sugary drinks
☐ swapped saturated fats for good fats

move
☐ walked _____ minutes / _____ steps
☐ performed Sugar Buster exercises
☐ got other exercise _____

choose
☐ got enough sleep (_____ hours)
☐ kept TV time under 2 hours
☐ found time for relaxation and/or socializing

My attitude today:

☐ excellent
☐ pretty good
☐ not my best day; I'll do better tomorrow

(12) saturday

My numbers:

weight _____

blood sugar (time/level) _____ / _____

_____ / _____ • _____ / _____

Servings I ate today:

vegetables 0 1 2 3 4 **5 6 7**
fruit 0 1 2 **3**
whole grains 0 1 2 3 **4 5 6**
calcium-rich foods 0 1 **2 3**

Times I ate out of boredom, stress, or habit:

0 1 2 3 4 5

How I took charge:

eat
☐ ate a healthy breakfast
☐ had protein at every meal
☐ avoided refined carbohydrates
   and sugary drinks
☐ swapped saturated fats for good fats

move
☐ walked _____ minutes / _____ steps
☐ performed Sugar Buster exercises
☐ got other exercise _____

choose
☐ got enough sleep (_____ hours)
☐ kept TV time under 2 hours
☐ found time for relaxation and/or socializing

My attitude today:

☐ excellent
☐ pretty good
☐ not my best day; I'll do better tomorrow

smart tip When you exercise, treat your feet well. People with diabetes are at an increased risk of skin infections, particularly in the feet. Make sure your sneakers fit properly and don't pinch. Wear cushiony socks. And check your feet after each exercise session for cuts, sores, blisters, ulcers, or redness.

12 sunday

My numbers:

weight _____

blood sugar (time/level) _____ / _____

_____ / _____ • _____ / _____

Servings I ate today:

vegetables 0 1 2 3 4 **5 6 7**

fruit 0 1 2 **3**

whole grains 0 1 2 3 **4 5 6**

calcium-rich foods 0 1 **2 3**

Times I ate out of boredom, stress, or habit:

0 1 2 3 4 5

How I took charge:

eat
☐ ate a healthy breakfast
☐ had protein at every meal
☐ avoided refined carbohydrates
   and sugary drinks
☐ swapped saturated fats for good fats

move
☐ walked _____ minutes / _____ steps
☐ performed Sugar Buster exercises
☐ got other exercise _____

choose
☐ got enough sleep (_____ hours)
☐ kept TV time under 2 hours
☐ found time for relaxation and/or socializing

My attitude today:

☐ excellent
☐ pretty good
☐ not my best day; I'll do better tomorrow

> "If taking vitamins doesn't keep you healthy enough, try more laughter."
> —Nicolas-Sebastien Chamfort

12 the week in review

Successes and confessions

_____
_____
_____
_____
_____
_____

My numbers:

weight loss: _____ pounds
waist measurement: _____ inches

Next week's goals

eat
Keep your lunches to 350–450 calories. Make sure you ___ e your sandwich on whole-grain bread (the ___ "whole" must appear in the first ingredient), ___ nd bulk it up with plenty of lettuce, tomatoes, or cucumber slices.

move
Keep up your new habits of walking for 45 minutes a day on most days of the week, doing the Sugar Buster Routine twice a week, and looking for ways to fit other fitness into your day. This should be all the exercise you need.

choose
Really focus this week on getting enough sleep. If you're waking up tired, keep going to bed 15 minutes earlier until you're waking up refreshed.

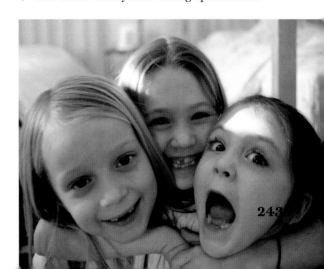

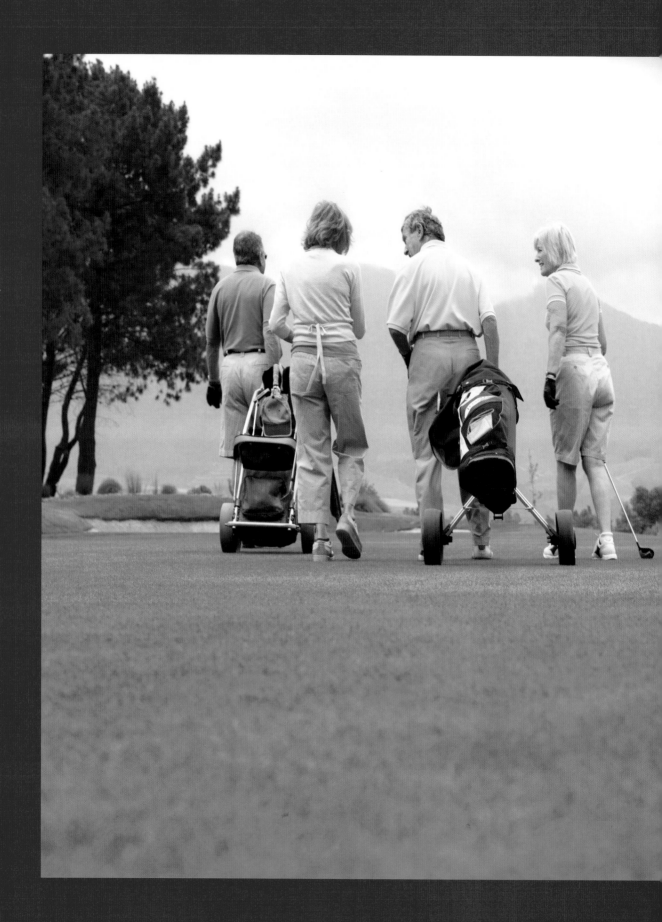

5

reverse diabetes
TOOLS

- Food Diary
- Nutritional Counters
- Shopping Help

- Better Health

Your Seven-Day Food Diary

On the Eat portion of the Eat, Move, Choose Plan we ask you to keep track of everything you eat and drink for one week before you start the plan. Write down what you've eaten or drunk, the estimated portion size, and the estimated calories (check the calorie counts starting on page 256 or at www.caloriecontrol.org). At the end of the week, look over your diary for patterns and opportunities. Do you never eat a fruit or vegetable at breakfast or lunch? Do you snack late at night? Where are you overdoing the calories?

EXAMPLE	WHAT I ATE/DRANK	ESTIMATED PORTION SIZE	CALORIES	NOTES
Breakfast	Coffee with 2 sugars	1 cup	35	Not enough sleep!
	Cornflakes w/	2 cups	300	
	2% milk	1 cup	120	
Lunch	Ham and cheese sandwich	1	360	Ate at meeting
	Chips - single serving	1 oz	160	
	Diet Cola	12 oz	0	

DAY 1	WHAT I ATE/DRANK	ESTIMATED PORTION SIZE	CALORIES	NOTES
Breakfast				
Lunch				
Dinner				
Snacks				

DAY 2	WHAT I ATE/DRANK	ESTIMATED PORTION SIZE	CALORIES	NOTES
Breakfast				
Lunch				
Dinner				
Snacks				

DAY 3	WHAT I ATE/DRANK	ESTIMATED PORTION SIZE	CALORIES	NOTES
Breakfast				
Lunch				
Dinner				
Snacks				

continued >>>

DAY 4	WHAT I ATE/DRANK	ESTIMATED PORTION SIZE	CALORIES	NOTES
Breakfast				
Lunch				
Dinner				
Snacks				

DAY 5	WHAT I ATE/DRANK	ESTIMATED PORTION SIZE	CALORIES	NOTES
Breakfast				
Lunch				
Dinner				
Snacks				

DAY 6	WHAT I ATE/DRANK	ESTIMATED PORTION SIZE	CALORIES	NOTES
Breakfast				
Lunch				
Dinner				
Snacks				

DAY 7	WHAT I ATE/DRANK	ESTIMATED PORTION SIZE	CALORIES	NOTES
Breakfast				
Lunch				
Dinner				
Snacks				

Reverse Diabetes Kitchen Makeover

A well-stocked, well-organized kitchen is your greatest Reverse Diabetes ally. Keeping the right foods at your fingertips means you'll be ready to put together fast, blood-sugar friendly dinners, build delicious lunches and breakfasts, and grab healthy treats when you want a snack. You'll be able to enjoy food without guilt, worry, fear—and without the danger of being sidetracked by temptations that make blood sugar spike and pack on pounds.

Ready to begin? The first step isn't shopping; it's clearing your kitchen of foods that pack too many calories or refined carbohydrates, too much fat, or too much sugar. Grab a trash bag and a box for items you can give away. (If there are items that other family members eat, consider putting them in a designated area of the pantry, refrigerator, or freezer, and leave yourself plenty of room for healthy stuff!) The second step: Use our "Stock Up" list to put the right edibles in place. No need to overspend the grocery budget; you can add a few to your shopping list each week.

PANTRY

Toss, give away, or move to a designated spot:

- ☐ Boxed mashed potato mix
- ☐ Breakfast cereals high in sugar or that don't list a whole grain as the first ingredient
- ☐ Cornflakes (the glycemic load is too high)
- ☐ Butter-flavored microwave popcorn
- ☐ Candy
- ☐ Canned fruit in heavy syrup
- ☐ Cereal bars (except those that are low sugar, contain no hydrogenated oil, and list a whole grain as the first ingredient)
- ☐ Cookies
- ☐ Corn and sunflower oil

- ☐ Crackers that contain hydrogenated oil or don't have a whole grain as the first ingredient
- ☐ Cream soups
- ☐ Non-diet soda and juice drinks
- ☐ Packaged and snack foods that list hydrogenated oils or trans fats
- ☐ Sugar-sweetened iced tea or lemonade mix
- ☐ Shortening
- ☐ Chips
- ☐ White bread
- ☐ White rice

Stock

- ☐ Applesauce, jars (use in place of oil for baking)
- ☐ Barley (use in soup and as a side dish)

- ☐ Broth—low-sodium chicken or vegetable, canned
- ☐ Cereal, whole-grain, with at least 3 grams of fiber per serving
- ☐ Cocoa powder, unsweetened
- ☐ Cooking spray
- ☐ Couscous, whole-grain
- ☐ Fruit, canned in juice or light syrup
- ☐ Garlic, fresh
- ☐ Legumes (kidney beans, chickpeas, black beans, etc.), canned or dried
- ☐ Mushrooms, dried
- ☐ Oatmeal (rolled oats)
- ☐ Oils—olive, canola
- ☐ Onions
- ☐ Pasta, whole-grain
- ☐ Peanut butter
- ☐ Popcorn kernels

- ☐ Potatoes, baking or roasting, and sweet potatoes or yams
- ☐ Raisins, other dried fruit
- ☐ Rice, brown
- ☐ Salmon, canned
- ☐ Sugar substitute
- ☐ Soups—low-sodium broth-based soups, especially vegetable and bean soups
- ☐ Tomatoes, canned
- ☐ Tomato sauce, no salt added
- ☐ Tuna, canned in water
- ☐ Vegetables, canned
- ☐ Vinegars
- ☐ Whole-grain bread, mini bagels, and rolls
- ☐ Whole-grain crackers
- ☐ Whole-wheat flour

REFRIGERATOR

Toss, give away, or move to a designated spot:

☐ Full-fat cheddar, jack, and other cheeses (or cut the cheese the recipe calls for in half)

☐ Full-fat mayonnaise

☐ Full-fat milk, half-and-half, and cream

☐ Full-fat sour cream

☐ Full-fat yogurt

☐ Sugary drinks—sodas, sweetened teas, fruit juice "drinks"

☐ Butter (or use very sparingly)

☐ Margarines that contain trans fats

Stock

☐ Margarine

(with 0 trans fats and saturated fat)

☐ Hard cheese for grating, such as Parmesan

☐ Eggs and/or egg substitute

☐ Milk—low-fat or nonfat

☐ Yogurt, plain—low-fat or nonfat, sweetened with a no-calorie sweetener if desired

☐ Nonfat or low-fat sour cream

☐ Lean beef, chicken, turkey, or pork

☐ Fruit, assorted fresh

☐ Vegetables, assorted fresh—plus "staples" such as onions and celery

☐ Carrot sticks

FREEZER

Toss, give away, or move to a designated spot:

☐ Breaded fish sticks, fish fillets, and chicken

☐ French fries and potato nuggets

☐ Full-fat ice cream

☐ Vegetables in butter or cream sauces

☐ Frozen snack foods (such as pizza pockets)

☐ Frozen waffles (except whole-grain)

☐ Frozen dinners containing more than 15 grams of fat per serving

☐ Bacon and full-fat breakfast sausage

Stock

☐ Breads—whole-wheat and whole-grain pita

☐ Berries and other fruit, frozen without added sugar

☐ Sugar-free frozen fruit pops or bars

☐ Chicken breasts, individually portioned

☐ Edamame

☐ Fish fillets (unbreaded), shelled shrimp, scallops

☐ Ground turkey or lean ground beef

☐ Meatless burgers

☐ Vegetables, frozen without sauces

KITCHEN EQUIPMENT

☐ Good-quality nonstick skillet (it will allow you to sauté foods with very little oil)

☐ Heat-proof rubber spatula

☐ Salad spinner

☐ Vegetable steamer

☐ Nonstick stir-fry pan

☐ Pot (with lid) large enough to cook soup, rice, or pasta

☐ Vegetable scrubber

☐ Microwave-safe food storage containers

☐ Opaque storage containers for "treat" foods for other family members (so you

won't be tempted by the sight of the contents!)

☐ Zipper-lock bags

☐ Plastic wrap

☐ Aluminum foil

☐ Freezer bags and containers

☐ Sharp kitchen knives

☐ 2 dishwasher-safe cutting boards (reserve one for vegetables and fruit, one for meat)

251

Weekly Shopping List

Make a dozen copies of this list and post one each week on your refrigerator. Use the check-off boxes to note what you need so that grocery shopping's a breeze.

FRUITS
- ☐ Apples
- ☐ Bananas
- ☐ Berries
- ☐ Grapes
- ☐ Kiwifruit
- ☐ Lemons/limes
- ☐ Mangoes
- ☐ Melons
- ☐ Oranges
- ☐ Peaches/nectarines/ apricots
- ☐ Pears
- ☐ Plums
- ☐ Other:

———————————————
———————————————
———————————————

VEGETABLES
- ☐ Asparagus
- ☐ Bell peppers
- ☐ Broccoli
- ☐ Carrots
- ☐ Cauliflower
- ☐ Celery
- ☐ Corn
- ☐ Cucumber
- ☐ Eggplant
- ☐ Garlic
- ☐ Green beans
- ☐ Kale, collards, and other greens for cooking
- ☐ Mushrooms
- ☐ Onions
- ☐ Potatoes (sweet and white)
- ☐ Salad greens
- ☐ Spinach
- ☐ Tomatoes
- ☐ Winter Squash
- ☐ Zucchini/Summer Squash
- ☐ Other:

———————————————
———————————————
———————————————

MEAT AND SEAFOOD
- ☐ Chicken or turkey breast
- ☐ Lean beef (round, sirloin, flank steak, tenderloin)
- ☐ Lean pork (ham, tenderloin, center loin chop)
- ☐ Fresh fish or seafood
- ☐ Other:

———————————————
———————————————
———————————————

DAIRY AISLE
- ☐ Eggs
- ☐ Low-fat cheeses
- ☐ Low-fat tofu
- ☐ Low-fat yogurt
- ☐ Margarine
- ☐ Skim milk

GRAINS
- ☐ Barley
- ☐ Bulgur
- ☐ Oatmeal
- ☐ Rice, brown or converted
- ☐ Whole-grain cereal
- ☐ Whole-grain bread
- ☐ Whole-grain crackers
- ☐ Whole-grain pasta
- ☐ Other:

———————————————
———————————————
———————————————

NONPERISHABLES
- ☐ Cooking spray
- ☐ Gelatin
- ☐ Nuts (almonds, walnuts, peanuts)
- ☐ Oils (olive, canola)
- ☐ Peanut butter and other nut butters
- ☐ Splenda or other sugar substitute

CANNED GOODS
- ☐ Beans (black, kidney, navy, etc.)
- ☐ Soup (low-sodium, bean/vegetable)
- ☐ Tomatoes
- ☐ Other vegetables (artichoke hearts, roasted peppers)
- ☐ Tuna packed in water

- ☐ Canned fruit in juice or light syrup

FREEZER AISLE
- ☐ Frozen fish fillets (without breading or sauce)
- ☐ Frozen shrimp and/or scallops
- ☐ Frozen vegetables
- ☐ Frozen fruit (without added sugar)
- ☐ Veggie burgers
- ☐ Sugar-free frozen fruit pops or bars
- ☐ Other:

———————————————
———————————————
———————————————

OTHER

———————————————
———————————————
———————————————
———————————————
———————————————
———————————————
———————————————
———————————————
———————————————
———————————————
———————————————

Diabetes Testing and Management Schedule

At Every Doctor's Visit (usually 4 times per year)

TEST	DATE	RESULT	DATE	RESULT	DATE	RESULT	DATE	RESULT
A1C (goal is lower than 7)								
Blood pressure (goal is lower than 130/80)								
Foot check								

Twice a Year

TEST	DATE	DATE
Dental cleaning and exam		

Yearly (on anniversary of last test)

TEST	LAST YEAR'S DATE	LAST YEAR'S RESULT	THIS YEAR'S DATE	THIS YEAR'S RESULT
Microalbumin urine test (for kidney function)				
Eye exam (with dilation)				
LDL cholesterol*				
HDL cholesterol**				
Triglycerides***				
Foot exam (from a podiatrist)				
Flu shot				

*goal is lower than 100 mg/dl or lower than 70 mg/dl if you have known cardiovascular disease

**goal is higher than 40 mg/dl for men and higher than 50 mg/dl for women

***goal is lower than 150 mg/dl

253

daily food and exercise log

If cutting portion sizes and carbs at one meal still leaves your blood sugar levels high before the next meal, try adding exercise to bring those levels down further.

Day:_____   Date:_____

MORNING

Breakfast Time:_____   Blood sugar before eating:_____

ITEM	AMOUNT	CARBS*

Blood sugar two hours after eating:_____

Snack Time:_____   Blood sugar before eating:_____

ITEM	AMOUNT	CARBS*

Exercise Time:_____

ACTIVITY

DURATION

MIDDAY

Lunch Time:_____   Blood sugar before eating:_____

ITEM	AMOUNT	CARBS*

Blood sugar two hours after eating:_____

Snack Time:_____   Blood sugar before eating:_____

ITEM	AMOUNT	CARBS*

Exercise Time:_____

ACTIVITY

DURATION

EVENING

Dinner Time:_____   Blood sugar before eating:_____

ITEM	AMOUNT	CARBS*

Blood sugar two hours after eating:_____

Snack Time:_____   Blood sugar before eating:_____

ITEM	AMOUNT	CARBS*

Exercise Time:_____

ACTIVITY

DURATION

*choices or grams

Handy Numbers to Know

GENERAL BLOOD SUGAR TARGETS

Fasting or before meal glucose	90–130 mg/dl
After-meal glucose (two hours after the start of your meal)	>180 mg/dl
Bedtime glucose	100–140 mg/dl

HOW TO TRANSLATE A1C NUMBERS

A1C	Blood Glucose Level	
6.0%	135 mg/dl	7.5 mmol/l*
6.5%	153 mg/dl	8.5 mmol/l*
7.0%	170 mg/dl	9.5 mmol/l*
7.5%	188 mg/dl	10.5 mmol/l*
8.0%	205 mg/dl	11.4 mmol/l*
8.5%	223 mg/dl	12.4 mmol/l*
9.0%	240 mg/dl	13.3 mmol/l*
9.5%	258 mg/dl	14.3 mmol/l*
10.0%	275 mg/dl	15.3 mmol/l*
10.5%	293 mg/dl	16.3 mmol/l*
11.0%	310 mg/dl	17.2 mmol/l*
11.5%	328 mg/dl	18.2 mmol/l*
12.0%	345 mg/dl	19.1 mmol/l*

* Millimoles per liter, used outside the U.S.

HEALTHY WAIST CIRCUMFERENCE

Men	up to 40 inches
Women	up to 35 inches

If your waist is bigger than this, you are at increased risk for type 2 diabetes, high blood pressure, high cholesterol, and cardiovascular disease.

Calories, Carbohydrates, and Fiber in Common Foods

Item	Amount	Calories	Carb grams	Fiber grams
BEEF				
Beef, chuck	3 oz	293	0	0
Corned beef	3 oz	213	0.8	0
Ground beef, 75% lean	3 oz	236	0	0
Ground beef, 85% lean	3 oz	213	0	0
Beef, rib	3 oz	304	0	0
Beef, bottom round	3 oz	210	0	0
Beef, top sirloin	3 oz	207	0	0
BEVERAGES				
Beer, light	12 fl oz	103	5.2	0
Beer, regular	12 fl oz	138	10.7	0
Chocolate milk	1 cup	226	31.7	1.1
Club soda	12 fl oz	0	0	0
Coffee	6 fl oz	2	0	0
Cola	12 fl oz	155	39.8	0
Diet cola	12 fl oz	4	0.4	0
Espresso	2 fl oz	1	0	0
Fruit punch	8 fl oz	117	29.7	0.5
Hot cocoa	1 cup	113	24	1
Ginger ale	12 fl oz	124	32.1	0
Instant coffee	6 fl oz	4	0.6	0
Lemonade	8 fl oz	112	34.1	0.2
Liquor (rum, gin, vodka, whiskey)	1.5 fl oz	110	0	0
Piña colada	4.5 fl oz	245	32	0.4
Soy milk	1 cup	127	12.08	3.2
Tea	6 fl oz	2	0.5	0
Wine, red	3.5 fl oz	74	1.8	0
Wine, white	3.5 fl oz	70	0.8	0
BREAD, BAGELS, ROLLS				
Bagel, plain	4"	245	48	2
Bagel, cinnamon raisin	4"	244	49	2
Bagel, egg	4"	247	47.2	2
Biscuit, buttermilk	4"	358	45.1	1.5
Bread, French	1/2" slice	69	13	0.8

Item	Amount	Calories	Carb grams	Fiber grams
Bread, Italian	1 slice	54	10	0.5
Bread, white	1 slice	67	12.7	0.6
Bread, wheat	1 slice	69	12.9	1.9
Bread, rye	1 slice	83	15.5	1.9
Bread, pumpernickel	1 slice	80	15.2	2.1
Bread, raisin	1 slice	71	13.6	1.1
Croissant	1	231	26.1	1.5
Corn bread	1 piece	173	28.3	1.4
Pita	4"	77	15.6	0.6
CEREALS				
All Bran	1/2 cup	79	23	9.7
Apple Cinnamon Cheerios	3/4 cup	118	25	1.6
Cap'n Crunch	3/4 cup	108	22.9	0.7
Cheerios	1 cup	111	22.2	3.6
Chex, Corn	1 cup	112	25.8	0.6
Chex, Honey Nut	3/4 cup	117	26	0.4
Chex, Multi-Bran	1 cup	165	41	6.4
Cornflakes	1 cup	101	24.4	0.7
Cream of Wheat	1 cup	126	26.9	1
Froot Loops	1 cup	118	26.2	0.8
Frosted Flakes	3/4 cup	114	28	1
Frosted Mini-Wheats	1 cup	173	42	5.5
Honey Nut Cheerios	1 cup	115	24	1.6
Life	3/4 cup	121	25	2
Oatmeal, regular	1 cup	147	25.3	4
Oatmeal, instant, apples and cinnamon	1 packet	130	26.5	2.7
Puffed Rice	1 cup	56	12.6	0.2
Puffed Wheat	1 cup	44	10	0.5
Raisin Bran	1 cup	195	46.5	7.3
Rice Krispies	1 1/4 cups	119	28	0.1
Special K	1 cup	117	22	0.7
Shredded Wheat	2 biscuits	155	36.2	5.5
Total	3/4 cup	105	24	2.6

Item	Amount	Calories	Carb grams	Fiber grams
Trix	1 cup	122	26	0.7
Wheaties	1 cup	107	26.7	3

DAIRY AND EGGS

Item	Amount	Calories	Carb grams	Fiber grams
Butter	1 Tbsp	102	0	0
Cheese food, American	1 oz	94	2.2	0
Cheese spread	1 oz	82	2.5	0
Cheese, blue	1 oz	100	0.7	0
Cheese, cheddar	1 oz	114	0.4	0
Cheese, cottage, regular	1 cup	216	5.6	0
Cheese, cottage, 2% milk fat	1 cup	203	8.2	0
Cheese, cottage, 1% milk fat	1 cup	163	6.2	0
Cheese, cream	1 Tbsp	51	0.4	0
Cheese, feta	1 oz	75	1.2	0
Cheese, mozzarella, part skim milk	1 oz	72	0.79	0
Cheese, mozzarella, whole milk	1 oz	85	0.6	0
Cheese, Muenster	1 oz	104	0.3	0
Cheese, Parmesan	1 Tbsp	22	0.2	0
Cheese, American	1 oz	106	0.5	0
Cheese, provolone	1 oz	100	0.6	0
Cheese, ricotta, part skim milk	1 cup	339	12.6	0
Cheese, ricotta, whole milk	1 cup	428	7.5	0
Cheese, Swiss	1 oz	108	1.5	0
Cream, half and half	1 Tbsp	20	0.7	0
Cream, heavy whipping	1 Tbsp	52	0.4	0
Cream, light	1 Tbsp	29	0.6	0
Cream, sour	1 Tbsp	26	0.5	0
Cream, sour, reduced-fat	1 Tbsp	20	0.6	0
Cream, sour, fat-free	1 Tbsp	12	2	0
Egg, whole	large	74	0.8	0
Egg, white	large	17	0.2	0
Egg, yolk	large	53	0.6	0
Eggnog	1 cup	343	34.3	0
Ice cream, chocolate	1/2 cup	143	18.6	0.8

Item	Amount	Calories	Carb grams	Fiber grams
Ice cream, vanilla, soft-serve	1/2 cup	191	19.1	0.6
Ice cream, vanilla	1/2 cup	133	15.6	0.5
Milkshake, vanilla	11 fl oz	351	55.6	0
Buttermilk	1 cup	98	11.7	0
Milk, condensed, sweetened	1 cup	982	166.5	0
Milk, evaporated, nonfat	1 cup	200	29.1	0
Milk, nonfat	1 cup	83	12.1	0
Milk, 1% milk fat	1 cup	102	12.2	0
Milk, 2% milk fat	1 cup	102	11.4	0
Milk, whole	1 cup	146	11	0
Yogurt, fruit, low-fat	8 oz	232	43.2	0
Yogurt, plain, low-fat	8 oz	143	16	0

FATS AND OIL

Item	Amount	Calories	Carb grams	Fiber grams
Lard	1 Tbsp	115	0	0
Margarine	1 Tbsp	102	0.1	0
Margarine-like spread	1 Tbsp	51	0	0
Mayonnaise, regular	1 Tbsp	99	0	0
Mayonnaise, fat-free	1 Tbsp	12	2	0.6
Oil, canola	1 Tbsp	124	0	0
Oil, olive	1 Tbsp	119	0	0
Oil, peanut	1 Tbsp	119	0	0
Oil, sesame	1 Tbsp	120	0	0
Oil, vegetable or corn	1 Tbsp	120	0	0
Shortening	1 Tbsp	113	0	0

FISH AND SHELLFISH

Item	Amount	Calories	Carb grams	Fiber grams
Catfish, breaded and fried	3 oz	195	6.8	0.6
Crab	3 oz	82	0	0
Flounder	3 oz	99	0	0
Haddock, baked	3 oz	95	0	0
Halibut	3 oz	119	0	0
Lobster	3 oz	83	1.1	0
Ocean perch	3 oz	103	0	0
Orange roughy	3 oz	76	0	0

continued >>>

Item	Amount	Calories	Carb grams	Fiber grams
Pollock	3 oz	96	0	0
Rainbow trout	3 oz	144	0	0
Raw clams	3 oz	63	2.2	0
Raw oysters	6 med	57	3.3	0
Salmon, baked or broiled	3 oz	184	0	0
Salmon, canned	3 oz	118	0	0
Sardines	3 oz	177	0	0
Scallops, breaded	6 large	200	9.4	0
Shrimp, breaded	3 oz	206	5.2	0.2
Swordfish	3 oz	132	0	0
Tuna, baked or broiled	3 oz	118	0	0
Tuna, chunk white	3 oz	109	0	0

FRUIT AND JUICES

Item	Amount	Calories	Carb grams	Fiber grams
Apple juice	1 cup	117	29	0.2
Apple	1	72	19.1	3.3
Applesauce, sweetened	1 cup	194	51	3.1
Applesauce, unsweetened	1 cup	108	28	2.9
Apricot	1	17	3.9	0.7
Apricots, dried	1/4 cup	96	25	3.6
Apricots, canned in heavy syrup	1 cup	214	55	4.1
Apricots, canned in juice	1 cup	117	30	3.9
Apricot nectar, canned	1 cup	141	36	1.5
Asian pear	1 small	51	13	4.4
Avocado	1 oz	47	2.5	1.9
Banana	1	105	27	3.1
Blackberries	1 cup	75	18	7.6
Blueberries	1 cup	83	21	3.5
Cantaloupe	1 cup	107	28	3
Cherries, sour	1 cup	88	22	2.7
Cherries, sweet	10	49	11	1.6
Cranberries, dried, sweetened	1/4 cup	92	24	2.5
Cranberry juice cocktail	8 fl oz	144	36.4	0.3
Cranberry sauce, canned	1 slice	86	22	0.6
Currants, dried	1/4 cup	102	26.7	2.4

Item	Amount	Calories	Carb grams	Fiber grams
Dates, chopped	1/4 cup	122	32.7	3.3
Figs, dried	1/4 cup	127	32.5	5.8
Figs, fresh	1	37	9.6	1.7
Grape juice	1 cup	154	37.9	0.3
Grapefruit	1/2	39	9.9	1.3
Grapefruit juice	1 cup	96	22.7	0.2
Grapes, red or green	1 cup	110	29	1.4
Kiwi	1	46	11.1	2.3
Honeydew melon	1 cup	60	16	1
Lemon juice	juice of 1 lemon	12	4	0.2
Lime juice	juice of 1 lime	10	3.2	0.2
Mandarin oranges, canned in light syrup	1 cup	154	41	1.8
Mango	1 cup	107	28	3.7
Nectarine	1	67	16.0	2.2
Orange juice	1 cup	112	25.8	0.5
Orange	1	62	15.4	3.1
Papaya	1 cup	55	29.8	2.5
Peach	1	38	9.4	1.5
Peaches, canned in heavy syrup	1 cup	194	52	3.4
Peaches, canned in juice	1 cup	109	29	3.2
Pear	1 pear	96	25.7	5.1
Pears, canned in heavy syrup	1 cup	197	51	4.3
Pears, canned in juice	1 cup	124	32	4
Pineapple juice	1 cup	140	34.5	0.5
Pineapple	1 cup	74	19.6	2.2
Pineapple, canned in heavy syrup	1 cup	198	51	2
Pineapple, canned in juice	1 cup	149	39	2
Plantain, raw	1	218	57	4.1
Plantain, cooked slices	1 cup	179	48	3.5
Plum	1	30	7.5	0.9

Item	Amount	Calories	Carb grams	Fiber grams
Plums, canned in heavy syrup	1 cup	230	60	2.6
Plums, canned in juice	1 cup	146	38	2.5
Prunes, dried	5	100	26	3
Prunes, stewed	1 cup	265	70	16.4
Prune juice	1 cup	182	44.7	2.6
Raisins	1/4 cup	108	28.7	1.3
Raspberries	1 cup	64	14.7	8
Strawberries	1 cup	53	12.8	3.3
Tangerine	1	31	7.8	1.6
Watermelon	1 cup	56	11.5	0.6

GRAINS AND PASTAS

Item	Amount	Calories	Carb grams	Fiber grams
Couscous	1 cup	176	36.5	2.2
Barley, pearled and cooked	1 cup	193	44	6
Bulgur	1 cup	151	33	8.2
Cornmeal	1 cup	444	94	8.9
Egg noodles	1 cup	213	39.7	1.8
Kasha (buckwheat groats)	1 cup	155	33	4.5
Oat bran (raw)	1 cup	231	62.3	14.5
Rice, brown	1 cup	216	45	3.5
Rice, white	1 cup	205	45	0.6
Rice, instant	1 cup	162	35	1
Rice, wild	1 cup	166	35	3
Pasta, regular	1 cup	197	40	2.4
Pasta, whole-wheat	1 cup	174	37	6.3
Wheat flour, bleached (white)	1 cup	455	95	3.4
Wheat flour, whole-grain	1 cup	407	87	14.6
Wheat germ	1 Tbsp	27	3	0.9

LAMB, VEAL, AND GAME

Item	Amount	Calories	Carb grams	Fiber grams
Lamb, leg	3 oz	219	0	0
Lamb, loin	3 oz	265	0	0
Lamb, shoulder	3 oz	294	0	0
Veal, leg	3 oz	179	0	0
Duck	1/2 duck	144	0	0

LEGUMES

Item	Amount	Calories	Carb grams	Fiber grams
Baked beans	1 cup	239	53.9	10.4
Black beans	1 cup	227	40.8	15
Chickpeas	1 cup	185	32.7	7.9
Great northern beans	1 cup	209	37.3	12.4
Lentils	1 cup	230	39.9	15.6
Navy beans	1 cup	255	47.4	19.1
Pinto beans	1 cup	245	44.8	15.4
Red kidney beans	1 cup	225	40.4	13.1

NUTS AND SEEDS

Item	Amount	Calories	Carb grams	Fiber grams
Almonds	1 oz	164	5.6	3.3
Brazil nuts	1 oz	186	3.5	2.1
Cashews	1 oz	163	9.3	1
Chestnuts	1 cup	350	75.7	7.3
Hazelnuts	1 oz	178	4.7	2.7
Macadamia nuts	1 oz	203	3.6	2.3
Peanuts	1 oz	166	6.1	2.3
Pecans	1 oz	196	3.9	2.7
Pistachios	1 oz	161	7.6	2.9
Pumpkin seeds	1 oz	148	3.8	1.1
Sesame seeds	1 Tbsp	47	1.2	1
Sunflower seeds	1 oz	165	6.8	2.9
Walnuts	1 oz	185	3.9	1.9

PORK

Item	Amount	Calories	Carb grams	Fiber grams
Pork sausage	1 patty	92	0	0
Bacon	3	103	0.3	0
Ham, roasted	3 oz	207	0	0
Pork, loin chops	3 oz	235	0	0
Pork, roast	3 oz	217	0	0
Pork, shoulder	3 oz	280	0	0
Pork, spareribs	3 oz	337	0	0

continued >>>

Item	Amount	Calories	Carb grams	Fiber grams
POULTRY				
Chicken roll	2 slices	87	1.4	0
Chicken, breast w/o skin	1/2 breast	142	0	0
Chicken, dark meat w/o skin	1 drum-stick	76	0	0
Chicken, thigh w/o skin	1 thigh	109	0	0
Chicken, breast w/ skin, batter-fried	1/2 breast	364	12.6	0.4
Chicken, dark meat w/ skin, batter-fried	1 drum-stick	193	6	0.2
Chicken, thigh w/ skin, batter-fried	1 thigh	238	7.8	0.3
Turkey, roasted, dark	3 oz	157	0	0
Turkey, roasted, light	3 oz	132	0	0
SAUSAGE AND LUNCH MEAT				
Bologna	2 slices	175	3.1	0
Chicken, white meat	2 slices	72	1.3	0
Chicken breast, roasted, fat free	2 slices	48	0.9	0
Cooked salami	2 slices	142	1.3	0
Ham, regular	2 slices	91	2.1	0.7
Ham, extra lean	2 slices	60	0.4	0
Hard salami	2 slices	77	0.8	0
Sausage, pork or beef	2 links	103	0.7	0
Turkey breast	2 slices	55	1.8	0
Turkey breast, fat free	2 slices	47	2.52	0
Vienna sausage	1	37	0.4	0
SNACKS				
Chex Mix	1 oz	120	8.5	1.6
Cheese puffs	1 oz	157	15.3	0.3

Item	Amount	Calories	Carb grams	Fiber grams
Crackers, saltine	4	51	8.5	0.4
Granola bar, plain	1 bar	134	18.3	1.5
Olives	5 large	25	1.4	0.7
Pickles, dill	1	12	2.7	0.8
Popcorn, air-popped	1 cup	31	6.2	1.2
Popcorn, oil-popped	1 cup	55	6	1.1
Potato chips	1 oz	155	14.5	1
Pretzels	10	229	47.5	1.9
Rice cakes	1 cake	35	7.3	0.4
Tortilla chips	1 oz	142	17.8	1.8
SOUPS, GRAVIES, AND SAUCES				
Barbecue sauce	1 Tbsp	12	2	0.2
Beef bouillon	1 cup	29	1.8	0
Beef gravy	1/4 cup	31	2.8	0.2
Cheese sauce	1/4 cup	110	4.3	0.3
Chicken gravy	1/4 cup	47	3.2	0.2
Chicken noodle soup	1 cup	75	9.4	0.7
Country sausage gravy	1/4 cup	96	3.9	0.4
Cream of mushroom soup	1 cup	129	9.3	0.5
Hot pepper sauce	1 tsp	1	0.1	0
Lentil soup	1 cup	126	20.3	5
Manhattan clam chowder	1 cup	78	12.2	1.5
Minestrone	1 cup	82	11.2	1
Mushroom gravy	1/4 cup	30	3.3	0.2
New England clam chowder	1 cup	164	16.7	1.5
Onion soup	1 cup	27	5.1	1
Pasta sauce	1 cup	185	28.2	1
Pea soup	1 cup	165	26.5	2.8
Salsa	1 Tbsp	4	1	0.3
Teriyaki sauce	1 Tbsp	15	2.9	0
Tomato soup	1 cup	85	16.6	0.5

Item	Amount	Calories	Carb grams	Fiber grams
Turkey gravy	1/4 cup	30	3	0.2
Vegetable beef soup	1 cup	78	10.2	0.5

SWEETS

Item	Amount	Calories	Carb grams	Fiber grams
Brownies	1	227	35.8	1.2
Chocolate chip cookies	1 cookie	49	9.3	0.4
Cinnamon roll	1 roll	223	30.5	1.4
Cake, pound	1 piece	109	13.7	0.1
Cake, chocolate w/o frosting	1 piece	340	50.7	1.5
Coffee cake, crumb-type	1 piece	263	29	1.3
Doughnut, plain	1	198	23.4	0.7
Doughnut, glazed	1	242	26.6	0.7
Fudge	1 piece	70	13	0.3
Graham crackers	2	59	10.8	0.2
Hard candy	1 small piece	12	2.9	0
Jellybeans	10 large	106	26.5	0.1
Marshmallows	1 cup	159	40.7	0.1
Milk chocolate	1 bar	235	26.2	1.5
Pie, apple	1 piece	411	57.5	1.9
Pie, pecan	1 piece	503	63.7	4
Pie, pumpkin	1 piece	316	40.9	2.9
Pineapple upside down cake	1 piece	267	58	0.9
Pudding, chocolate	1/2 cup	154	27.8	0.6
Semisweet chocolate pieces	1 cup	805	106.1	9.9
Snickers	1 bar	266	36.8	1.4

VEGETABLES

Item	Amount	Calories	Carb grams	Fiber grams
Asparagus	4 spears	13	3.5	2.9
Beets	1 cup	75	16.9	3.4
Broccoli	1 cup	55	5.8	2.3
Brussels sprouts	1 cup	56	11	4.1
Cabbage	1 cup	17	3.9	1.6
Carrots	1 carrot	30	10.5	3.1
Cauliflower	1 cup	25	5.3	2.5
Celery	1 cup	17	3.6	1.9
Collard greens	1 cup	92	9	5.3
Corn	1 cup	133	31.7	3.9
Cucumbers	1 cup	16	3.8	0.8
Eggplant	1 cup	28	7	2.5
Endive	1 cup	9	2	1.6
Kale	1 cup	39	7	2.6
Leeks	1 cup	32	8	1
Lettuce, iceberg	1 cup	8	1.6	0.7
Lima beans	1 cup	170	32	9.9
Mushrooms	1 cup	15	2.3	0.8
Mustard greens	1 cup	21	3	2.8
Okra	1 cup	52	11	5.2
Onions	1 cup	67	16.2	2.2
Parsnips	1 cup	111	26.5	5.6
Potato w/ skin	1	118	27.4	2.4
Peas	1 cup	125	22.8	8.8
Peppers, green	1 cup	30	6.9	2.5
Radishes	1 radish	1	0.2	0.1
Red hot chili pepper	1	18	4	0.7
Romaine lettuce	1 cup	10	1.8	1.2
Soybeans	1 cup	254	20	7.6
Scallions	1 cup	32	7.3	2.6
Spinach	1 cup	7	1.1	0.7
Squash, summer	1 cup	18	3.8	2.5
Squash, winter	1 cup	76	18.1	2.5
Sweet potato	1	131	30.2	4.8
Tomatoes	1 cup	32	7.1	2.2
Turnips	1 cup	34	7.9	3.1
Water chestnuts	1 cup	70	17.2	3.5

Glycemic Loads of Common Foods

The glycemic load (GL) is a scale used to indicate how much one serving of a particular food raises a person's blood sugar. A GL of 10 or less is considered low. Check your blood sugar two hours after eating a food to find out how it affects your blood sugar, since your reaction might be different. The GL is closely tied to portion size; if you eat twice as much as the portion size indicated, the food will have double the effect on your blood sugar. (Keep in mind that these portion sizes aren't necessarily the same as those used in the diabetic exchange system.) Work with your registered dietitian to figure out how to fit more low-GL foods into your eating plan.

LOW (GL = 10 OR LESS)

Breads, Tortillas, Grains	Serving size	GL
Coarse barley bread (75% intact kernels)	2 slices	10
Soy and flaxseed bread	2 slices	10
Whole-grain pumpernickel bread	2 slices	10
Pearled barley	1 cup	8
Popcorn	2 cups	8
Wheat tortillas	2 6-inch	6

Breakfast Cereals	Serving size	GL
Alpen Muesli	1/3 cup (1 oz)	10
Oatmeal, instant 1 cup prepared	(1 oz)	10
All-Bran	1/2 cup (1 oz)	9
Bran Buds	1/3 cup (1 oz)	7
Oatmeal made from rolled oats 1 cup prepared	(1 oz)	7

Beans and Peas	Serving size	GL
Lima beans	1 cup	10
Pinto beans	1 cup	10
Chickpeas	1 cup	8
Baked beans	1 cup	7
Kidney beans	1 cup	7
Navy beans	1 cup	7
Butter beans	1 cup	6
Green peas	1 cup	6
Split peas, yellow	1 cup	6
Lentils, green or red	1 cup	5

Dairy and Soy Drinks	Serving size	GL
Low-fat yogurt with fruit and sugar	7 oz	9
Soy milk	1 cup (8 oz)	7
Low-fat chocolate milk, sweetened with aspartame	1 cup (8 oz)	3
Low-fat yogurt with fruit, sweetened with aspartame	7 oz	2

Fruits and Vegetables	Serving size	GL
Prunes, pitted, chopped	1/3 cup (2 oz)	10
Apricots, dried, chopped	1/3 cup (2 oz)	9
Peaches, canned in light syrup	1/2 cup (4 oz)	9
Grapes, medium bunch	(about 50) 4 oz	8
Mango, sliced	2/3 cup (4 oz)	8
Pineapple, diced	2/3 cup (4 oz)	7
Apple	1 small	6
Kiwifruit, sliced	2/3 cup (4 oz)	6
Beets, sliced	1/2 cup	5
Orange	1 small	5
Peach	1 small	5
Plums	2 small	5
Pear	1 small	4
Strawberries	about 6 medium	4
Watermelon, chopped	2/3 cup (4 oz)	4
Carrots, raw	1 large	3
Cherries	about 16 (4 oz)	3
Grapefruit	1/2	3

Beverages	Serving size	GL
Orange juice, unsweetened	3/4 cup (6 oz)	10
Grapefruit juice, unsweetened	3/4 cup (6 oz)	7
Tomato juice	3/4 cup (6 oz)	4

Sweets	Serving size	GL
M&Ms with peanuts	25 (1 oz)	6
Nutella (chocolate hazelnut spread)	4 Tbsp	4

Nuts	Serving size	GL
Mixed nuts, roasted	1/3 cup (1.5 oz)	4
Cashew nuts	about 13 (1.5 oz)	3
Peanuts	1/3 cup (1.5 oz)	1

MEDIUM (GL = 11–19)

Bread, Tortillas, Crackers, Chips	Serving size	GL
Coarse barley bread (50% intact kernels)	2 slices	18
High-fiber white bread	2 slices	18
Corn chips	2 oz	17
100% whole-grain bread	2 slices	14
Sourdough rye bread	2 slices	12
Stone-ground wheat thins	4	12
Corn tortillas	2 6-inch	11

Grains	Serving size	GL
Converted long-grain white rice	2/3 cup cooked	16
Brown rice	2/3 cup cooked	18
Quinoa	2/3 cup cooked	16
Wild rice	2/3 cup cooked	18
Bulgur	2/3 cup cooked	12

Pasta	Serving size	GL
Spaghetti (cooked 15 minutes)	1 cup	17
Whole-wheat spaghetti	1 cup	13
High-protein spaghetti	1 cup	12

Beverages	Serving size	GL
Low-fat chocolate milk	8 oz	12
Pineapple juice, unsweetened	6 oz	12
Apple juice	8 oz	8

Fruits, Vegetables, Beans	Serving size	GL
Sweet corn	1 cup	18
Sweet potato	1 medium (5 oz)	17
Figs, dried, chopped	1/3 cup (2 oz)	16
Banana	1 small (4 oz)	11
Black-eyed peas	1 cup	11

Breakfast Cereals	Serving size	GL
Nabisco Cream of Wheat, regular	1 cup prepared (1 oz)	17
Post Grape-Nuts	1/2 cup (1 oz)	16
Cheerios	1 cup (1 oz)	15
Life	3/4 cup (1 oz)	15
Special K	1 cup (1 oz)	14

HIGH (GL = 20 OR HIGHER)

Potatoes	Serving size	GL
Baked russet Burbank potato	1 medium	26
French fries	5 oz	22

Grains	Serving size	GL
Sticky white rice	2/3 cup cooked	31
Couscous	2/3 cup cooked	23
Long-grain white rice	2/3 cup cooked	23

Pasta	Serving size	GL
Udon Japanese noodles	1 cup cooked	25
Spaghetti (cooked 20 minutes)	1 cup	22

Breads	Serving size	GL
French baguette	2 slices	30
Middle Eastern flatbread	1 large	30
Italian white bread	2 slices	22
Hamburger roll	1	21
Mini-bagel (Lender's)	1	20
Wonder Bread	2 slices	20

Breakfast Cereals	Serving size	GL
Kellogg's Cornflakes	1 cup (1 oz)	24
Rice Chex	1 1/4 cups (1 oz)	23
Nabisco Cream of Wheat, instant	1 cup prepared (1 oz)	22
Rice Krispies	3/4 cup (1 oz)	22
Corn Chex	1 cup (1 oz)	21

Dried Fruit	Serving size	GL
Raisins	1/3 cup	28
Dates, dried, chopped	1/3 cup	25

Beverages	Serving size	GL
Ocean Spray Cranberry Juice Cocktail	12 oz	36
Coca-Cola	12 oz	24

Sweets	Serving size	GL
Mars Bar	2 oz	26
Jelly beans	20	22

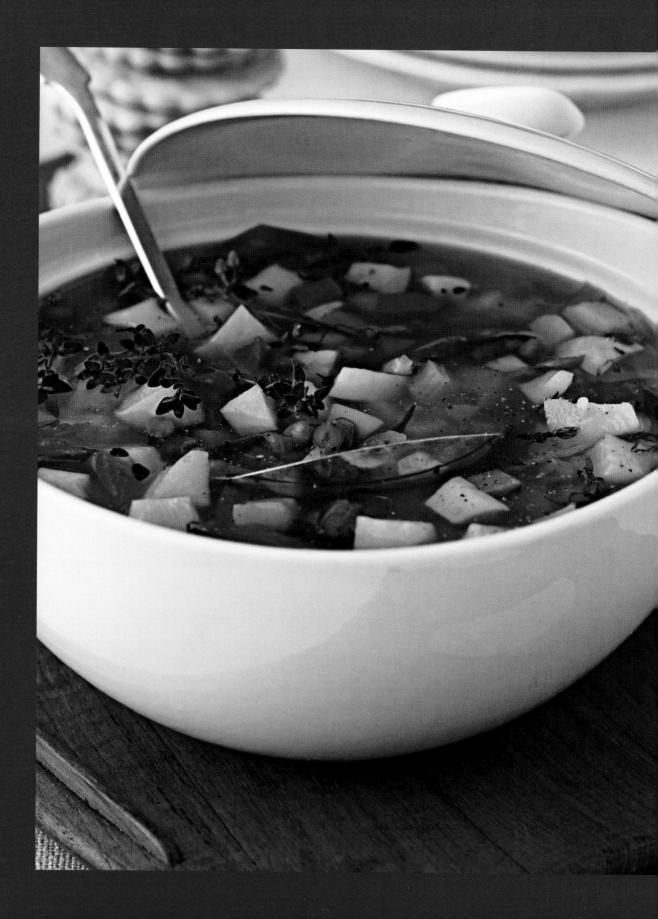

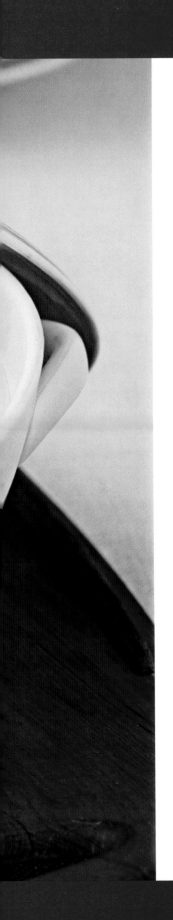

6

reverse diabetes
RECIPES

- Easy-to-Make Meals
- Diabetes-Friendly Dishes
- Full-of-Flavor Nutrition

- Better Health

breakfasts

Summer Greens Scramble

Serves 2

- 2 cups shredded, stemmed fresh kale
- 5 large eggs
- 5 large egg whites
- 1/4 teaspoon ground cumin
- 1/4 teaspoon salt
- 1/4 cup chopped lean ham from the deli
- 2 scallions, trimmed and thinly sliced

- ONE In large saucepan of boiling salted water, cook fresh kale until tender, 3 to 5 minutes. Drain. Rinse under cold water. Drain well.

- TWO In large bowl, whisk together eggs, egg whites, cumin, and salt.

- THREE Coat large nonstick skillet with nonstick cooking spray. Heat over medium heat. Add egg mixture. Stir until eggs start to thicken slightly, 2 to 3 minutes. Stir in kale, ham, and scallions. Cook, stirring occasionally, until eggs are soft-scrambled, 2 to 3 minutes.

Per serving: 145 calories, 7 g total fat, 2 g saturated fat, 270 mg cholesterol, 385 mg sodium, 5 g carbohydrates, 1g fiber, 15 g protein

"Mostly Whites" Spinach Omelet with Tomato-Mushroom Sauce

Serves 2

- 1 1/2 teaspoons olive oil
- 4 ounces mushrooms, sliced (about 3/4 cup)
- 1 can (8 ounces) no-salt added tomato sauce
- 4 large egg whites
- 1 large egg
- 1/4 teaspoon black pepper
- 1 small onion, chopped
- 1/2 cup packed cooked chopped spinach (about 5 ounces)
- 2 teaspoons grated Parmesan cheese

- ONE In small nonstick saucepan over medium-high heat, heat 1/2 teaspoon oil. Add mushrooms. Cook until softened, 4 minutes, stirring once. Add tomato sauce. Simmer until thickened, about 5 minutes. Remove from heat. Cover.

- TWO In small bowl, beat egg whites, egg, and pepper until blended.

- THREE In large nonstick skillet over medium heat, heat remaining teaspoon oil. Add onion. Sauté until softened, 4 minutes. Stir in spinach. Cook until heated through. Stir half of spinach mixture into egg mixture. Reserve remaining spinach mixture.

- FOUR Coat same skillet with nonstick cooking spray. Heat over medium heat. Pour spinach-egg mixture into skillet, spreading evenly. Cook, without stirring, until eggs begin to thicken slightly around edge of skillet, about 1 minute. Run thin spatula around edge of skillet, lifting eggs so uncooked portion flows under cooked portion. Repeat until center of omelet is still moist but no longer runny, about 3 minutes total.

- FIVE Spread reserved spinach mixture over half of omelet. Sprinkle with cheese. Fold omelet to cover filling. Reduce heat to low. Cover and cook until eggs are set but still soft, 3 to 4 minutes. Slide omelet onto serving plate. Top with mushroom sauce.

Per serving: 205 calories, 7 g total fat, 2 g saturated fat, 108 mg cholesterol, 229 mg sodium, 22 g carbohydrates, 6 g fiber, 17 g protein,

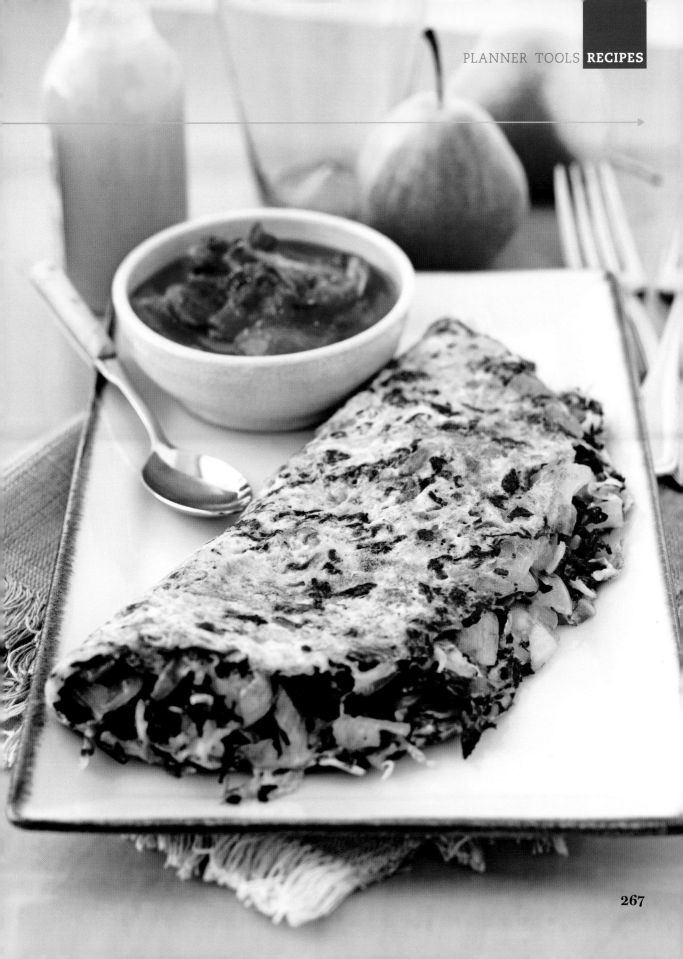

breakfasts

Multigrain Pancakes

Serves 8

- 2 cups low-fat buttermilk
- 1/2 cup old-fashioned rolled oats
- 2/3 cup whole-wheat flour
- 2/3 cup all-purpose flour
- 1/4 cup toasted wheat germ
- 1 1/2 teaspoons baking powder
- 1/2 teaspoon baking soda
- 1/4 teaspoon salt
- 1 teaspoon cinnamon
- 2 large eggs
- 1/4 cup firmly packed brown sugar
- 1 tablespoon canola oil
- 2 teaspoons vanilla extract
- 1 cup maple syrup, warmed
- 1 1/2 cups sliced strawberries or blueberries

ONE Mix the buttermilk and oats in a small bowl. Let stand for 15 minutes.

TWO Whisk the whole-wheat flour, all-purpose flour, wheat germ, baking powder, baking soda, salt, and cinnamon in a large bowl.

THREE Whisk the eggs, sugar, oil, and vanilla in a medium bowl. Add the buttermilk mixture. Add this mixture to the flour mixture and mix with a rubber spatula just until flour mixture is moistened.

FOUR Coat a large nonstick skillet with cooking spray. Heat over medium heat. Spoon about 1/4 cup batter for each pancake into the skillet and cook until bottoms are golden and small bubbles start to form on top, about 3 minutes. Flip the pancakes and cook until browned and cooked through, 1 to 2 minutes. (Adjust the heat as necessary for even browning.) Keep the pancakes warm in a 200°F oven while you finish cooking the remaining batter.

FIVE Top with maple syrup and strawberries (or blueberries). One serving is 2 pancakes. Wrap any leftover pancakes individually in plastic wrap and refrigerate for up to 2 days or freeze for up to 1 month. Reheat in a toaster or toaster oven.

Per serving: 292 calories, 3 g total fat, 1 g saturated fat, 56 mg cholesterol, 331 mg sodium, 60 g carbohydrates, 3 g fiber, 8 g protein

Oatmeal with Apple and Flaxseeds

Serves 4

- 2 cups low-fat (1%) milk or vanilla soy milk
- 3/4 cup old-fashioned rolled oats (not quick oats)
- 1 medium apple, peeled, cored and chopped
- 1/3 cup dried cranberries or raisins
- 1/2 teaspoon cinnamon
- 1/4 cup whole flaxseeds, ground, or 1/3 cup flaxseed meal
- 1/4 cup nonfat plain or vanilla yogurt
- 1/4 cup maple syrup, warmed, or 2 tablespoons brown sugar

ONE Combine the milk, rolled oats, apple, dried cranberries (or raisins), and cinnamon in a heavy medium saucepan. Bring to a simmer over medium-high heat, stirring almost constantly.

TWO Reduce the heat to medium-low and cook, stirring often, until creamy and thickened, 3 to 5 minutes.

THREE Stir in the flaxseeds. Spoon the cereal into individual bowls and top each serving with a dollop of yogurt and a drizzle of maple syrup. One serving is 2/3 cup. Leftovers will keep, covered, in the refrigerator for up to 2 days. Reheat in the microwave.

Per serving: 282 calories, 7 g total fat, 1 g saturated fat, 8 mg cholesterol, 84 mg sodium, 47 g carbohydrates, 6 g fiber, 10 g protein

appetizers

Cheesy Zucchini Bites

Makes 35 appetizers

- 5 medium zucchini (about 6 inches long)
- 4 ounces blue cheese, crumbled
- 3 tablespoons grated Parmesan cheese
- 1 teaspoon dried basil
- 1/8 teaspoon pepper
- 1 pint cherry tomatoes, thinly sliced

● **ONE** Cut zucchini into 3/4-inch slices. Using a melon baller or small spoon, scoop out the insides and discard, leaving the bottom intact. Place zucchini on an ungreased baking sheet; spoon 1/2 teaspoon crumbled blue cheese into each.

● **TWO** Combine the Parmesan cheese, basil, and pepper; sprinkle half over blue cheese. Top each with a tomato slice; sprinkle with the remaining Parmesan mixture. Bake at 400°F until cheese is melted, 5-7 minutes. Serve warm.

Per serving (one appetizer): 19 calories, 1 g total fat, 1 g saturated fat, 3 mg cholesterol, 58 mg sodium, 1 g carbohydrate, 0 fiber, 1 g protein

Asparagus Guacamole

Makes 2 cups

- 1 pound fresh asparagus, trimmed and cut into 1-inch pieces
- 1/3 cup chopped onion
- 1 garlic clove
- 1/3 cup chopped seeded tomato
- 2 tablespoons reduced-fat mayonnaise
- 1 tablespoon lemon juice
- 1/2 teaspoon salt
- 3/4 teaspoon minced fresh cilantro or parsley
- 1/4 teaspoon chili powder
- 6 drops hot pepper sauce
    Assorted raw vegetables and baked tortilla chips

● **ONE** Place 1/2 inch of water and asparagus in a saucepan; bring to a boil. Reduce heat; cover and simmer until tender, about 5 minutes. Drain; place asparagus in a blender or food processor. Add onion and garlic; cover and process until smooth.

● **TWO** In a bowl, combine tomato, mayonnaise, lemon juice, salt, cilantro, chili powder, and hot pepper sauce. Stir in the asparagus mixture until blended. Serve with vegetables and chips. Refrigerate leftovers; stir before serving.

Per serving (1/3 cup guacamole): 42 calories, 2 g total fat, 0 saturated fat, 2 mg cholesterol, 240 mg sodium, 5 g carbohydrate, 1 g fiber, 3 g protein

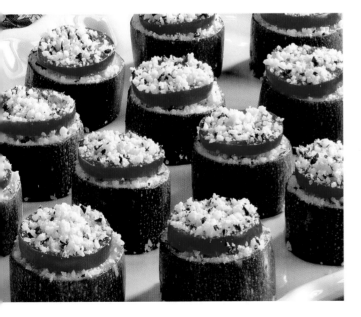

appetizers

Tomato Black Bean Salsa

Serves 8

3	medium tomatoes, seeded and chopped
1	can (15 ounces) black beans, rinsed and drained
3/4	cup fresh or frozen corn
1/2	cup finely chopped red onion
1/2	cup chopped roasted red pepper
1	jalapeño pepper, finely chopped*
2	tablespoons minced fresh cilantro or parsley
1/4	cup lime juice
1	garlic clove, minced
1	teaspoon dried oregano
1	teaspoon ground cumin
1/2	teaspoon salt
1/2	teaspoon ground coriander
	Baked tortilla chips

● In a large bowl, combine the first 13 ingredients. Cover and refrigerate for at least 2 hours before serving. Serve with tortilla chips. Yield: 4 cups.

Per serving (1/2 cup salsa): 80 calories, 1 g total fat, 0 saturated fat, 0 cholesterol, 318 mg sodium, 15 g carbohydrate, 4 g fiber, 4 g protein

Editor's Note: When cutting or seeding hot peppers, use rubber or plastic gloves to protect your hands. Avoid touching your face.

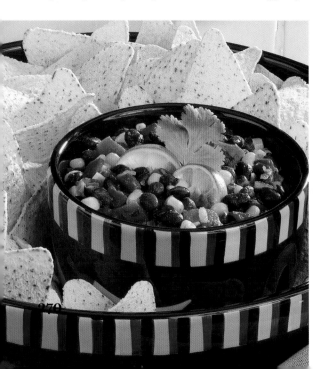

Pita Pizzas

Serves 4

1/2	cup thinly sliced roasted red bell peppers
1/4	teaspoon crushed fennel seeds or dried oregano, crumbled
1/4	teaspoon salt
1/8	teaspoon black pepper
1	ounce reduced-fat mozzarella cheese, shredded (about 1/4 cup)
1/2	ounce Gruyère or Jarlsberg cheese, shredded (about 2 tablespoons)
2	whole-wheat pita breads (4 inches)
8	teaspoons bottled tomato sauce or pizza sauce
1/2	small red onion, thinly sliced

● **ONE** Preheat broiler.

● **TWO** In small bowl, combine red peppers, fennel or oregano, salt, and pepper. In second bowl, combine mozzarella and Gruyère.

● **THREE** Separate each pita bread into 2 flat rounds. Place rounds, rough side up, on baking sheet. Broil 4 inches from heat until golden brown around edges, about 1 minute. Remove from broiler.

● **FOUR** Spread 2 teaspoons sauce over each pita, covering edges. Spoon 2 tablespoons red pepper mixture over each pita. Sprinkle with cheese, dividing equally, then add onion in rings.

● **FIVE** Broil until cheese is melted and pizzas are hot, about 2 minutes.

Per serving: 137 calories, 3 g total fat, 2 g saturated fat, 7 mg cholesterol, 475 mg sodium, 23 g carbohydrate, 3 g fiber, 7 g protein

Bean and Vegetable Tostadas

Makes 6

- 6 corn tortillas (6 inches)
  Nonstick cooking spray
- 1 can (15 ounces) black beans,
  drained and rinsed
- 1 can (11 ounces) canned corn kernels,
  drained and rinsed
- 1 small tomato, cored and chopped
  (about 1/2 cup)
- 2 tablespoons finely chopped red onion
- 1 small jalapeño pepper, seeded and
  finely chopped*
- 2 tablespoons chopped cilantro
- 1 tablespoon fresh-squeezed lime juice
- 1/2 teaspoon salt
- 1/8 to 1/4 teaspoon hot red pepper sauce
- 1 small ripe avocado, pitted, peeled,
  and chopped

● **ONE** Preheat oven to 450°F. Place tortillas in single layer on baking sheets. Coat both sides of tortillas with cooking spray. Bake until lightly browned and crisp, about 10 minutes, flipping tortillas over halfway through. Transfer to wire racks and let cool.

● **TWO** In large bowl, stir together beans, corn, tomato, onion, jalapeño, cilantro, lime juice, salt, and hot sauce. Gently fold in avocado. Spoon 1/2 cup onto each tortilla.

Per serving (1 tostada): 130 calories, 1 g total fat, 0 g saturated fat , 0 mg cholesterol, 390 mg sodium, 26 g carbohydrate, 5 g fiber, 5 g protein

Editor's Note: When cutting or seeding hot peppers, use rubber or plastic gloves to protect your hands. Avoid touching your face.

Steamed Vegetable Platter with Peanut Dip

Serves 8

- 2/3 cup water
- 1/3 cup creamy peanut butter
- 1 clove garlic, minced
- 2 teaspoons grated fresh ginger
- 2 medium scallions, chopped
- 2 tablespoons packed brown sugar
- 2 tablespoons soy sauce
- 1/8 teaspoon chili powder
- 1 tablespoon fresh-squeezed lemon juice
- 6 large carrots, peeled, halved lengthwise,
  cut in 3 x 1/4-inch sticks or 16 baby carrots,
  scraped
- 2 large red or yellow bell peppers, halved,
  seeded, sliced 1/4-inch thick
- 1/2 pound snow peas, trimmed, or 1/2 pound
  green beans, trimmed
- 8 radishes, sliced thin

● **ONE** For peanut dip: In small saucepan, bring water to boil. Stir in peanut butter, garlic, ginger, scallions, sugar, soy sauce, and chili powder. Simmer 2 minutes. Remove from heat. Stir in lemon juice. Set aside to cool slightly or refrigerate until ready to serve.

● **TWO** In a large saucepan with a steaming basket, bring water to a boil. Fill a sink with ice water. Steam carrots for 3 minutes, lift out and plunge into ice water to cool. Steam bell peppers for 1 minute, lift out, and plunge into ice water to cool. Steam snow peas or beans for 2 minutes, lift out, and plunge into ice water to cool. Drain vegetables and dry with paper towels.

● **THREE** On serving platter, arrange carrots, bell peppers, and snow peas or green beans with peanut dip in small bowl in center. Add radishes for garnish and contrast.

Per serving: 136 calories, 6 g total fat, 1 g saturated fat, 0 mg cholesterol, 305 mg sodium, 19 g carbohydrates, 5 g fiber, 5 g protein

soups, salads, and light bites

Creamy Greens Soup

Serves 8

- 2 teaspoons olive oil
- 2 leeks, pale green and white parts only, rinsed and coarsely chopped
- 1 medium onion, coarsely chopped
- 2 cloves garlic, minced
- 1 small bunch collard greens, stemmed and coarsely chopped
- 1 small bunch Swiss chard, stemmed and coarsely chopped
- 2 medium Yukon Gold or all-purpose potatoes, unpeeled and coarsely chopped
- 1 carrot, peeled and coarsely chopped
- 2 cans (14 1/2 ounces each) reduced-sodium, fat-free chicken broth
- 1 teaspoon salt
- 4 cups water
- 1/2 cup half-and-half

ONE In large pot over medium heat, heat oil. Add leeks and onion. Sauté until softened, about 5 minutes. Add garlic; sauté 2 minutes. Add collard greens, Swiss chard, potatoes, and carrot. Stir in broth, 4 cups water, and salt. Simmer, partially covered, 50 minutes.

TWO In blender or food processor, puree soup in small batches. Return to pot. Stir in half-and-half. Heat just until warmed through.

Per serving: 124 calories, 4 g total fat, 2 g saturated fat, 7 mg cholesterol, 459 mg sodium, 20 g carbohydrate, 5 g fiber, 5 g protein

Carrot Soup with Dill

Serves 4

- 1 tablespoon vegetable oil
- 1 onion, coarsely chopped
- 1 clove garlic, minced
- 2 cans (14 1/2 ounces each) reduced-sodium, fat-free chicken broth
- 1 1/4 pounds carrots, peeled and coarsely chopped (4 cups)
- 1/2 teaspoon dried thyme, crumbled
- 1/4 teaspoon salt
- 1/4 teaspoon white pepper
- 1/4 cup plain low-fat yogurt
- 1 tablespoon finely chopped dill

ONE In medium saucepan over medium heat, heat oil. Add onion and garlic. Sauté until softened, 5 minutes. Add broth, carrots, and thyme. Simmer, uncovered, until vegetables are very tender, about 40 minutes.

TWO In batches, puree soup in blender. Add salt and pepper. To serve hot, ladle into bowls and garnish each bowl with yogurt and dill. To serve cold, remove from heat and let cool to room temperature. Cover and refrigerate until cold. Garnish just before serving.

Per serving: 135 calories, 4 g total fat, 0 g saturated fat, 1 mg cholesterol, 773 mg sodium, 20 g carbohydrate, 5 g fiber, 6 g protein

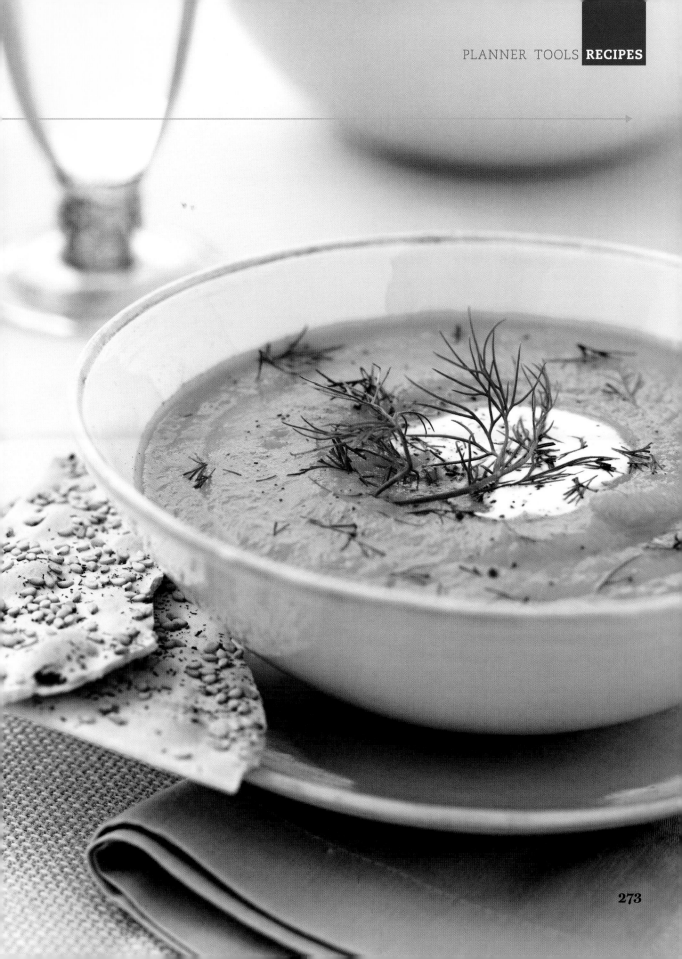

soups, salads, and light bites

Golden Squash Soup

Serves 8

    3   cups coarsely chopped onion
  1/4   teaspoon ground nutmeg
  1/4   teaspoon ground cinnamon
  1/4   teaspoon dried thyme
    2   bay leaves
1 1/2   cups water
    2   celery stalks, chopped
    1   medium carrot, chopped
    2   cups mashed cooked butternut squash, divided
1 1/2   cups tomato juice, divided
    1   cup apple juice, divided
    1   cup orange juice, divided
        Pepper to taste

● ONE In a large saucepan or Dutch oven coated with nonstick cooking spray, sauté onion with nutmeg, cinnamon, thyme, and bay leaves until onion is tender. Add water, celery, and carrot; cover and simmer until carrot is tender. Discard bay leaves.

● TWO In a blender container, place half of the squash and half of the tomato, apple and orange juices; add half of the vegetable mixture. Puree; return to pan. Repeat with the remaining squash, juices, and vegetable mixture; return to pan. Add pepper; heat through.

Per serving (1 cup): 86 calories, 0 g total fat, 0 g saturated fat, 0 mg cholesterol, 45 mg sodium, 21 g carbohydrate, 2 g fiber, 1 g protein

Summer Garden Soup

Serves 6

    2   teaspoons olive oil
    1   medium onion, finely chopped
    1   large stalk celery, finely chopped
    2   teaspoons finely chopped, peeled fresh ginger
  1/4   pound green beans, cut into 1/2-inch pieces
    2   medium potatoes, unpeeled and cut into 1/2-inch cubes
    1   large carrot, peeled and cut into 1/2-inch cubes
    1   medium yellow summer squash, quartered lengthwise, seeded, and cut into 1/2-inch cubes
    8   cups water
    1   bay leaf
  3/4   teaspoon salt
  3/4   cup fresh or frozen green peas
    2   plum tomatoes, seeded and coarsely chopped
    2   tablespoons finely chopped fresh basil leaves
1 1/2   teaspoons finely chopped fresh thyme leaves

● ONE In large pot over medium heat, heat oil. Add onion, celery, and ginger. Sauté until very tender, about 10 minutes. Add green beans, potatoes, carrot, squash, water, bay leaf, and salt. Simmer, covered, 20 minutes.

● TWO Uncover soup. Simmer 15 minutes. For last 5 minutes, add peas, tomatoes, basil, and thyme. Remove bay leaf before serving.

Per serving: 88 calories, 2 g total fat, 0 g saturated fat, 0 mg cholesterol, 307 mg sodium, 17 g carbohydrate, 4 g fiber, 3 g protein

Turkey, Spinach, and Rice in Roasted Garlic Broth

Serves 4

- 2 medium whole heads garlic, unpeeled
- 2 tablespoons tomato paste
- 2 cans (14 1/2 ounces each) reduced-sodium, fat-free chicken or turkey broth
- 1 cup cooked turkey cubes
- 1 cup cooked long-grain white rice
- 3/4 pound spinach, stemmed and coarsely chopped
- 1/4 teaspoon black pepper
- 1/4 teaspoon hot pepper flakes, or to taste
- 1 tablespoon fresh-squeezed lemon juice

ONE Preheat oven to 400°F.

TWO Cut top third off garlic heads. Wrap each head in foil. Bake until very soft, about 50 minutes. Let cool. Remove foil. Squeeze out pulp into small bowl.

THREE In large saucepan, stir together garlic pulp and tomato paste. Stir in broth. Bring to a boil. Add turkey, rice, spinach, pepper, and pepper flakes. Simmer, uncovered, 8 minutes. Just before serving, stir in lemon juice.

Per serving: 197 calories, 4 g total fat, 1 g saturated fat, 30 mg cholesterol, 208 mg sodium, 24 g carbohydrate, 3 g fiber, 19 g protein

Round Steak Chili

Serves 10

- 1 pound beef round steak, trimmed and cut into 1/2-inch cubes
- 1 large onion, chopped
- 2 garlic cloves, minced
- 1 can (46 ounces) V8 juice
- 1 can (28 ounces) crushed tomatoes
- 2 cups sliced celery
- 1 medium green pepper, chopped
- 1 bay leaf
- 2 tablespoons chili powder
- 1 teaspoon dried oregano
- 1 teaspoon brown sugar
- 1/2 teaspoon each celery seed, paprika, ground mustard, and cumin
- 1/4 teaspoon cayenne pepper
- 1/4 teaspoon dried basil
- 1 can (1 ces) kidney beans, rinsed and dra d

In a large kettle or Dutch oven coated with nonstick cooking spray, brown meat, onion, and garlic. Add V8, tomatoes, celery, green pepper, and seasonings; bring to a boil. Reduce heat; simmer, uncovered, for 3 hours. Add kidney beans; heat. Remove bay leaf before serving.

Per serving (1 cup): 200 calories, 3 g total fat, 1 g saturated fat, 40 mg cholesterol, 240 mg sodium, 22 g carbohydrate, 7 g fiber, 22 g protein

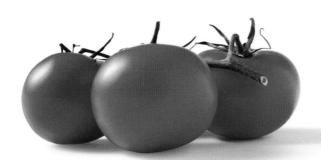

soups, salads, and light bites

Chicken-Tomato Soup with Tortillas

Serves 6

1	whole bone-in chicken breast, skin removed
8	cups reduced-sodium, fat-free chicken broth
3	cloves garlic
1	teaspoon salt
1	teaspoon black pepper
1	teaspoon dried oregano, crumbled
1	tablespoon olive oil
5	scallions, coarsely chopped
1	can (4 1/2 ounces) green chiles, drained
4	medium tomatoes, coarsely chopped
1/2	cup fresh-squeezed lime juice
4	corn tortillas (6 inches), sliced into 3 x 1/4-inch strips, toasted
3	tablespoons chopped cilantro

ONE Place chicken, broth, 2 cloves garlic, salt, pepper, and oregano in medium saucepan. Simmer, uncovered, 25 minutes.

TWO Remove chicken from pot. Remove and discard bones. Cut chicken into large chunks. Strain and reserve broth.

THREE In large saucepan over medium heat, heat oil. Mince remaining garlic. Add to saucepan along with scallions. Sauté until softened, 5 minutes. Add chiles, tomatoes, and strained broth. Simmer, partially covered, 15 minutes. (Recipe can be made ahead up to this point.)

FOUR Add chicken chunks, lime juice, and toasted tortilla strips. Simmer 5 minutes. Garnish with cilantro.

Per serving: 200 calories, 5 g total fat, 1 g saturated fat, 60 mg cholesterol, 550 mg sodium, 11 g carbohydrate, 2 g fiber, 25 g protein

Avocado, Jicama, and Orange Salad

Serves 6

3	tablespoons olive oil
1	tablespoon fresh-squeezed lime juice
1	clove garlic, minced
1 1/2	teaspoons white-wine vinegar
1/4	teaspoon ground cumin
1/8	teaspoon salt
	Pinch chili powder
8	ounces jicama, peeled and cut into 3 x 1/4-inch strips
2	oranges, peeled and cut into sections
1	avocado, pitted, peeled, and cut into chunks
1/2	small red onion, thinly sliced crosswise
8	cups torn romaine lettuce

ONE In small bowl, whisk together oil, lime juice, garlic, vinegar, cumin, salt, and chili powder to make vinaigrette. In large bowl toss together jicama, oranges, avocado, onion, and vinaigrette. Refrigerate 15 minutes.

TWO Serve salad on bed of romaine leaves.

Per serving: 156 calories, 12 g total fat, 2 g saturated fat, 0 mg cholesterol, 57 mg sodium, 14 g carbohydrates, 7 g fiber, 3 g protein

soups, salads, and light bites

Bulgur with Spring Vegetables

Serves 6

1 1/4   cups bulgur
3 1/2   cups boiling water
  2   tablespoons olive oil
  3   tablespoons fresh lemon juice
1/8   teaspoon salt
1/2   teaspoon pepper
  2   leeks, halved lengthwise, cut crosswise into 1-inch pieces, and well washed
  2   cloves garlic, minced
12   asparagus spears, cut into 2-inch lengths
  1   cup frozen peas
1/4   cup chopped fresh mint

ONE In large heatproof bowl combine bulgur and boiling water. Let stand until bulgur is tender, about 30 minutes; stir after 15 minutes. Drain bulgur in large fine-meshed sieve to get rid of any remaining liquid.

TWO In large bowl whisk together 1 tablespoon of oil, the lemon juice, salt, and pepper. Add drained bulgur and fluff with a fork.

THREE In medium skillet over low heat, heat remaining 1 tablespoon oil. Add leeks and garlic to skillet and cook until leeks are tender, about 5 minutes. Transfer to bowl with bulgur.

FOUR In steamer set over a pan of boiling water, steam asparagus until tender, about 4 minutes. Add peas during final 30 seconds of steaming. Add vegetables to bowl of bulgur along with mint and toss to combine. Serve at room temperature or chilled.

Per serving: 188 calories, 5 g total fat, 0.5 g saturated fat, 0 mg cholesterol, 330 mg sodium, 32 g carbohydrates, 8 g fiber, 6 g protein

Garlic Green and Wax Beans

Serves 12

1 1/2   pounds fresh green beans
1 1/2   pounds fresh wax beans
  7   garlic cloves, minced, divided
1/4   cup reduced-fat sour cream
1/4   cup fat-free milk
  1   teaspoon white wine vinegar or cider vinegar
  1   teaspoon olive or canola oil
1/2   teaspoon salt
1/8   teaspoon pepper
  1   cup shredded part-skim mozzarella cheese
    Minced fresh parsley

ONE In a large saucepan, place beans and 6 garlic cloves in a steamer basket over 1 inch of boiling water. Cover and steam until beans are crisp-tender, 8-10 minutes. Transfer to a large bowl; set aside.

TWO In a small bowl, combine sour cream, milk, and vinegar; let stand for 1 minute. Whisk in the oil, salt, pepper, and remaining garlic. Pour over beans and toss.

THREE Cover and chill for at least 2 hours. Just before serving, sprinkle with cheese and parsley.

Per serving (3/4 cup): 76 calories, 2 g total fat, 1 g saturated fat, 7 mg cholesterol, 157 mg sodium, 9 g carbohydrate, 4 g fiber, 5 g protein

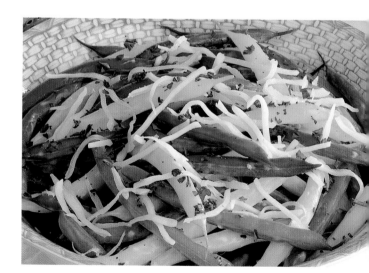

Green Vegetable Salad with Garlic and Ginger

Serves 4

1/2	pound broccoli
1/2	pound small bok choy, or other Chinese leaves
4	scallions
1/4	pound sugar snaps, trimmed
1	small clove garlic, crushed
1	teaspoon finely grated ginger
1	teaspoon dark-brown sugar
1	tablespoon Thai fish sauce

ONE Fill steamer pot with water to just below basket. Bring water to a boil.

TWO Cut broccoli into small florets, trimming stalks to about 1/2 inch. Peel remaining stalk and cut diagonally into 1/2-inch slices. Trim bok choy and slice stems. Trim scallions and cut diagonally into thin slices.

THREE In large bowl, combine broccoli, bok choy, scallions, and sugar snaps. Add garlic and ginger and toss well. Transfer to steamer basket, cover and steam until vegetables are tender-crisp, 3-4 minutes.

FOUR In small cup, combine sugar and fish sauce, stirring until sugar dissolves. Arrange vegetables in serving dish and drizzle with this dressing. Serve hot, or let cool, then refrigerate until 10 minutes before serving.

Per serving: 50 calories, 0 g total fat, 0 g saturated fat, 0 mg cholesterol, 400 mg sodium, 9 g carbohydrate, 3 g fiber, 4 g protein

Endive, Apple, and Watercress Salad with Almonds

Serves 6

1/3	cup plain low-fat yogurt
1	tablespoon reduced-fat mayonnaise
2	teaspoons honey
1	teaspoon Dijon mustard
1/4	teaspoon curry powder
1/8	teaspoon ground ginger
1	bunch watercress, tough stems removed
1	large endive, halved lengthwise and cut crosswise into 1/2-inch-thick slices
1	McIntosh apple, halved, cored, and thinly sliced
2	tablespoons sliced or slivered almonds, toasted

In small bowl, whisk together yogurt, mayonnaise, honey, mustard, curry powder, and ginger to make dressing. In large bowl toss together watercress, endive, apple, and dressing. Top with almonds.

Per serving: 54 calories, 2 g total fat, 0 g saturated fat, 2 mg cholesterol, 62 mg sodium, 54 g carbohydrate, 1 g fiber, 2 g protein

soups, salads, and light bites

Rainbow Fruit Salad

Serves 12

1/2 cup honey
1/3 cup orange juice
2 tablespoons lemon juice
1/4 teaspoon ground ginger
1/8 teaspoon ground nutmeg
5 cups cubed cantaloupe
1 cup fresh blueberries
2 large firm bananas, sliced
2 medium nectarines, peeled and sliced
2 cups sliced fresh strawberries
2 cups halved seedless grapes

● In a small bowl, combine the first five ingredients; mix well. In a large bowl, combine the fruit. Add dressing and toss to coat. Serve immediately with a slotted spoon.

Per serving (1 cup): 126 calories, 1 g total fat, 0 g saturated fat, 0 mg cholesterol, 8 mg sodium, 32 g carbohydrate, 3 g fiber, 1 g protein

Cucumber, Radish, and Snow Pea Salad

Serves 4

6 ounces snow peas, trimmed
1 tablespoon rice vinegar
2 teaspoons sugar
2 teaspoons soy sauce
1 teaspoon dark sesame oil
1/8 teaspoon salt
2 cucumbers, scored and thinly sliced
2 bunches radishes, thinly sliced
1 tablespoon sesame seeds, toasted (optional)

● ONE In saucepan of lightly salted boiling water, cook snow peas until crisp-tender, 2-3 minutes. Drain. Rinse under cold running water.

● TWO In small bowl, whisk together vinegar, sugar, soy sauce, sesame oil, and salt until sugar and salt are dissolved to make vinaigrette.

● THREE In large bowl, toss together snow peas, cucumbers, radishes, and vinaigrette. Sprinkle with sesame seeds, if using.

Per serving: 64 calories, 2 g total fat, 0 g saturated fat, 0 mg cholesterol, 247 mg sodium, 10 g carbohydrate, 3 g fiber, 3 g protein

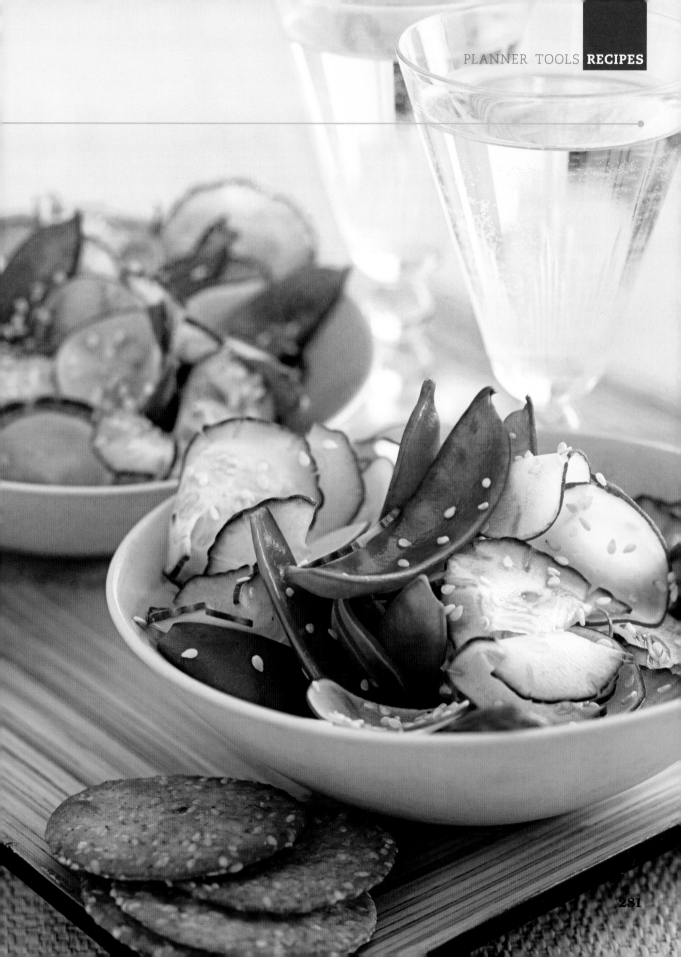

main meals

Chicken and Asparagus Bundles

Serves 4

4	boneless skinless chicken breast halves (1 pound)
20	fresh asparagus spears (about 1 pound), trimmed
4 1/2	teaspoons olive or canola oil
2	teaspoons lemon juice
1/2	teaspoon dried basil
1/4	teaspoon dried thyme
1/4	teaspoon pepper
1/8	teaspoon salt
1/4	cup chopped scallions
2	teaspoons cornstarch
1	cup chicken broth

ONE Flatten chicken breasts slightly. Wrap each around five asparagus spears; secure with toothpicks. Place in a 13 x 9 x 2-inch baking dish coated with nonstick cooking spray. Combine the oil, lemon juice, and seasonings; pour over bundles. Cover asparagus tips with foil.

TWO Cover and bake at 350°F for 15 minutes. Uncover; sprinkle with the scallions. Bake until the chicken juices run clear and asparagus is crisp-tender, 12-15 minutes longer. Remove bundles to a serving platter and keep warm.

THREE In a saucepan, combine cornstarch and broth until smooth; stir in pan juices. Bring to a boil; cook and stir until thickened, about 2 minutes. Remove toothpicks from bundles; top with sauce.

Per serving (1 bundle with about 1/3 cup sauce): 207 calories, 7 g total fat, 1 g saturated fat, 66 mg cholesterol, 316 mg sodium, 6 g carbohydrate, 2 g fiber, 29 g protein

Caribbean Chicken

Serves 6

1/2	cup lemon juice
1/3	cup honey
3	tablespoons canola oil
6	scallions, sliced
3	jalapeño peppers, seeded and chopped*
3	teaspoons dried thyme
3/4	teaspoon salt
1/4	teaspoon ground allspice
1/4	teaspoon ground nutmeg
6	boneless skinless chicken breast halves (1 1/2 pounds)

ONE Place the first nine ingredients in a blender or food processor; cover and process until smooth. Pour 1/2 cup into a small bowl for basting; cover and refrigerate. Pour remaining marinade into a large resealable plastic bag; add chicken. Seal bag and turn to coat; refrigerate for up to 6 hours.

TWO Drain and discard marinade. Coat grill rack with nonstick cooking spray before starting the grill. Grill chicken, covered, over medium heat until juices run clear, 4-6 minutes on each side, basting frequently with the reserved marinade.

Per serving (1 chicken breast half): 205 calories, 6 g total fat, 1 g saturated fat, 66 mg cholesterol, 272 mg sodium, 11 g carbohydrate, 0 g fiber, 27 g protein

Editor's Note: When cutting or seeding hot peppers, use rubber or plastic gloves to protect your hands. Avoid touching your face.

Grilled Citrus Chicken

Serves 6

6   boneless skinless chicken breast halves
    (1 1/2 pounds)
1/2 cup packed brown sugar
1/4 cup cider vinegar
3   tablespoons lemon juice
3   tablespoons lime juice
3   tablespoons Dijon mustard
3/4 teaspoon garlic powder
1/4 teaspoon pepper

- Place chicken in a shallow glass dish. Combine remaining ingredients; pour over chicken. Cover and refrigerate 4 hours or overnight. Drain, discarding marinade. Grill chicken over medium-hot coals, turning once, until juices run clear, about 15-18 minutes.

Per serving: 200 calories, 2 g total fat, 1 g saturated fat, 20 mg cholesterol, 180 mg sodium, 20 g carbohydrate, 0 g fiber, 26 g protein

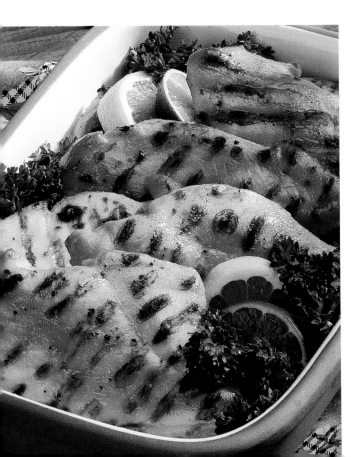

Curry Chicken Dinner

Serves 8

8   boneless, skinless chicken breast halves
    (2 pounds)
1/2 cup all-purpose flour
2   tablespoons cooking oil
2   medium onions, chopped
2   medium green peppers, chopped
1   garlic clove, minced
2   teaspoons curry powder
1/2 teaspoon white pepper
2   cans (14 1/2 ounces each) diced tomatoes, undrained
1   teaspoon chopped fresh parsley
1/2 teaspoon dried thyme
1   cup water
3   tablespoons raisins
    Hot cooked rice (optional)

- **ONE** Dust chicken with flour. In a Dutch oven over medium heat, brown the chicken in oil. Remove chicken and set aside.

- **TWO** Add onions, green peppers, and garlic to drippings; sauté until tender, 3-4 minutes. Add curry and pepper; mix well. Return chicken to the pan. Add tomatoes, parsley, thyme, and water.

- **THREE** Cover and bake at 375°F until chicken is tender and juices run clear, 45-50 minutes. Stir in raisins. Serve over rice if desired.

Per serving: 230 calories, 6 g total fat, 1 g saturated fat, 63 mg cholesterol, 233 mg sodium, 17 g carbohydrate, 2 g fiber, 25 g protein

main meals

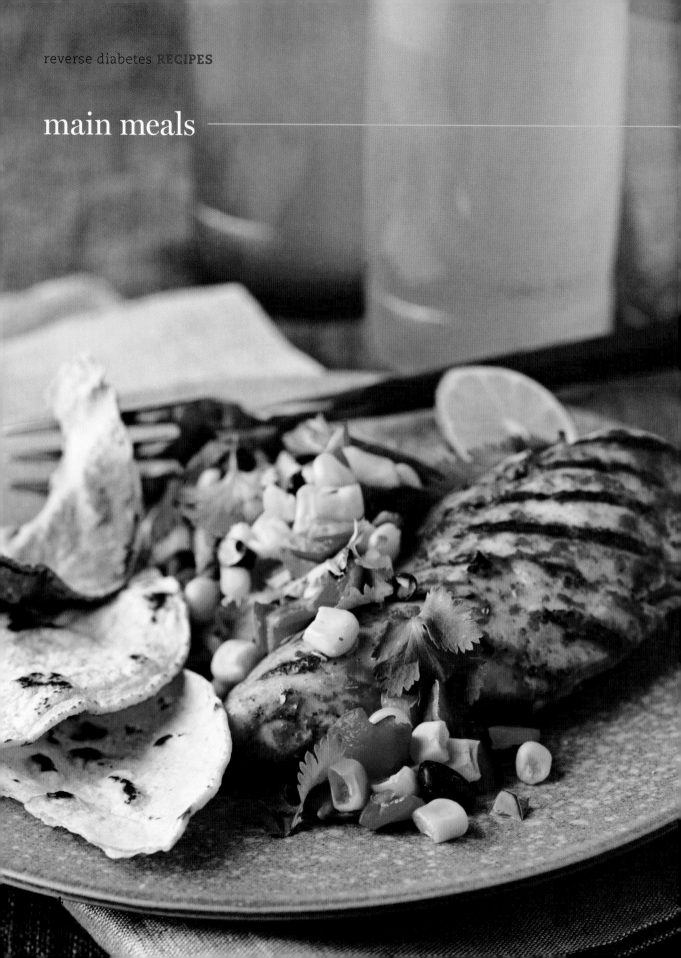

Grilled Chicken Breast with Corn and Pepper Relish

Serves 4

- 2 cloves garlic, minced
- 2 teaspoons chili powder
- 1/4 teaspoon salt
- 3 tablespoons fresh-squeezed lime juice
- 2 tablespoons vegetable oil
- 1 1/2 pounds boneless, skinless chicken breasts, pounded 3/8 inch thick
- 3/4 cup reduced-sodium, fat-free chicken broth
- 1 1/2 cups fresh, drained canned, or thawed frozen corn kernels
- 1 cup diced, seeded, roasted red bell pepper
- 2/3 cup canned black beans, drained and rinsed
- 2 tablespoons coarsely chopped red onion
- 1 jalapeño pepper, seeded and finely chopped*
- 1/4 teaspoon salt
- 3 tablespoons chopped cilantro

ONE In medium bowl, stir together garlic, chili powder, salt, 2 tablespoons lime juice, and oil. Add chicken and rub with marinade. Let stand at room temperature no more than 15 minutes.

TWO Preheat grill to medium-hot or preheat broiler.

THREE Grill or broil chicken 3 inches from heat just until cooked through, 3-4 minutes per side.

FOUR To make relish: In large skillet, heat broth. Add corn kernels, bell pepper, black beans, onion, jalapeño, and salt. Heat through. Just before serving, stir in cilantro and remaining lime juice. Serve chicken topped with relish.

Per serving: 375 calories, 12 g total fat, 2 g saturated fat, 95 mg cholesterol, 521 mg sodium, 29 g carbohydrate, 5 g fiber, 40 g protein

Editor's Note: When cutting or seeding hot peppers, use rubber or plastic gloves to protect your hands. Avoid touching your face.

Orange Beef with Broccoli

Serves 4

- 2 teaspoons cornstarch
- 1/4 cup dry sherry
- 2 tablespoons reduced-sodium soy sauce
- 1/4 teaspoon baking soda
- 12 ounces flank steak, cut into thin strips
- 4 teaspoons olive oil
- 4 tablespoons finely slivered orange zest
- 1/4 teaspoon crushed red pepper flakes
- 5 cups broccoli florets and stems
- 1 red bell pepper, cut into matchsticks
- 4 scallions, thinly sliced
- 3 cloves garlic, minced
- 1 cup jicama matchsticks

ONE In medium bowl, whisk together cornstarch, sherry, soy sauce, and baking soda. Add steak, tossing to coat. Refrigerate 30 minutes.

TWO In large nonstick skillet over medium heat, heat 3 teaspoons oil. Reserving marinade, add beef, half of orange zest, and pepper flakes to skillet. Stir-fry until beef is just cooked, 3 minutes. Transfer to plate.

THREE Add remaining oil, broccoli, bell pepper, scallions, and garlic to skillet. Cook 3 minutes. Add 1/2 cup water. Cook until broccoli is crisp-tender, 2 minutes.

FOUR Stir 1/3 cup water and reserved marinade into skillet. Bring to boil. Cook, stirring, 1 minute. Return beef to skillet. Add jicama. Cook until beef is heated through, 1 minute. Garnish with remaining orange zest.

Per serving: 284 calories, 14 g total fat, 4.4 g saturated fat, 16 g cholesterol, 473 mg sodium, 16 g carbohydrates, 5.3 g fiber, 21 g protein

main meals

Honey-Lime Pork Chops

Serves 6

Chops

1/2	cup lime juice
1/2	cup reduced-sodium soy sauce
2	tablespoons honey
2	garlic cloves, minced
6	boneless pork loin chops (4 ounces each)

Sauce

3/4	cup reduced-sodium chicken broth
1	garlic clove, minced
1 1/2	teaspoons honey
1/2	teaspoon lime juice
1/8	teaspoon browning sauce
	Dash pepper
2	teaspoons cornstarch
2	tablespoons water

ONE In a large resealable plastic bag, combine the lime juice, soy sauce, honey, and garlic. Add pork chops. Seal bag and turn to coat; refrigerate for 8 hours or overnight. Drain and discard marinade. Grill chops, covered, over medium heat or broil 4 inches from the heat until juices run clear, 6-7 minutes on each side.

TWO For sauce, combine the broth, garlic, honey, lime juice, browning sauce, and pepper in a small saucepan. Bring to a boil. Combine the cornstarch and water until smooth; stir into the broth mixture. Return to a boil; cook and stir until thickened, 1-2 minutes. Serve with the pork chops.

Per serving (1 chop with 2 tablespoons sauce): 200 calories, 5 g total fat, 2 g saturated fat, 71 mg cholesterol, 884 mg sodium, 11 g carbohydrate, 0 g fiber, 26 g protein

New Mexican Green Chili

Serves 4

1	tablespoon olive oil
1	pound well-trimmed pork tenderloin, cut into 1-inch chunks
5	scallions, thinly sliced
4	cloves garlic, minced
2	large green bell peppers, cut into 1/2-inch squares
2	pickled jalapeño peppers, seeded and minced*
2	teaspoons ground cumin
2	teaspoons ground coriander
1/2	teaspoon salt
1	cup water
1	can (15 ounces) chickpeas, rinsed and drained
1/2	cup chopped cilantro

ONE Heat oil in nonstick Dutch oven over medium-high heat. Add pork, and brown, about 4 minutes. With slotted spoon, transfer pork to plate.

TWO Reduce heat to medium. Add scallions and garlic and cook until scallions are tender, about 2 minutes. Stir in all peppers and cook until bell peppers are tender, about 4 minutes. Return pork to pan. Add cumin, coriander, and salt. Stir. Add water and bring to a boil. Reduce to simmer, cover, and cook 20 minutes. Stir in chickpeas. Cover and cook until chickpeas are heated, about 5 minutes Stir in cilantro before serving.

Per serving: 300 calories, 10 g total fat, 2 g saturated fat, 74 mg cholesterol, 565 mg sodium, 24 g carbohydrate, 7 g fiber, 31 g protein

Editor's Note: When cutting or seeding hot peppers, use rubber or plastic gloves to protect your hands. Avoid touching your face.

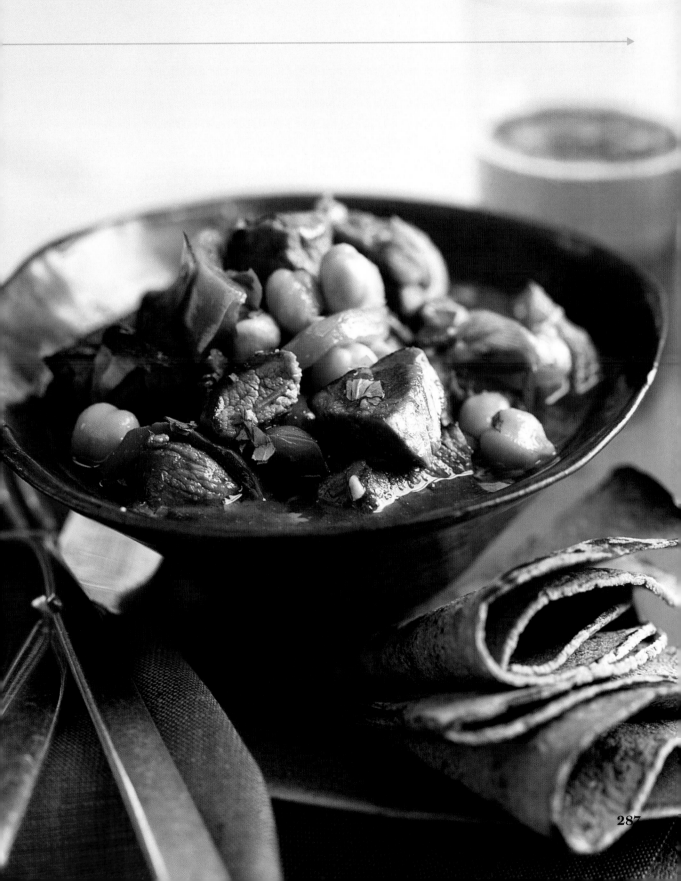

main meals

Pork Tenderloin with Honey-Mustard Sauce

Serves 4

1	tablespoon chopped fresh rosemary or 1 teaspoon dried
2	garlic cloves, minced
1	teaspoon grated lemon zest
1/2	teaspoon salt
1	pork tenderloin (about 1 pound), trimmed
1/3	cup fresh lemon juice
1/4	cup honey
3	tablespoons coarse Dijon mustard
1/2	cup nonfat half-and-half
1	tablespoon all-purpose flour

ONE Preheat oven to 400°F. Line small roasting pan with foil. Combine rosemary, garlic, lemon zest, and salt in small bowl and rub evenly over pork tenderloin; transfer pork to pan. Mix lemon juice, honey, and mustard in small bowl. Transfer half to small saucepan and set aside.

TWO Brush pork with 2 tablespoons honey-mustard sauce. Roast pork until glazed and golden brown or until instant-read thermometer reads 160°F, about 25 minutes, basting 2 or 3 times with remaining sauce.

THREE Meanwhile, put half-and-half in small bowl and whisk in flour until smooth. Warm reserved honey-mustard sauce in small saucepan over low heat. Gradually whisk in half-and-half mixture and cook, whisking constantly, until sauce thickens, about 3 minutes. Serve over the pork.

Per serving: 247 calories, 5 g total fat, 1 g saturated fat, 74 mg cholesterol, 525 mg sodium, 25 g carbohydrate, 1 g fiber, 25 g protein

Sea Scallops and Cherry Tomato Sauté

Serves 4

1	pound sea scallops
4	teaspoons cornstarch
2	teaspoons olive oil
3	cloves garlic, minced
1	pint cherry tomatoes
2/3	cup dry vermouth, white wine, or chicken broth
1/2	teaspoon salt
1/3	cup chopped fresh basil
1	tablespoon cold water

ONE Dredge scallops in 3 teaspoons of the cornstarch, shaking off excess. In large nonstick skillet over medium heat, heat oil. Add scallops and sauté until golden brown and cooked through, about 3 minutes. With slotted spoon, transfer scallops to bowl.

TWO Add garlic to pan and cook 1 minute. Add tomatoes and cook until they begin to collapse, about 4 minutes. Add vermouth, salt, and basil to pan. Bring to a boil and cook for 1 minute.

THREE Meanwhile, stir together remaining 1 teaspoon cornstarch and cold water in small bowl. Add cornstarch mixture to pan and cook, stirring, until sauce is slightly thickened, about 1 minute.

FOUR Return scallops to pan, reduce to a simmer, and cook just until heated through, about 1 minute.

Per serving: 176 calories, 4 g total fat, 1 g saturated fat, 37 mg cholesterol, 483 mg sodium, 10 g carbohydrate, 1 g fiber, 20 g protein

Asian Steamed Fish Fillets with Vegetable Sticks

Serves 4

1 1/2 pounds halibut or other firm-fleshed white fish fillets, in 4 pieces
2 tablespoons soy sauce
2 tablespoons white wine or sake
1 thin slice fresh ginger, peeled and cut in thin sticks
2 medium carrots, peeled and cut into 3 x 1/4-inch sticks
2 ounces snow peas, cut in half lengthwise
1/2 yellow bell pepper, seeded and cut into thin sticks

ONE Place fillets in baking dish that will fit inside large steamer basket or on rack that will fit into large skillet. In small cup, stir together soy sauce and white wine. Pour over fish. Top with ginger and carrots.

TWO Fill skillet with 1 inch of water. Bring to a simmer. Place steamer basket or wire rack in skillet. Place baking dish containing fish in basket or on rack. Cover skillet or basket. Steam 5-6 minutes. Add snow peas and yellow pepper to baking dish. Cover. Steam until fish flakes when touched with fork and vegetables are crisp-tender, about 5 minutes. Serve at once.

Per serving: 175 calories, 3 g total fat, 0 g saturated fat, 45 mg cholesterol, 558 mg sodium, 7 g carbohydrate, 2 g fiber, 32 g protein

Baked Cod Casserole with Potatoes, Tomatoes, and Arugula

Serves 4

1 pound red potatoes, unpeeled and cut in 1/2-inch-thick slices
1 onion, thinly sliced
1 tablespoon olive oil
1/2 teaspoon salt
4 plum tomatoes, seeded and coarsely chopped
3 cloves garlic, minced
1/2 teaspoon dried oregano, crumbled
1 1/2 cups arugula leaves
1 pound cod, scrod, halibut, or other thick, firm-fleshed white fish steaks, cut into 2-inch chunks

ONE Preheat oven to 350°F. In 13 x 9 x 2-inch baking dish, combine potatoes, onion, oil, and 1/4 teaspoon salt.

TWO Bake 20 minutes, stirring mixture once.

THREE Stir tomatoes, garlic, and oregano into potato mixture. Spread arugula on top in even layer. Top with cod. Sprinkle with remaining 1/4 teaspoon salt.

FOUR Bake, covered with aluminum foil, just until fish is cooked through, 15-18 minutes. Transfer fish and vegetable mixture to serving plates. Spoon pan juices over each serving.

Per serving: 213 calories, 5 g total fat, 1 g saturated fat, 43 mg cholesterol, 363 mg sodium, 21 g carbohydrate, 4 g fiber, 22 g protein

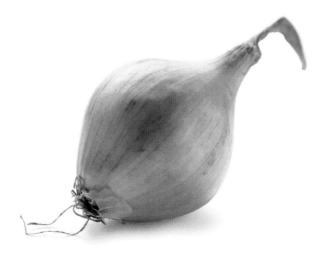

main meals

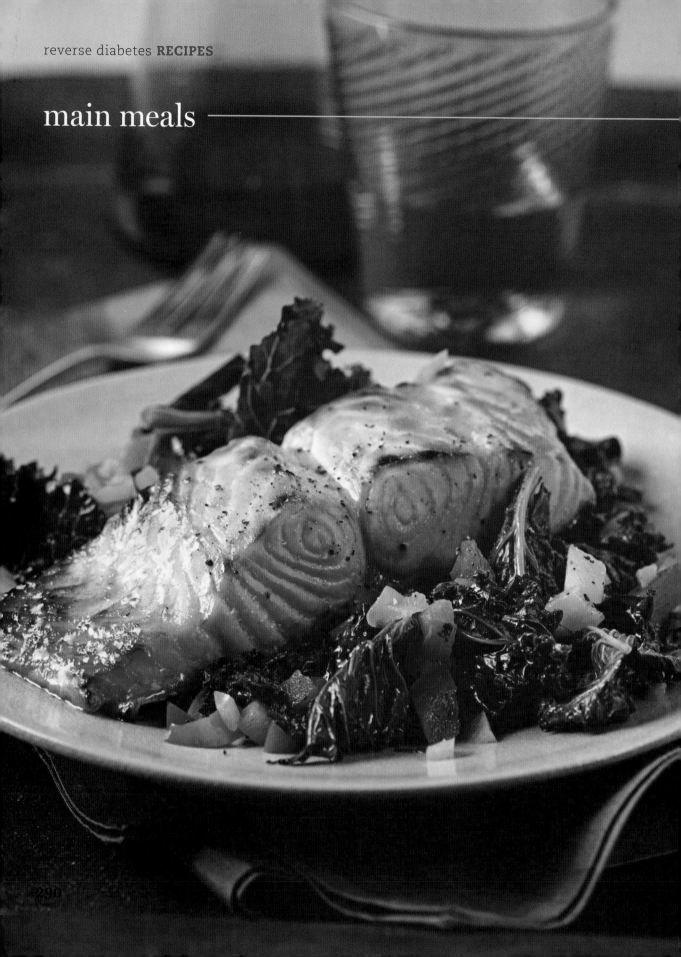

Salmon on a Bed of Greens

Serves 4

1/4	cup grapefruit juice
1 1/2	tablespoons mustard
1 1/2	tablespoons honey
1/4	teaspoon red pepper flakes
4	salmon fillets (6 ounces each)
1 1/2	pounds kale, large stems removed and leaves chopped
3	tablespoons olive oil
1/2	red bell pepper, seeded and finely chopped
1/2	yellow pepper, seeded and finely chopped

ONE In baking dish large enough to hold fish fillets in single layer, combine grapefruit juice, mustard, honey, and pepper flakes. Add salmon to dish, turning to coat both sides with marinade. Refrigerate, covered, 30 minutes.

TWO Preheat broiler.

THREE In large pot, bring 2 quarts of water to a boil. Add kale. Return water to boil and cook 5 minutes. Drain well. Squeeze out excess water.

FOUR Heat olive oil in large skillet over medium heat. Add red and yellow bell peppers. Sauté 1 minute. Add kale. Sauté until peppers and kale are tender, about 3 minutes. Remove skillet from heat and keep warm.

FIVE Remove salmon from marinade. Place, skin side down, on rack in foil-lined broiler pan. Reserve marinade.

SIX Broil salmon 4 inches from heat for 3 minutes. Brush on remaining marinade. Broil until fish is opaque and flakes when touched with knife, 3 to 4 minutes. (If fish begins to brown too much, drop to lower rack in broiler.) Serve salmon on bed of kale and peppers.

Per serving: 402 calories, 18 g total fat, 3 g saturated fat, 97 mg cholesterol, 21 g carbohydrates, 233 mg sodium, 3 g fiber, 41 g protein

Sunshine Halibut

Serves 4

1/3	cup chopped onion
1	garlic clove, minced
2	tablespoons minced fresh parsley
1/2	teaspoon grated orange peel
4	halibut steaks (4 ounces each)
1/4	cup orange juice
1	tablespoon lemon juice
1/4	teaspoon salt
1/4	teaspoon lemon-pepper seasoning

ONE In a nonstick skillet coated with nonstick cooking spray, sauté onion and garlic until tender; remove from the heat. Stir in parsley and orange peel.

TWO Place halibut in an 8-inch square baking dish coated with nonstick cooking spray. Top with onion mixture.

THREE Combine orange and lemon juices; pour over fish. Sprinkle with salt and lemon-pepper. Cover and bake at 400°F until fish flakes easily with a fork, 15-20 minutes.

Per serving: 142 calories, 3 g total fat, 0 g saturated fat, 36 mg cholesterol, 237 mg sodium, 4 g carbohydrate, 0 g fiber, 24 g protein

main meals

Zippy Shrimp

Serves 8

1 1/4	cups chicken or vegetable broth
10	medium pitted ripe olives, finely chopped
1	red chile pepper, finely chopped*
2	tablespoons lemon juice
1	tablespoon minced fresh rosemary or 1 teaspoon dried rosemary, crushed
4	garlic cloves, minced
2	teaspoons Worcestershire sauce
1	teaspoon paprika
1/2	teaspoon salt
1/4-1/2	teaspoon pepper
2	pounds fresh or frozen uncooked shrimp, peeled and deveined

- In a large nonstick skillet, combine the first 10 ingredients. Bring to a boil; cook until mixture is reduced by half. Add shrimp. Simmer, uncovered, until shrimp turn pink, stirring occasionally, 3-4 minutes.

Per serving (1/2 cup): 141 calories, 3 g total fat, 0 g saturated fat, 172 mg cholesterol, 520 mg sodium, 3 g carbohydrate, 0 g fiber, 24 g protein

Note: When cutting or seeding hot peppers, use rubber or plastic gloves to protect your hands. Avoid touching your face.

Eggplant Lasagna

Serves 12

2	tablespoons olive oil
1	large onion, chopped
2	cloves garlic, minced
1	tablespoon Italian seasoning
2	cans (14 ounces each) diced tomatoes
1	can (28 ounces) tomato sauce
1	small eggplant, peeled and cut into 1-inch pieces
1/4	teaspoon salt
1	container (16 ounces) lite silken tofu, drained
2	large eggs
1	cup grated Parmesan cheese
9	no-boil lasagna noodles
1	package (8 ounces) shredded part-skim mozzarella cheese

- ONE Preheat the oven to 400°F. Heat the oil in a large saucepan over medium-high heat. Add the onion and cook until tender, about 5 minutes. Add the garlic and Italian seasoning and cook for 1 minute. Add the tomatoes and tomato sauce and bring to a simmer. Reduce the heat to low and simmer until the flavors are blended, 40 minutes.

- TWO Meanwhile, coat a baking sheet with sides with cooking spray. Add the eggplant, coat with cooking spray, and sprinkle with the salt. Roast, turning occasionally, until browned, 30 minutes.

- THREE In a food processor, combine the tofu, eggs, and Parmesan and puree until smooth.

- FOUR Coat a 9 x 13-inch baking dish with cooking spray. Spread 1 cup sauce in the dish and arrange 3 lasagna noodles on top. Spread half of the tofu filling over the noodles, followed by half of the eggplant. Top with 1 1/2 cups sauce and 1/2 cup mozzarella. Repeat with another layer, then top with the remaining noodles, sauce, and mozzarella.

- FIVE Cover with foil and bake for 1 hour. Remove the foil and bake until heated through, about 15 minutes. Let cool slightly before serving.

Per serving: 229 calories, 10 g total fat, 4 g saturated fat, 51 mg cholesterol, 852 mg sodium 23 g carbohydrate, 3 g fiber, 15 g protein

Barley Risotto with Asparagus and Mushrooms

Serves 4

- 2 cans (14 1/2 ounces each) reduced-sodium, fat-free chicken broth
- 2 tablespoons olive oil
- 1 onion, finely chopped
- 8 ounces mushrooms, preferably mixture of wild varieties, coarsely chopped
- 2 cloves garlic, minced
- 1 cup pearl barley
- 8 ounces asparagus, trimmed, and cut into bite-size pieces, leaving tips whole
- 1/2 cup grated Parmesan cheese

ONE In medium saucepan, heat broth and 2 cups water to just below a simmer. Cover; keep at a simmer.

TWO In large deep nonstick skillet over medium heat, heat oil. Sauté onion until slightly softened, about 3 minutes. Add mushrooms and garlic. Sauté until mushrooms are softened, about 5 minutes. Stir in barley. Stir in 2 cups hot broth mixture. Simmer, covered, 15 minutes.

THREE Meanwhile, blanch asparagus tips in the pot of hot broth for 2 minutes. Transfer with slotted spoon to plate.

FOUR Add more hot broth to barley mixture, 1/2 cup at a time, stirring frequently. Let each batch of liquid be absorbed before adding more. When adding the last batch of liquid, stir in asparagus stem pieces. Stir in Parmesan. Serve risotto topped with asparagus tips.

Per serving: 329 calories, 10 g total fat, 2 g saturated fat, 23 mg cholesterol, 743 mg sodium, 49 g carbohydrate, 10 g fiber, 15 g protein

Couscous-Stuffed Peppers

Serves 6

- 6 large bell peppers (red, yellow, orange, or green)
- 1 tablespoon vegetable oil
- 1 small zucchini, finely chopped
- 2 cloves garlic, minced
- 1 tablespoon fresh-squeezed lemon juice
- 2 cups cooked couscous
- 1 can (15 ounces) chickpeas, drained and rinsed
- 1 ripe tomato, seeded and finely chopped
- 1 teaspoon dried oregano, crumbled
- 1/2 teaspoon salt
- 1/4 teaspoon black pepper
- 1/2 cup crumbled feta cheese

ONE Slice tops off peppers to make lids. Scoop out membranes and seeds and discard. In large saucepan of lightly salted boiling water, simmer peppers and lids covered, 5 minutes. Drain.

TWO Preheat oven to 350°F.

THREE Heat oil in medium saucepan over medium heat. Add zucchini and garlic. Sauté 2 minutes. Stir in lemon juice. Cook 1 minute and remove from heat. Stir in couscous, chickpeas, tomato, oregano, salt, and pepper. Stir in cheese. Fill each pepper with couscous mixture. Place upright in shallow baking dish. Cover with pepper tops.

FOUR Bake just until filling is heated through, about 20 minutes.

Per serving: 207 calories, 4 g total fat, 1 g saturated fat, 3 mg cholesterol, 307 mg sodium, 36 g carbohydrate, 7 g fiber, 8 g protein

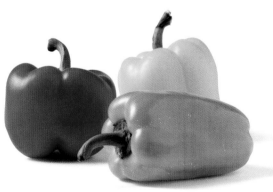

side dishes

Steamed Sesame Spinach

Serves 4

- 1 pound spinach, stems removed
- 1/8 teaspoon red pepper flakes
- 1/2 teaspoon dark sesame oil
- 1 teaspoon salt
- 1 teaspoon fresh-squeezed lemon juice
- 1 tablespoon sesame seeds, toasted

ONE In medium saucepan, steam spinach with pepper flakes until tender, 3 to 5 minutes. Transfer to serving bowl.

TWO Add sesame oil, salt, and lemon juice to spinach. Toss to mix. Sprinkle with sesame seeds. Serve at once.

Per serving: 38 calories, 2 g total fat, 0 g saturated fat, 0 mg cholesterol, 43 mg sodium, 4 g carbohydrates, 3 g fiber, 3 g protein

Baked Sweet Potato "Fries"

Serves 4

- 1 pound sweet potatoes, peeled and cut into 1/2-inch-thick "fries"
- 1 tablespoon vegetable oil
- 1/4 teaspoon salt
- 1/4 teaspoon black pepper

ONE Preheat oven to 425°F. Lightly coat baking sheet with nonstick cooking spray.

TWO In large bowl, combine sweet potatoes, oil, salt, and pepper. Toss to coat. Spread fries in single layer on baking sheet.

THREE Bake 10 minutes. Turn fries over. Continue baking until tender and lightly browned, about 10 minutes longer.

Per serving: 102 calories, 4 g total fat, 0 g saturated fat, 0 mg cholesterol, 152 mg sodium, 17 g carbohydrates, 2 g fiber, 1 g protein

Zippy Green Beans

Serves 6

- 4 cups fresh or frozen green beans, cut into 2-inch pieces
- 2 bacon strips, diced
- 1 medium onion, thinly sliced
- 1/2 cup white wine or apple juice
- 3 tablespoons sugar
- 3 tablespoons tarragon vinegar or cider vinegar
- 1/4 teaspoon salt
- 2 teaspoons cornstarch
- 1 tablespoon cold water

ONE Place beans in a saucepan and cover with water; bring to a boil. Cook, uncovered, until crisp-tender, 8-10 minutes. Meanwhile, in a large nonstick skillet, cook bacon over medium heat until crisp. Remove with a slotted spoon to paper towels. Drain, reserving 1 teaspoon drippings.

TWO In the drippings, sauté onion until tender. Add wine or apple juice, sugar, vinegar, and salt. Combine cornstarch and cold water until smooth; add to the skillet. Bring to a boil; cook and stir until thickened, about 2 minutes. Drain beans; top with onion mixture. Sprinkle with bacon; toss to coat.

Per serving (3/4 cup): 98 calories, 2 g total fat, 1 g saturated fat, 3 mg cholesterol, 140 mg sodium, 16 g carbohydrate, 3 g fiber, 2 g protein

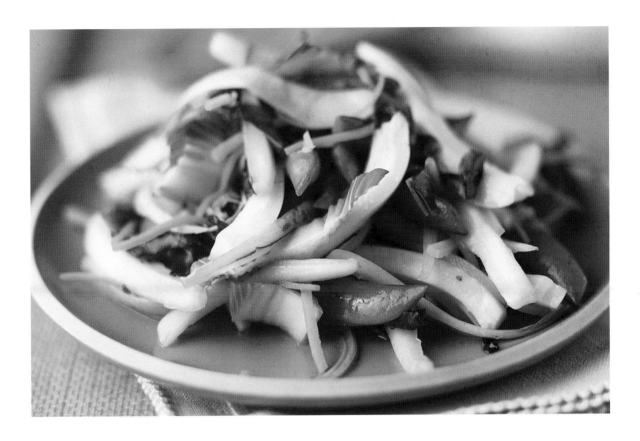

Stir-Fried Bok Choy with Sugar Snap Peas

Serves 4

2   teaspoons olive oil
1   carrot, cut into matchsticks
2   tablespoons slivered fresh ginger
1   pound bok choy, cut into 1/2-inch-wide slices
8   ounces sugar snap peas, trimmed
3   tablespoons orange juice concentrate
1   tablespoon light-brown sugar
1   tablespoon reduced-sodium soy sauce
1/2 teaspoon salt
1   teaspoon cornstarch blended with
    1 tablespoon water

ONE In large nonstick skillet over medium heat, heat 1/4 cup water and oil. Add carrot and ginger, and cook, stirring frequently, until carrot is crisp-tender, about 3 minutes.

TWO Add bok choy, sugar snap peas, orange juice concentrate, brown sugar, soy sauce, and salt. Cover and cook until bok choy begins to wilt, about 3 minutes.

THREE Uncover and cook, stirring frequently, until bok choy is crisp-tender, about 2 minutes. Stir in cornstarch mixture and cook, stirring constantly, until vegetables are evenly coated, about 1 minute.

Per serving: 109 calories, 3 g total fat, 1 g saturated fat, 0 mg cholesterol, 630 mg sodium, 19 g carbohydrate, 3 g fiber, 4 g protein

side dishes

Roasted Carrots with Rosemary

Serves 6

- 1   pound large carrots, peeled and cut into 2 x 1/4-inch sticks
- 1/4   teaspoon salt
- 1 1/2   teaspoons olive oil
- 1   teaspoon minced fresh rosemary leaves or 1/2 teaspoon dried, crumbled

ONE Preheat oven to 400°F.

TWO Mound carrot sticks on baking sheet. Sprinkle with salt and drizzle with oil. Gently toss. Spread out on sheet into single layer.

THREE Roast 10 minutes. Stir in rosemary. Roast until crisp-tender and lightly browned in spots, 7-10 minutes.

Per serving: 44 calories, 1 g total fat, 0 g saturated fat, 0 mg cholesterol, 136 mg sodium, 8 g carbohydrate, 2 g fiber, 1 g protein

Roast Asparagus and Red Pepper with Parmesan

Serves 4

- 1   pound asparagus, trimmed and bottom half of stalks thinly peeled
- 1   red bell pepper, seeded and cut lengthwise into thin strips
- 1   tablespoon olive oil
- 1   tablespoon balsamic vinegar
- 1   ounce Parmesan cheese, in one piece
- 1/4   teaspoon black pepper

ONE Preheat oven to 500°F.

TWO Place asparagus and bell pepper strips in large shallow baking pan. Drizzle with oil. Toss to coat.

THREE Roast until crisp-tender, 10 to 12 minutes, turning occasionally. Transfer to serving dish.

FOUR Sprinkle with vinegar. Toss to coat. Using a vegetable peeler, shave cheese into thin curls over vegetables. Season with pepper.

Per serving: 86 calories, 6 g total fat, 2 g saturated fat, 6 mg cholesterol, 140 mg sodium, 5 g carbohydrates, 2 g fiber, 5 g protein

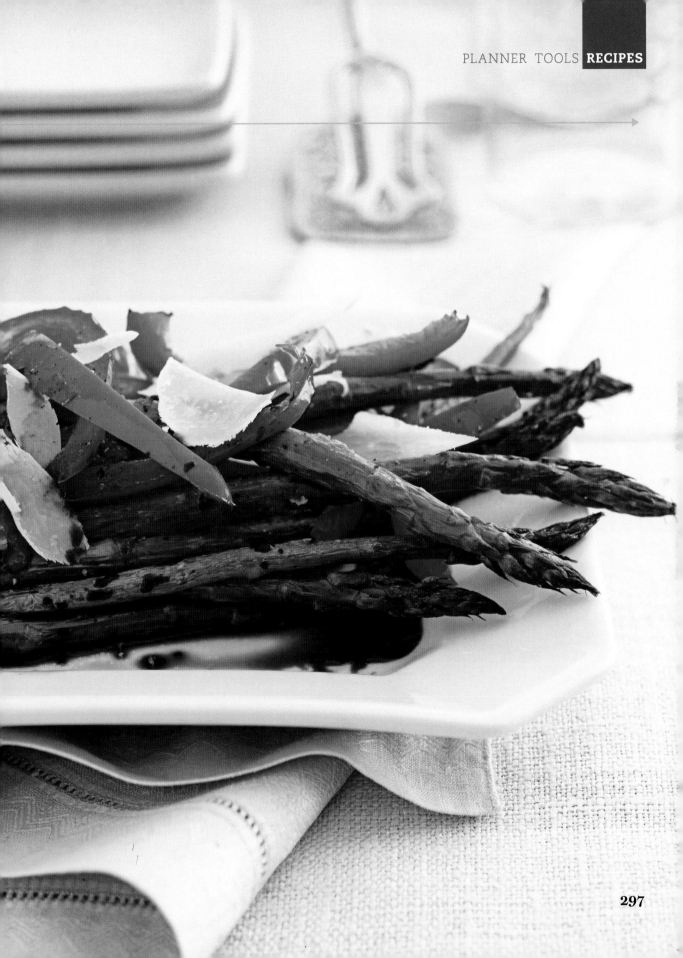

side dishes

Whole Baked Cauliflower with Yogurt-Chive Sauce

Serves 6

- 1/2 cup plain low-fat yogurt
- 1/4 cup loosely packed minced fresh chives
- 1 1/2 tablespoons Dijon mustard
- 1 head cauliflower
- 2 teaspoons olive oil
- 1 large shallot, minced
- 1/4 teaspoon dried oregano, crumbled
- 1 1/4 cups fresh bread crumbs

ONE In blender, puree yogurt, chives, and mustard to make sauce. Refrigerate.

TWO Preheat oven to 350°F. Trim leaves from base of cauliflower. Remove bottom stem. In large pot of salted boiling water, cook cauliflower, fully submerged, until barely crisp-tender, about 6 minutes. Drain. Let cool slightly.

THREE Heat oil in medium nonstick skillet over medium heat. Add shallot and oregano. Sauté 2 minutes. Stir in bread crumbs, mixing well. Cook, stirring, until lightly browned, about 2 minutes. Place cauliflower, stem end up, in dish. Fill with crumb mixture. Bake until bread crumbs are golden and cauliflower is fork-tender, 20-25 minutes. Serve with sauce.

Per serving: 83 calories, 3 g total fat, 1 g saturated fat, 1 mg cholesterol, 289 mg sodium, 12 g carbohydrate, 3 g fiber, 4 g protein

Sweet-and-Sour Red Cabbage

Serves 8

- 1 cup water
- 1/4 cup packed brown sugar
- 3 tablespoons vinegar
- 1 tablespoon vegetable oil
- Dash pepper
- 4 cups shredded red cabbage
- 2 tart apples, peeled and sliced

In a large skillet, combine water, brown sugar, vinegar, oil, and pepper. Cook until hot, 2-3 minutes, stirring occasionally. Add cabbage; cover and cook for 10 minutes over medium-low heat, stirring occasionally. Add apples; cook, uncovered, until tender, stirring occasionally, about 10 minutes more.

Per serving: 69 calories, 2 g total fat, 1 g saturated fat, 0 mg cholesterol, 15 mg sodium, 14 g carbohydrate, 2 g fiber, 1 g protein

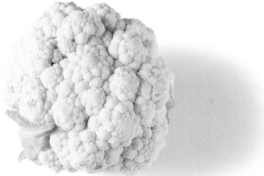

dessert

Watermelon Ice

Serves 4

- 1 teaspoon unflavored gelatin
- 2 tablespoons water
- 4 cups seeded, cubed watermelon, divided
- 2 tablespoons lime juice
- 2 tablespoons honey

ONE In a microwave-safe bowl, sprinkle gelatin over water; let stand for 2 minutes. Microwave on High for 40 seconds; stir. Let stand until gelatin is dissolved, about 2 minutes. Pour into a blender or food processor; add 1 cup watermelon, lime juice, and honey. Cover and process until smooth. Add remaining melon, a cup at a time, and process until smooth.

TWO Pour into a 9-inch square dish; freeze until almost firm. Transfer to a chilled bowl; beat with an electric mixer until mixture is bright pink. Pour into serving dishes; freeze until firm. Remove from the freezer 15-20 minutes before serving.

Per serving (3/4 cup): 85 calories, 1 g total fat, 0 g saturated fat, 0 mg cholesterol, 5 mg sodium, 20 g carbohydrate, 1 g fiber, 2 g protein

Old-Fashioned Fruit Cobbler

Serves 8

Filling
- 3 cups chopped (1/2-inch pieces) rhubarb
- 2 cups halved strawberries
- 1/4 cup granulated sugar
- 3 tablespoons cornstarch
- 1 1/2 teaspoons grated orange zest

Topping
- 1/4 cup whole flaxseed
- 1/3 cup whole-wheat flour
- 1/3 cup all-purpose flour
- 1/4 cup plus 1 teaspoon sugar
- 1 teaspoon baking soda
- 1/2 teaspoon baking powder
  pinch of salt
- 2 ounces (1/4 cup) reduced-fat cream cheese
- 2 tablespoons canola oil
- 1/4 cup low-fat buttermilk
- 3 tablespoons sliced almonds

ONE Preheat the oven to 400°F. Coat an 8 x 8-inch baking dish with cooking spray.

TWO To make the filling: In a large bowl, combine the rhubarb, strawberries, sugar, cornstarch, and orange zest and mix. Spread in the baking dish.

THREE To make the topping: Grind the flaxseed into a coarse meal in a spice grinder or blender. Transfer to a large bowl. Add the flour, 1/4 cup sugar, baking soda, baking powder, and salt and whisk to blend. Add the cream cheese and blend with a pastry blender or your fingers, until the mixture resembles coarse crumbs. Add the oil and toss with a fork. Gradually add the buttermilk, stirring with a fork until the dough clumps. Transfer to a lightly floured surface and knead several times. Pat into a 1/2-inch-thick square and cut into 9 pieces. Arrange the pieces over the fruit, leaving a little space between them. Sprinkle with the almonds and remaining 1 teaspoon sugar.

FOUR Bake until the fruit is bubbly and the biscuit is golden and firm, 35 to 40 minutes.

Per serving: 213 calories, 9 g total fat, 1 g saturated fat, 4 mg cholesterol, 258 mg sodium, 31 g carbohydrate, 4 g fiber, 4 g protein

dessert

Homemade Pumpkin Spice Ice Cream

Serves 6

1 1/4 cups evaporated low-fat (2%) milk
1 large egg
1/2 cup packed light-brown sugar
2/3 cup canned solid-pack pumpkin puree
1 teaspoon vanilla extract
1/2 teaspoon ground ginger
1/2 teaspoon cinnamon
 Large pinch ground nutmeg
 Pinch salt

ONE In medium saucepan, bring milk to a boil.

TWO In large bowl, whisk together egg and sugar. Gradually whisk in boiling milk. Stir in pumpkin, vanilla, ginger, cinnamon, nutmeg, and salt. Refrigerate until thoroughly chilled.

THREE Freeze in ice-cream maker, following manufacturer's directions. Soften slightly before serving.

Per serving (1/2 cup): 141 calories, 1 g total fat, 1 g saturated fat, 40 mg cholesterol, 102 mg sodium, 26 g carbohydrate, 1 g fiber, 5 g protein

Lemon Blueberry Cheesecake

Serves 12

1 package (3 ounces) lemon gelatin
1 cup boiling water
2 tablespoons butter or stick margarine, melted
1 tablespoon canola oil
1 cup graham cracker crumbs (about 16 squares)
1 carton (24 ounces) fat-free cottage cheese
1/4 cup sugar

Topping:
2 tablespoons sugar
1 1/2 teaspoons cornstarch
1/4 cup water
1 1/3 cups fresh or frozen blueberries, divided
1 teaspoon lemon juice

ONE In a bowl, dissolve gelatin in boiling water; cool. Combine butter and oil; add crumbs and blend well. Press onto the bottom of a 9-inch springform pan. Chill. In a blender, process cottage cheese and sugar until smooth. While processing, slowly add cooled gelatin. Pour into crust; chill overnight.

TWO For topping, combine sugar and cornstarch in a saucepan; stir in water until smooth. Add 1 cup blueberries. Bring to a boil; cook and stir until thickened, about 2 minutes. Stir in lemon juice; cool slightly. Process in a blender until smooth. Refrigerate until completely cooled. Carefully run a knife around edge of pan to loosen cheesecake; remove sides of pan. Spread the blueberry mixture over the top. Top with remaining blueberries. Refrigerate leftovers.

Per serving: 171 calories, 4 g total fat, 1 g saturated fat, 8 mg cholesterol, 352 mg sodium, 27 g carbohydrate, 1g fiber, 8 g protein

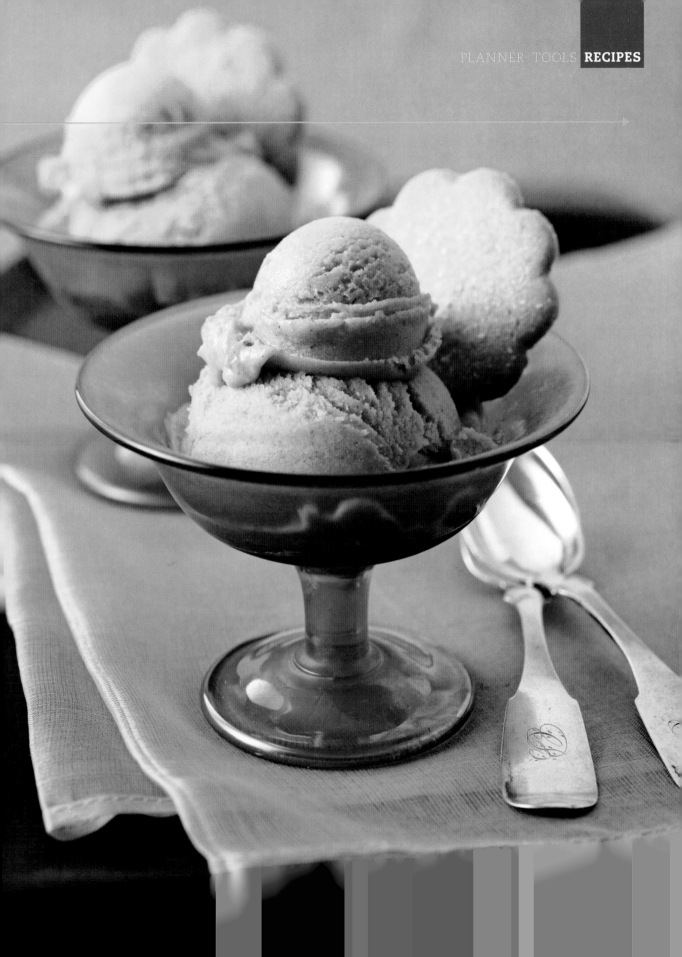

dessert

Grilled Peaches with Berry Sauce

Serves 4

1/2 cup sweetened frozen raspberries, partially thawed

1 1/2 teaspoons lemon juice

2 medium fresh peaches, peeled and halved

5 teaspoons brown sugar

1/4 teaspoon ground cinnamon

1/2 teaspoon vanilla extract

1 teaspoon margarine

ONE In a blender or food processor, process raspberries and lemon juice until pureed. Strain and discard seeds. Cover and chill.

TWO Place the peach halves, cut side up, on a large piece of heavy-duty foil (about 18 x 12 inches). Combine brown sugar and cinnamon; sprinkle into peach centers. Sprinkle with vanilla; dot with margarine. Fold foil over peaches and seal tightly. Grill over medium-hot coals until heated through, about 15 minutes. Open foil carefully to allow steam to escape. To serve, spoon the raspberry sauce over peaches.

Per serving: 80 calories, 1 g total fat, 0 g saturated fat, 0 mg cholesterol, 5 mg sodium, 18 g carbohydrate, 1 g fiber, 1 g protein

Five-Star Cookies

Makes 16 cookies

2 tablespoons hazelnuts, finely chopped

2 tablespoons sunflower seeds, finely chopped

1/4 cup dried apricots, finely chopped

1/4 cup stoned dried dates, finely chopped

1 tablespoon light brown sugar

1/2 cup barley flakes

1/2 cup whole-wheat flour

1/2 teaspoon baking soda

2 tablespoons canola oil

4 tablespoons apple juice

ONE Preheat the oven to 350°F. Mix the chopped hazelnuts, sunflower seeds, apricots, and dates together in a bowl. Add the sugar, barley flakes, flour, and baking soda, and stir to combine.

TWO Mix together the canola oil and apple juice, and pour over the dry mixture. Stir until the dry ingredients are just moistened.

THREE Drop the batter by rounded teaspoonfuls onto a baking sheet coated with cooking spray. Using the back of a fork dipped in flour, gently flatten each ball and neaten the edges with your fingers.

FOUR Bake until golden brown, about 10 minutes. Transfer to a wire rack and cool. These can be kept in an airtight container for up to 4 days.

Per cookie: 61 calories, 3 g total fat, 0 g saturated fat, 0 mg cholesterol, 41 mg sodium, 9 g carbohydrates, 1 g fiber, 1 g protein

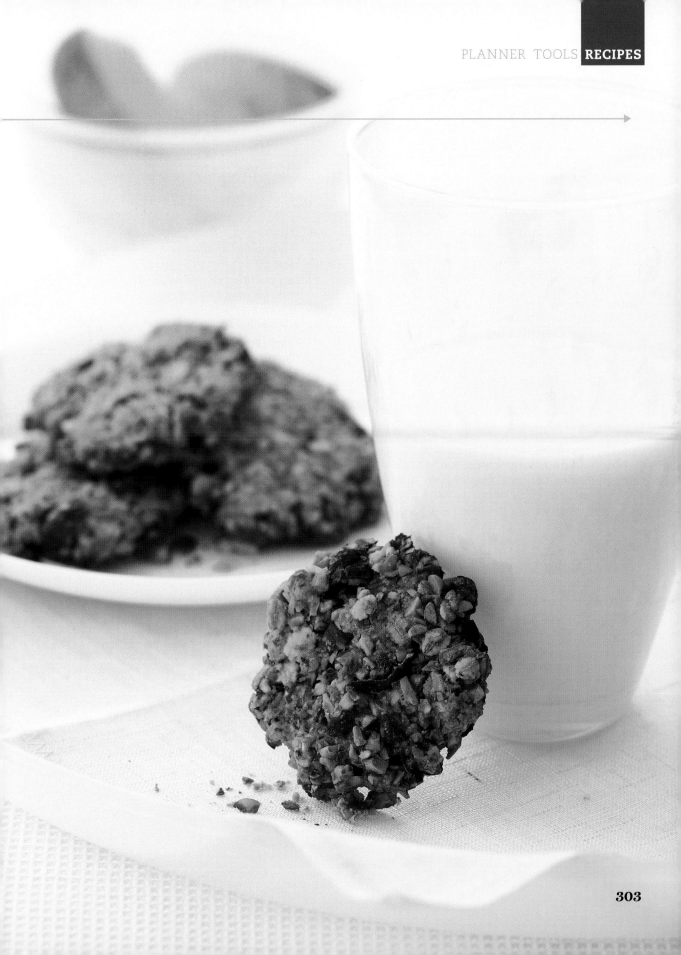

dessert

Slow-Cooker Apple and Pear Compote

Serves 8

- 2 pounds firm cooking apples, such as Granny Smith, Empire, Northern Spy, or Rome, peeled, cored, and sliced (7 cups)
- 1 pound ripe but firm pears, such as Bosc or Anjou, peeled, cored, and sliced (2 1/2 cups)
- 1/4 cup granulated sugar
- 1 tablespoon fresh lemon juice
- 2 strips (about 3/4" x 2 1/2") lemon zest
- 1 teaspoon grated fresh ginger
- 1 teaspoon vanilla extract
- 1/4 cup sliced almonds
- 1/2 cup low-fat plain or vanilla yogurt

ONE Coat a 4-quart or larger slow cooker with cooking spray. Add the apples, pears, sugar, lemon juice, lemon zest, and ginger and toss to mix well. Cover and cook until the fruit is very tender and almost translucent but not pureed, 2 1/2 to 3 1/2 hours on high or 6 to 7 hours on low. Discard the lemon zest. Gently stir in the vanilla. Transfer to a medium bowl and let cool slightly. Cover and refrigerate until chilled. The compote will keep, covered, in the refrigerator for up to 4 days or in the freezer for up to 4 months.

TWO Meanwhile, toast the almonds in a small dry skillet over medium-low heat, stirring constantly, until golden and fragrant, 3 to 4 minutes.

THREE Top each serving with a dollop of yogurt and sprinkle with almonds. One serving is 1/2 cup of compote, 1 tablespoon of yogurt, and 1/2 tablespoon of almonds.

Per serving: 131 calories, 2 g fat, 0 g saturated fat, 1 mg cholesterol, 11 mg sodium, 29 g carbohydrates, 3 g fiber, 2 g protein

Bulgur Pudding with Golden Raisins and Pistachios

Serves 6

- 1/3 cup fine or medium bulgur, rinsed
- 1/4 teaspoon ground cardamom
- 1 1/4 cups 1% milk
- 2/3 cup seedless golden raisins or dark seedless raisins
- 1/4 cup granulated sugar
- 1 large egg
- 2 teaspoons freshly grated lemon zest
- 1/2 teaspoon vanilla extract
- 1/3 cup chopped peeled pistachios or slivered almonds

ONE In a medium saucepan, combine the bulgur, cardamom, and 2 cups water. Bring to a simmer over medium-high heat. Immediately remove from the heat, cover, and let stand until the bulgur is tender, about 20 minutes. Drain and press out excess water. Return the bulgur to the pan.

TWO Add the milk, raisins, and sugar and bring to a simmer, stirring often, over medium-high heat. Reduce the heat to medium-low and cook, stirring, for 2 minutes.

THREE Whisk the egg in a medium bowl. Gradually stir in the bulgur mixture. Return to the pan and cook, stirring, over medium-low heat, until slightly thickened, 1 to 2 minutes. (Do not boil. You can use an instant-read thermometer to gauge readiness; the pudding should reach a temperature of 160°F.) Transfer to a clean bowl and stir in the lemon zest and vanilla. Let cool slightly, then cover and refrigerate until chilled. Sprinkle each serving with a scant 1 tablespoon pistachios. The pudding will keep, covered, in the refrigerator for up to 2 days. One serving is 1/3 cup.

Per serving (1/3 cup): 195 calories, 5 g total fat, 1 g saturated fat, 37 mg cholesterol, 76 mg sodium, 33 g carbohydrates, 3 g fiber, 6 g protein

Index

exercise (*continued*)
in morning vs. evening, 106
and quitting smoking, 139
relaxation, 14, 137, 142, 147–53
sleep improved with, 99, 141
snacks for, 56, 102–3, 234
"stealth" moves of, 125–26, 128–29
weight loss and, *see* weight management
see also Move plan; walking
exotic fruits, 58–59, 258, 262

F

fast food, 29, 89
fat, 18, 30, 32, 60
"bad" forms of, *see* saturated fat; trans fats
nutritional tables on, 257
trimming of, from meat or poultry, 60, 196, 202
fats, good, 12, 25, 30, 61, 67–72
diabetes-related benefits of, 12, 15, 30–32, 42–44, 63, 67, 69, 70–72
fish as source of, 30, 32, 43, 63–64, 67, 87, 164
nutritional table on, 257
secondary health benefits of, 12, 32, 43, 63, 67, 71, 164
snack options with, 12, 25, 30, 32, 42, 44–45, 67, 70–72, 83
substituting "bad" fats with, 12, 25, 32, 63–64, 68–70, 72, 87, 235
weight management with, 12, 32, 45, 67, 71, 235
fiber, 24, 31, 33–34, 47, 54, 71, 211, 232
"bean cuisine" options high in, 53, 64–65, 81
breakfast options with, 47, 48–49, 52, 79, 232, 233
"good" fat sources of, 44, 45, 70–71
nutritional counter tables of, 256–61
top produce sources of, 37, 42–43, 45, 53, 57–58, 179, 197
weight loss aided with, 24, 33, 34, 52, 53, 65
whole-grain sources of, 42, 44, 48–53, 173, 190, 233
see also soluble fiber

fish, 72, 77, 82, 86, 190, 205, 220
grilling of, 63, 64, 67, 220
health benefits of, 32, 43, 63, 67
healthy toppings for, 41, 56, 58, 214
lean protein options of, 24, 63–64
mood-elevating properties of, 164
nutritional table on, 257–58
recipes for, 220, 289–91
as source of "good" fat, 25, 30, 32, 43, 63, 164
fish oil capsules, 33, 164
Five-Star Cookies, 302
flaxseed, 25, 30, 49, 71–72, 79, 262
health benefits of, 44, 71–72
recipes with, 268, 299
food diaries, 25, 29, 246–49
food exchange system, 73–74, 262
foot problems, 16, 20, 139
traveling care kit for, 169
workout precautions and, 20, 92, 100, 103–4, 106, 174, 242
Frisbee, 127
fruit, 15, 32, 46, 54–59, 85, 211
aiming for variety in, 57–59
blood-sugar levels and, 24, 53, 54, 56, 57–58, 102, 197, 234
breakfast ideas for, 48–50, 52, 54–56, 75, 79, 232
canned, 54, 59, 77, 258, 259
dessert options with, 52–53, 56–59, 72, 83, 86, 89, 299–304
health benefits of, 11, 24, 31, 42, 43, 53, 57–58, 197
juice, *see* juice, fruit
lunch or dinner ideas for, 56–57, 71, 80, 82
nutritional and GL tables on, 258, 262, 263
Plate Approach and, 74–75
recipes with, 268, 277, 279, 280, 299
serving sizes of, 53, 54, 56, 77, 262, 263
shopping for, 57, 58
snack ideas for, 55–56, 58, 59, 72, 175, 234
weight loss aided with, 24, 33, 54, 55, 57

Credits

PAGES 262–263: "International Table of Glycemic Index and Glycemic Load Values 2002," Kaye Foster-Powell, Susanna H. A. Holt, and Janette C. Brand-Miller, *American Journal of Clinical Nutrition*, vol. 76, no. 1 (2002), 5–56. Additional data from www.glycemicindex.com, www.mypyramid.gov, and www.ars.usda.gov.

PHOTOS: Courtesy of Jupiter Images (AbleStock.com, BananaStock, Big Cheese Photo, Blend Images, BrandX Pictures, Comstock Images, Corbis, Creatas Images, Dynamic Graphics, Goodshoot, Image Source Black, Image Source Pink, Image Source White, Image100, PhotoAlto Agency, PhotoObjects.com, Photos.com, Pixland, Polka Dot Images, Tetra Images, ThinkStock Images)